ENDOSCOPICALLY ASSISTED AESTHETIC PLASTIC SURGERY

Endoscopically Assisted Aesthetic Plastic Surgery

Peter Bela Fodor, M.D., F.A.C.S
Assistant Clinical Professor of Plastic Surgery
University of California, Los Angeles
Medical Director
EsthetiCare Center for Plastic Surgery
Midway Hospital
Medical Center
Los Angeles, California

Nicanor G. Isse, M.D.
Clinical Attendee
UCLA Medical Center
University of California
Los Angeles, California
Director of Endoscopic Plastic Surgery
Department of Plastic Surgery
Premier Surgical Center
Burbank, California

Timothy C. Hengst
Medical Illustrator

with 312 *illustrations*

Mosby

St. Louis Baltimore Boston Carlsbad Chicago Naples New York Philadelphia Portland
London Madrid Mexico City Singapore Sydney Tokyo Toronto Wiesbaden

Mosby
Dedicated to Publishing Excellence

A Times Mirror
Company

Publisher: Anne Patterson
Executive Editor: Robert Hurley
Associate Developmental Editor: Christine Pluta
Project Manager: Linda Clarke
Production Editor: Deborah Ann Cicirello
Designer: Carolyn O'Brien
Electronic Production Coordinator: Terri Bovay
Manufacturing Supervisor: Karen Lewis
Cover Design: Carolyn O'Brien
Part Opener Photographs: The Bettmann Archive

Printed in the United States of America
Composition by Mosby Electronic Production—St. Louis
Printing/binding by Walsworth

Mosby–Year Book, Inc.
11830 Westline Industrial Drive
St. Louis, Missouri 63146

Library of Congress Cataloging in Publication Data
Endoscopically assisted aesthetic plastic surgery / [edited by] Peter Bela Fodor, Nicanor G. Isse; Timothy C. Hengst, medical illustrator.
p. cm.
Includes bibliographical references and index.
ISBN 0-8151-3389-8
1. Surgery, Plastic. 2. Endoscopic surgery. I. Fodor, Peter Bela. II. Isse, Nicanor G.
[DNLM: 1. Surgery, Plastic—methods. 2. Endoscopy—methods. WO 600 E57 1996]
RD118.8.E55 1996
617.9′5—dc20
DNLM/DLC
for Library of Congress 95-593
CIP

96 97 98 99 00 / 9 8 7 6 5 4 3 2 1

CONTRIBUTORS

Shirley A. Anain, M.D.
Clinical Instructor of Surgery
University of Buffalo Medical School
Buffalo, New York

Ewaldo Bolivar de Souza Pinto, M.D.
Faculdade Federal Fluminense
Centro Científico Brasileiro de Cirurgia Plástica
Santos, São Paulo, Brazil

Gustavo A. Colon, M.D.
Clinical Professor of Plastic Surgery
Tulane University
New Orleans, Lousiana

Richard V. Dowden, M.D., C.M., F.A.C.S.
Assistant Clinical Professor of Plastic Surgery
Case Western Reserve University
Cleveland, Ohio

Patricia J. Erazo I., M.D.
Facultad de Medicina
Universidad de Guayaquil
Centro Científico Brasileiro de Cirurgia Plástica
São Paulo, Brazil

Antonio Fuente del Campo, M.D., F.A.C.S.
Professor of Plastic and Craniofacial Surgery
Hospital Angeles del Pedregal
Mexico City, Mexico

Joseph P. Hunstad, M.D.
Assistant Clinical Professor, Department of Plastic Surgery
University of North Carolina
Chapel Hill, North Carolina;
Chief, Department of Plastic Surgery
University Hospital;
Director, The Hunstad Center for Cosmetic Plastic Surgery
Charlotte, North Carolina

Gerald W. Johnson, M.D.
Founder
Tops Surgical Specialty Hospital
Houston, Texas

Maria Fernanda Lopez, M.D.
Universidad del Valle
Facultad de Medicina
Centro Científico Brasileiro de Cirurgia Plástica
São Paulo, Brazil

G. Patrick Maxwell, M.D.
Assistant Professor of Plastic Surgery
Vanderbilt University School of Medicine;
Director
Institute of Aesthetic and Reconstructive Surgery
Baptist Hospital
Nashville, Tennessee

Richard A. Mladick, M.D., F.A.C.S.
Director
Center for Cosmetic Plastic Surgery
Virginia Beach, Virginia

Paul H. Rosenberg, M.D.
Community Hospital at Dobbs Ferry
Dobbs Ferry, New York

Gordon H. Sasaki, M.D., F.A.C.S.
Clinical Associate Professor of Surgery
University of Southern California Medical School
Los Angeles, California;
Active Member
Huntington Medical Hospital
Pasadena, California

Luiz S. Toledo, M.D., F.I.C.S.
Private Practice
São Paulo, Brazil

M. Dean Vistnes, M.D.
Stanford University Medical Center
Stanford, California

To Barbara, Now and Always

P.B.F.

To My Mother, My Children and Christina

N.G.I.

FOREWORD

What a pleasure it is for me to write the Foreword for this very timely book by Peter Bela Fodor, Nicanor Isse, and their colleagues. Both Dr. Fodor and Dr. Isse have contributed so very much to this field of endoscopic plastic surgery (E.P.S.), which has expanded so rapidly in the last year or two that it is hard to believe that its origins seem to be traced only to 1992, as far as bibliographic referencing is concerned.

As long as I have known Peter Bela Fodor as the associate editor of our journal *Aesthetic Plastic Surgery*, I have been especially aware of his enthusiastic interest in all aspects of both reconstructive and aesthetic plastic surgery. In the Spring of 1983 our journal published its first article on lipolysis entitled "Lipolysis: the Illouz technique. . ."; it was only 9 years later that the video "Coronal facelift with endoscopic techniques" was presented in Washington, D.C., in 1992 by Vasconez's group[1] and another related video was presented at the same meeting by Liang and Narayan.[2] One of the earliest presentations of Isse's "endoforehead" operative experiences took place at the November 1992 meeting of the Los Angeles Society of Plastic Surgery.[3]

As a medical historian, it has always interested me that it took only a decade or less following the introduction of aspirative lipoplasty for the plastic surgery community to suddenly be faced with the introduction of another entirely new aspect of aesthetic plastic surgery. Both these aspects, namely, lipolysis and endoscopic surgery, came quickly to the attention of Peter Bela Fodor, in particular.

Dr. Fodor, as one of the prime movers and developers of the Lipoplasty Society of North America (LSNA) of which he is a past president, soon recognized the similarities of liposuction and endoscopic plastic surgery: small incisions, small scars, and as such, minimally invasive surgical procedures. In 1993 plastic surgeons learned of a markedly expanding group of conferences contributed to and publications written by Aiache, Anain, Bostwick, Carlson, Christ, Dowden, Eaves, Hamas, Ho, Johnson, Nahai, O'Neal, Price, Ramirez, and Vasconez with his group. In this same year at the 12th Biennial Congress of the International Society of Aesthetic Plastic Surgery held in Paris in September, a separate session was devoted to endoscopy and included papers by Aiache, Chajchir, Mitz, and Toledo.

Dr. Fodor and Dr. Isse became especially involved from the very beginning in endoscopy starting with The Forum for Innovative Plastic Surgery held in Dallas, Texas, by The Lipoplasty Society, Inc., April 14-15, 1994.[4] It was at this very important forum that specific contributors, Fodor, Isse, Sasaki, de Souza Pinto, and Fuente del Campo, addressed the advances in E.P.S.[4] From this panel at the forum grew the idea that this book now presented by Peter Bela Fodor and Nicanor Isse should be forthcoming to help in the education of the entire field of plastic and reconstructive surgery at large.

From the very first issue of *Aesthetic Plastic Surgery* in 1994, and throughout the rest of the year, there were published 10 papers and two video reviews of endoscopic procedures, which included one paper on rhinoplasty, five papers on facelifting, two papers on forehead lifting, one paper on breast augmentation, and one major editorial (Fodor).[5-15]

In the editorial by Peter Bela Fodor entitled "Endoscopic plastic surgery, a new milestone in plastic surgery," with a great deal of foresight,Dr. Fodor stated the following[6]:

> It is my belief that the impact of E.P.S. on the reconstructive and cosmetic aspects of our specialty will soon be compared in magnitude to microvascular, craniofacial, and tissue expansion techniques. Interestingly enough, all of these aspects of plastic surgery have evolved primarily during times of relative peace and not at times of human upheaval when new techniques have generally been known to take off.

Peter Bela Fodor, in his editorial, historically emphasized that[6]

> . . . endoscopically assisted surgical techniques have already been successfully used in breast augmentation procedures via transaxillary, transumbilical, and other more conventional approaches, for diagnostic evaluation of breast implant wall integrity, for forehead and upper two-thirds rhytidectomy, for plication of abdominal wall musculature, for carpal tunnel release, and for placement of tissue expanders in the craniofacial region among other uses.

In the same 1994 editorial, Dr. Fodor once again stressed certain very important aspects of endoscopy[6]:

> . . . just as liposuction assisted techniques are currently used in the course of a variety of reconstructive and cosmetic procedures, incorporating endoscopic techniques with many different operations will soon beome commonplace. With these techniques, dissection in otherwise cumbersome areas is facilitated by better lighting and magnification. The small access incisions not only dramatically decrease post-operative incisional tenderness and scarring but also are less disruptive to vascular and lymphatic circulation and therefore are associated with less post-operative

edema . . . these already apparent advantages of E.P.S. represent only the beginning! Creative thinking coupled with the technical excellence characteristic of plastic surgeons will lead to the development of many other applications of E.P.S. for the benefit of our patients.

Dr. Fodor's editorial insight as to the future of endoscopy, together with the already well-documented surgical skill and imagination of Isse and the other contributors, should be obviously demonstrable to all of those readers who will open the pages of this book and learn much more about the field of endoscopy than they have ever known before.

REFERENCES

1. Core GB, Vasconez LO, Askrem C, Yamamoto Y, Gamboa M: Coronal facelift with endoscopic techniques, *Plast Surg Forum* XV:227, 1992.
2. Liang M, Narayan K: Endoscopic ablation of the frontalis and corrugator muscles—a clinical study, *Plast Surg Forum* XV:54, 1992.
3. Isse NG: Endoforehead. Presented at the Los Angeles Society of Plastic Surgery, Los Angeles, November 1992.
4. Fodor PB, Isse NG: Session II—body sculpting with endoscopy. The Forum for Innovative Plastic Surgery. Presented to The Lipoplasty Society, Inc., Dallas, April 13, 1994.
5. Isse NG: Endoscopic face rejuvenation: endoforehead, the functional lift. Case reports, *Aesth Plast Surg* 18:21, 1994.
6. Fodor PB: Editorial: Endoscopic plastic surgery, a new milestone in plastic surgery, *Aesth Plast Surg* 18:31, 1994.
7. Ramirez OM: Endoscopic techniques in facial rejuvenation: an overview, Part I, *Aesth Plast Surg* 18:141, 1994.
8. Toledo LS: Video-endoscopic facelift, *Aesth Plast Surg* 18:149, 1994.
9. Mitz V: Endoscopic control during rhinoplasty, *Aesth Plast Surg* 18:153, 1994.
10. Chajchir A: Endoscopic subperiosteal forehead lift, *Aesth Plast Surg* 18:269, 1994.
11. Aiache AE: Endoscopic facelift, *Aesth Plast Surg* 18:275, 1994.
12. Ramirez OM: Endoscopic full facelift, *Aesth Plast Surg* 18:363, 1994.
13. Honig J-F: The fiber endoscope with guidable and flexible working instruments for endofacelift: a new instrument in facial surgery, *Aesth Plast Surg* 18:373, 1994.
14. Chajchir A, Benzaquen I, Spagnolo N, Lusicic N: Endoscopic augmentation mastoplasty, *Aesth Plast Surg* 18:377, 1994.
15. Vasconez LO, Core GB, Gamboa M, Askrem C, Yamamoto Y: Endoscopic techniques in coronal facelifting (video reviews), *Aesth Plast Surg* 18:106, 1994.

Blair O. Rogers, M.D., F.A.C.S.
Editor-in-Chief, Aesthetic Plastic Surgery
Clinical Professor of Surgery (Plastic Surgery)
New York University Medical Center
New York New York
President, International Society of Aesthetic Plastic Surgery

FOREWORD

The only constant in plastic surgery is ongoing change. There is a plethora of new surgical approaches, refinements of techniques, and applications of new technology in the search for new and better ways to improve results for our patients. We are constantly challenged by these changes and must keep an open mind to potential advances. We need, however, to proceed carefully in evaluating new techniques and to include them in our own practices only if they represent an improvement over our traditional approaches.

Endoscopy is one of these areas of rapidly growing interest, development, and possible improvement. During my term as president of the American Society for Aesthetic Plastic Surgery, the need to create an endoscopic task force to study the potential of these techniques became apparent. The charge to this task force has been to objectively evaluate the outcomes of endoscopically assisted procedures in aesthetic plastic surgery, to educate plastic surgeons about these techniques, and to incorporate this new technology into the mainstream of plastic surgery. Many of the contributors to this book are original members of this now-joint ASAPS-ASPRS Task Force on Endoscopy.

Endoscopic techniques are now standard procedures in many surgical specialties such as gynecology, general surgery, and orthopedic surgery. Plastic surgeons waited until the technology improved before embracing it. There is now a wave of enthusiasm for information about applications in aesthetic surgery as evidenced by the standing-room-only attendance at education programs dealing with endoscopy at the recent ASAPS annual meetings.

As has occurred in the past with other new techniques, additional time and critical evaluation of the short- and long-term results of endoscopic procedures will result in the emergence of guidelines for the appropriate applications of this technology, There is a need for a book that reflects the current state of the art. Drs. Peter Bela Fodor and Nicanor Isse, the editors of this volume, invited several contributors to address the different endoscopic approaches of this emerging technology. I congratulate the editors and their contributors for the development of an up-to-date, comprehensive, yet succinct book on endoscopic assistance in aesthetic plastic surgery.

Robert Singer, M.D.
Immediate Past President
American Society for Aesthetic Plastic Surgery

PREFACE

Endoscopic assistance is a very exciting new development in aesthetic plastic surgery, replete with a potential never anticipated before with traditional approaches. Like many other important technical advances in surgery in recent decades, it does not replace existing techniques, rather it enriches tremendously the options and approaches available to the surgeon, helps refine existing procedures, and ultimately obtains better surgical and cosmetic results.

It was with this enthusiasm that we first conceived the idea of mapping the current landscape of endoscopically assisted aesthetic plastic surgery in a book devoted to the subject. New ideas, irrespective of their subsequent impact and despite all the colorful apocryphal anecdotes about their genesis that make the history of science entertaining, do not arise ex nihilo, when the originator is hit on the head by an apple. Neither do we often jump dripping wet out of the bathtub and tear through town crying "Eureka." New ideas are typically the product of observation, careful consideration, dialogue, trial and error, and also doubt.

My personal interest in endoscopic plastic surgery was ignited in 1993 when I had the good fortune to meet Dr. Nicanor Isse. At the time he was relatively unknown at the national level but was pursuing his strong interest in these techniques. Today, Dr. Isse is one of the specialty's most creative and technically accomplished plastic surgeons. We owe him a debt of gratitude for pioneering the application of endoscopic techniques and the development of a great deal of instrumentation necessary for plastic surgery.

In the Spring of 1994 I was gathering and selecting panelists for the Spring Meeting of the Lipoplasty Society of North America, which was the first panel of a national scientific meeting devoted to endoscopy in plastic surgery. At that time the idea of taking that effort to a new level took shape naturally because I realized that the need for organized information on endoscopically assisted plastic surgery went far beyond the radius of that meeting's attendees. Nevertheless, the very next question that came to mind was "Is it really timely, or is it too early to do this?"

After all, endoscopic procedures are a recent development in our specialty. Relatively little has been published on these techniques in the peer-reviewed literature, and as of yet there are no comparative studies and no guidelines. Quite a few pioneers in several countries are working out their personal techniques, accumulating data, and occasionally presenting both at scientific meetings. On the whole, however, communications are still sporadic and fragmentary.

Nevertheless, while the very individualistic nature of these independent efforts has contributed to producing an impressive variety of approaches, a systematic process of "comparing notes" has yet to come, as is a serious attempt to establish standards. This very realization provided the answer to our one question: "No, it is not too early." It is, in fact, the right time to gather in one place the record of some of the most interesting efforts of professional experts who have accumulated some experience with the endoscopic technique, precisely for the purpose of taking stock of where we are and mapping our future course.

Our editorial efforts have had the purpose of producing a book that can be used by any colleague who wishes to know what is best expressed in vernacular as "what's going on" in endoscopically assisted aesthetic plastic surgery today. We have also had a more ambitious goal, that is, to assemble the kind of record that will continue to be useful years after some of the approaches described in this book may have been modified beyond recognition by further refinements or, indeed, have even been rendered obsolete. Yet, the book should ideally remain useful because it is, as we hope, the comprehensive and detailed record of the techniques being used or experimented with today, which *prefigures* future advancements.

These goals have defined and shaped this book. It was not meant to be a definitive text, such as a treatise of physiology or anatomy, but a current guide and an accurate chronicle of evolution still unfolding in many parts of the world simultaneously. For this reason each author has been allowed to retain his distinct, individual voice. The contributors represent a cross-section of American and international surgeons, some well-known to the readers of this volume, others less so. The same surgical technique applied to the same anatomic region is described differently in chapters written by different authors, which is a reflection of the creative variation of each approach as well as of the author's personal style. We felt it important to respect and preserve this individuality of both substance and style, if we were to provide an accurate picture of the state of the art at this point in time. Befittingly, our editing has been as noninvasive as the technique to which the book is dedicated.

In some cases, however, we did not hesitate to eliminate details or descriptions we considered redundant; for example, when discussing the submuscular breast augmentation approach, we considered it unnecessary to have a detailed description of the submuscular implant pocket dissection in more than one chapter to avoid repetition of an identical dissection technique. We leave it up to the reader, however, to compare, find similarities and distinctions, evaluate, and finally become informed by the wealth and diversity of the material assembled herein.

Aesthetic plastic surgery is concerned with molding and reshaping the human face and the human body for the purpose of establishing (or recreating) a youthful appearance, harmony, proportion, symmetry, and ultimately beauty. This aspect of our professional endeavor, which represents its unifying concept, involves subjective judgment, feeling, and artistry and, as a result, is difficult to describe in technical terms. It is relatively easy, however, to describe and analyze the process, methods, and techniques used in our daily work, to quantify the results obtained with one procedure compared with another, or to determine the appropriateness of using a certain type of equipment in a given procedure. These are some of the essential topics of this book.

We hope that the descriptive survey we have provided of the status of various techniques employed in endoscopic aesthetic plastic surgery at this point in time will serve ably the multiple functions we had in mind: a red dot on the map that says "You are here," a baseline for future evaluation of further developments, and above all a practical guide for those colleagues who are interested in learning more about these new surgical approaches.

Finally, while stressing the importance and value of the new methods and techniques for which we share the enthusiasm of the distinguished experts whose contributions grace the pages of this volume, we wish to leave the reader with the reminder that beyond the most self-assured mastery of any new, sophisticated technique, the ultimate goal, the unifying concept of all we do professionally, remains as always on the next horizon, unattained yet worth striving for through personal talent and imagination.

Peter Bela Fodor, M.D., F.A.C.S.

ACKNOWLEDGMENTS

All coordinated efforts depend on the hard work and dedication of all involved. This volume has been no exception. In addition to all those whose names appear in these pages, my heartfelt thanks go to Rana Davidson, my assistant, for her patient, able and meticulous work on the manuscript from beginning to end; to Robert A. Hurley, whose editorial vision helped us turn a concept into concrete reality; to Chris Pluta, for her advice and attentive assistance; to Debbie Cicirello and the rest of the dedicated staff at Mosby who produced this beautiful volume.

P.B.F.

CONTENTS

Endoscopically Assisted Aesthetic Plastic Surgery

Introduction

A Historical Perspective

Peter Bela Fodor

Paul H. Rosenberg

The unprecedented pace of technologic advances and the rapidity with which the medical applications of these advances are diversified and refined are undoubtedly the hallmark of our time. Experience with the use of this new technology is also enhanced by the rapidity of peer contacts made possible, in turn, by the equally stupendous explosion in communication technology and by the facility of video demonstrations, which are more apt to create a sense of immediate experience than are discoursive descriptions aided by charts and static illustrations. This global concomitant accumulation of expertise explains why it is possible to evaluate new methodology much earlier in its chronologic development than was conceivable in the past. It also, in effect, mandates that such scientific evaluation be carried out periodically in a conscientious, timely manner to organize our knowledge as it accrues, comparing diverse experience, merging information, and refining all aspects of the clinical applications of the new technology.

Endoscopy, as we conceive of it today, is a "young" medical technique that has already revealed ample utility and benefit in the hands of the experienced physician and is fraught with promise in both diagnostic and therapeutic procedures. Like most "new" technologies that have preceded it in recent decades and have already taken their rightful place in medicine, it has a number of interesting features for the thinking physician. On closer inspection its novelty yields the realization that its entirety as a technique is actually constituted of a conglomerate of separate concept refinements and technologic advances with a history of their own. Looking back on these origins, one can discern incremental steps—sometimes continuous but more often discrete—that form the pathway to today's achievement. It is for this reason that we believe it useful to examine briefly such different aspects of its evolution as the invention of the endoscope, the development of the photoimaging technology, and endoscopic electrocautery.

Like other new technologies and techniques, endoscopy was not immediately nor uniformly embraced, or indeed contemplated, by all medical specialties that have turned out, so far, to benefit from its applications. For our specialty it may endure as a historical irony that, despite the distinguished pioneering efforts of plastic surgeons in virtually all relevant areas of surgery (not the least of which are microvascular surgery and organ transplantation), endoscopy languished in our peripheral vision at first.

Even as we begin to accumulate a record of experience with the applications of endoscopy in plastic surgery, it is important to realize the full complexity and richness of the roots of the concept.

Endoscopy

Parallel to the millenarian practice of open dissections in the quest to understand human anatomy, attempts to peer into the hidden recesses of the body through a small opening seeking to understand live physiology have their own long scientific pedigree.

Taken at face value of the term's Greek etymology (*endon,* within, and *skopein,* to view/to examine), examination of the internal environment of the human body goes as far back as Babylonian times. In fact, a precursor of the endoscope—crude by our standards but probably serviceable in its time—is described in the Babylonian Talmud (Niddah Treatise, section 65 b).[1] It consisted of a lead funnel with a bent mouthpiece connected to a wooden drainpipe, which was introduced into the vagina for direct visual examination of the uterine cervix. It obviously satisfied the first requirement of the concept of endoscopy, that is, access, albeit it was designed for use in an anatomic passage, not in a surgical stoma.

The second requirement, provision of a light source, took longer to fulfill. The first documented light source can be ascribed to Giulio Cesare Aranzi, who first described the medical application of the *camera obscura.* Not surprisingly for a genius as omnipresent in all the fields of knowledge of his time, Leonardo da Vinci also lent his imagination to this problem of visualization of dark recesses and, also unsurprisingly, his solution was from the realm of optics. He used a shutter to filter the sun's rays through a narrow chink, then focused the beam through the lens provided by a water-filled glass. This enhanced shaft of light was directed into the nasal cavity. We can speculate that the visual inspection afforded by this illumination was done rapidly, or the subjects of his experiments did not mind an occasional small burn from the unavoidable loupe effect.

Modern endoscopy, however, was truly born with the invention of the first light reflector by Bozzini in 1807. The reflector directed light rays into the cavities of a live animal's body and then refracted the rays to the observer's eye (Figure I-1).[2]

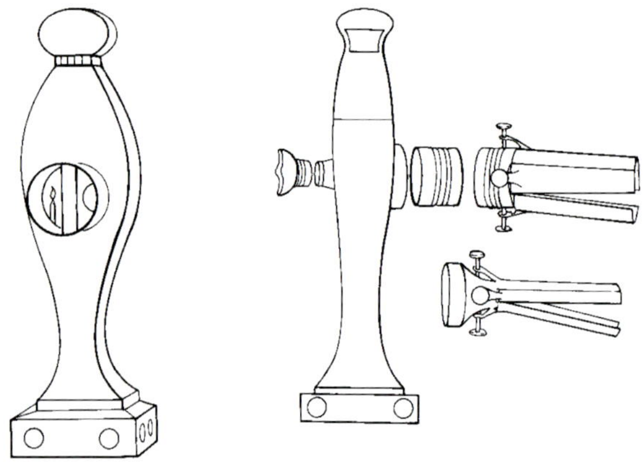

Bozzini's endoscope — The "lampholder" (early model)

Bozzini's endoscope — With rectal and vaginal tubes (later model)

FIGURE I-1
Early endoscope and light source attributed to Bozzini are shown.

Photoimaging

It was in 1874 that the first demonstration of photoimaging was given in Germany by Stein, who unveiled his *photo-endoscope.*[3] In 1901 Kelling used a cystoscope to explore the abdomen of a live dog into which air had been insufflated, a procedure that Kelling termed *koelioskopie.*[4] A decade later, Jacobaeus applied this technique to the examination of the human abdomen and termed the procedure *laparoscopy.*[5] Soon the applications of endoscopy were expanded from diagnosis to therapy, with the significant achievement of endoscopic lysis of intra-abdominal adhesions first carried out by Fervers in 1933.[5a] Tubal sterilization performed laparoscopically followed, as described by the Swiss physician Boesch.[6] Another pioneer was Ruddock, who documented his experience with 500 colonoscopy cases performed over a period of 4 years, of which 39 were associated with biopsies.

Important advancements were the invention of the 135-degree lens system and development of the dual-trocar technique, both of which were the contribution of the German physician Kalk, who in 1951 reported on his series of 2000 laparoscopies performed with zero mortality.[7] The dual-trocar technique led to further advancement in laparoscopic therapy. Dual instrumentation (triangulation) allowed for more complex movements and combined simultaneous efforts in minimal-access incision surgery.

Endoscopic Electrocautery

For a long time hemostasis was primarily obtained using the unipolar high-frequency device designed by Boesch in the 1930s. The invention of the fiberglass cable made it possible to discard the incandescent endoscopic tip and thus eliminate the burn hazard. The risk of burns had been significant due to the use of high-frequency current in fulguration procedures in the environment of a closed body cavity insufflated with oxygen. Endocoagulation, whose birth certificate reads "New Orleans, 1973," definitively ended the use of high-frequency current; monopolar and bipolar electrocautery through the endoscope ensured the achievement of hemostasis at much lower temperatures and without any contact between the electrical current and the patient's body.

Computerized Television Cameras

The early 1980s brought us the computer chip technology in television cameras, without which videolaparoscopy would not have been possible. Surgical specialties such as orthopedics and gastrointestinal surgery quickly incorporated laparoscopic techniques into their practices, of which perhaps the most frequently cited so far as a landmark clinical advance has been endoscopic cholecystectomy.

ENDOSCOPY IN PLASTIC SURGERY

As is to be expected in a new and rapidly advancing field whose landscape is changing every day as its frontiers are constantly being pushed farther and new landmarks are set, there are no "definitive" studies yet, and published reports in peer-reviewed journals are still few and far between. To evaluate the currently existing record we have performed a literature search using MEDLINE (an on-line segment of MEDLARS), specifying "endoscope," "endoscopy," and "plastic surgery" as key words used alone and in combination. To control for the time lag of article recording that is built into the MEDLARS (National Library of Medicine) system, which typically records an article 3 to 12 months after publication, we have manually searched individual issues for the corresponding period of the following journals: *Journal of Plastic and Reconstructive Surgery* (JPRS), *Aesthetic Plastic Surgery* (ASP), *Surgical Forum* (SF), *British Journal of Plastic Surgery* (BJPS), and *Scandinavian Journal of Plastic Surgery* (SJPS). There is, of course, the possibility that we may have missed some published reports; we trust, however, that the general picture which emerged from our search does justice to the existing record in its essential aspects, in terms of general trends as well as selected highlights.

In addition, we have evaluated the reports presented at meetings of scientific societies over the past few years (Table I-1), including the following: American Society of Plastic and Reconstructive Surgeons (ASPRS), American Society of Aesthetic Plastic Surgery (ASAPS), International Society of Aesthetic Plastic Surgery (ISAPS), Lipoplasty Society of North America (LSNA), and American Association of Plastic Surgeons (AAPS).

From this data collection of multiple disparate points an interesting pointillistic picture emerged, the pattern of which revealed a field replete with

TABLE I-1 PAPERS/INSTRUCTIONAL COURSES PRESENTED AT NATIONAL MEETINGS OF PLASTIC SURGICAL SOCIETIES

YEAR	ASPRS*	ASAPS†	ISAPS‡	LSNA§	OTHER	TOTAL
PRE 1992	0	0	0	0	2	2
1992	1	3	0	0	3	7
1993	8	2	7	0	5	22
1994	12	8	NA	26	16	62

*American Society of Plastic Reconstructive Surgeons
†American Society of Aesthetic Plastic Surgery
‡International Society of Aesthetic Plastic Surgery
§Lipoplasty Society of North America

TABLE I-2 PUBLICATIONS IN MAJOR PLASTIC SURGERY JOURNALS

YEAR	JPRS*	J AESTH SURG†	BJPS‡	OTHER	TOTAL
PRE 1992	1	0	0	0	1
1992	2	0	0	1	3
1993	3	1	1	2	7
1994	8	12	0	4	24

*Journal of Plastic and Reconstructive Surgery
†Aesthetic Plastic Surgery
‡British Journal of Plastic Surgery

individual pioneering work being done simultaneously, each variant bearing the imprint of the surgeon's creativity, personal preference, and specific experience with the technique. The reports published to date are amazingly diverse in the scope of the applications described, especially in view of their relatively small total number (Table I-2). They report on endoscopic techniques used in plastic surgery of the face, forehead, nose, breast, abdomen, and hand. In general, we found that the number of both presentations and published reports grew exponentially in the brief period evaluated, whereas growth of the number of articles published lagged behind considerably (Figure I-2). Of the total number of articles published we attempted to identify those representing pioneering efforts, despite the disadvantage of the foreshortened perspective available to us at this point. The chronology of the landmark reports, grouped by category or anatomic region, is summarized below.

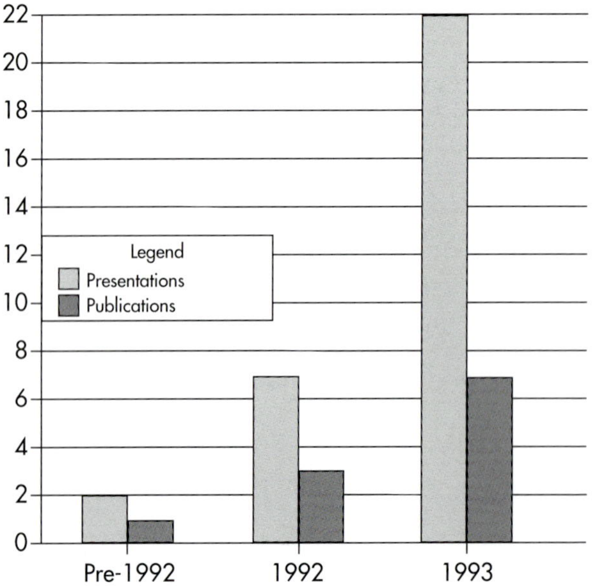

FIGURE I-2
Recent trends in endoscopy-related publications and presentations are shown.

Reconstructive Surgery

Reconstructive surgery is going through a phase of increased excitement owing to rapidly gained and continuously growing knowledge in several key areas, many of which will complement the achievements of minimally invasive surgery, in general, and endoscopic procedures, in particular. Currently there is strong interest in the significant clinical applications of growth factors, especially platelet-derived and transforming growth factors. Animal studies and preliminary clinical trials have shown that growth factors accelerate healing of surgical incisions and inhibit scar formation. Although approval from the Food and Drug Administration (FDA) for therapeutic use of growth factor preparations may be a few years away, one can anticipate the great potential synergies resulting from the combined use of minimal access surgery and growth factors.

At the same time, advanced work with microsurgical free flaps has led to highly sophisticated techniques of "prefabrication," whereby a free microvascular flap can be created before transfer to its intended location, viably furnished with its functioning angiostructures.[8] Tissue expansion techniques allow such flaps to be customized for size and thickness.[9]

Endoscopy has been incorporated into many creative applications in plastic surgery experiments as well as clinical procedures. Estes and co-workers described their experience with the creation and repair of cleft lip in lambs in utero,[10] and Rosenberg and co-workers[11,12] and Miller and co-workers[13] were able to harvest porcine jejunal segments and omentum in a dog model laparoscopically. Miller also reported his successful clinical experience with microvascular esophageal reconstruction using laparoscopically harvested jejunum.[14] Repair of a large soft tissue defect in a lower extremity was performed by Saltz by transfer of harvested omentum as a free flap to the repair site.[15] Pedicled flaps harvested from the omentum through 1-cm abdominal incisions were used by Boss in four reported cases of breast reconstruction following mastectomy.[16] Endoscopic tissue harvesting is being performed in numerous centers worldwide by many researchers (e.g., Miller and co-workers' reported harvesting of the rectus abdominis muscle[17]) and clinicians (e.g., Eaves and co-workers' harvested fascia lata femoris and latissimus dorsi in two and one patient, respectively[18]). Sasaki[19] and others[20,21] have performed endoscopically assisted dissection of the pocket prior to placement of tissue expanders to reduce the size of the incision, which, in turn, lessens the risk of subsequent extrusion of the expander. Sasaki's method allows tissue expansion to commence at the time of expander placement.

Aesthetic Plastic Surgery

LIPOPLASTY

In his 1984 landmark article Bahman Teimourian described a technique for endoscopic visualization of the subcutaneous area being treated with suction lipectomy. According to his article, endoscopy could thus be used to verify the integrity of vascular and neural structures at the site of liposuction and to provide direct visualization during the procedure. He went so far as to hypothesize that at some point in the future endoscopy could provide the means for evaluating the integrity of breast implants.[22] Even though he himself did not pursue these applications of endoscopy, Teimourian's paper constitutes a landmark in the conceptual pathway to their development.

BREAST IMPLANT

In his pioneering work begun in 1986, the late Frank Gerow[23] did, in fact, translate into clinical reality Teimourian's hypothesis. By 1993 he had reported on his use of endoscopy in the evaluation of breast implant integrity in more than 60 patients. Dowden and Anain,[24,25] Colon,[26] and others furthered and refined our knowledge and diagnostic skills with this modality, which has become an important auxiliary technique of benefit in the overall care of patients with silicone breast implants.

Rosenberg and co-workers,[27-29] Kompatscher,[30] and Dowden and Anain[31] described their technique of endoscopically assisted capsulotomy and capsulectomy to obtain release of periprosthetic capsular contracture. Rosenberg also devised a grading system to classify the status of the breast implant based on endoscopic examination of the breast.[32]

In 1991 Johnson and Christ reported on the endoscopically assisted technique of saline implant insertion through a periumbilical approach.[33] Using this method, Johnson has carried out more than 400 breast augmentation procedures to date.[34] In Ho's view, the direct visualization of the pocket provided by endoscopy adds an important degree of maneuver accuracy and control to the surgical performance of the procedure.[35]

ABDOMINOPLASTY AND BODY SCULPTING

A technique for endoscopically assisted abdominoplasty in patients with moderate tissue laxity and minimal skin excess was also developed by Johnson, who demonstrated it in January of 1992. To date he has performed this procedure in an additional 20 cases.[36]

The *Brazilian Journal of Plastic Surgery* records the early experience of Marco Faria-Correa with endoscopically assisted abdominoplasty, which he demonstrated at the ASPRS Conference held in Beverly Hills in March of 1993.[37]

RHINOPLASTY

Endoscopic evaluation of the results of rhinoplasty as well as endoscopically assisted rhinoplasty has been carried out by Mitz. Based on 35 initial cases of endoscopically assisted rhinoplasty, Mitz indicated that the new technique contributes to obtaining more precision in resections of cartilage and bony tissue, deep septal control, and refined precision in positioning the graft.[38]

FACIAL REJUVENATION

Core, Vasconez, and co-workers first described their endoscopically assisted coronal facelift technique in a video demonstration given at the 1992 ASPRS meeting held in Washington, DC.[39,40] At the time, their early results in seven cases indicated the advantages of using minimal access incisions placed in the hair-bearing scalp and those of endoscopic visualization during undermining of the glabellar region, brow, and scalp. While some of these advantages were intuitively obvious—for example, minimized scarring—others—such as reduced risk of alopecia frequently associated with conventional forehead lifting procedures—are now beginning to be clinically proved. The technique was based on using a skin excision in the temporal region and endoscopic muscle ablation in the brow to obtain wrinkle improvement. Although the follow-up was short term, the aesthetic results were impressive at postoperative evaluation.

Concomitantly, Liang and Narayanan gave a video presentation of their endoscopic technique of corrugator ablation used in combination with traditional rhytidectomy.[41] One year later, Hamas reported his experience with endoscopically assisted corrugator resection in 16 cases of patients treated for wrinkle improvement of the glabellar region.[42] The follow-up lasted only 3 to 7 months. This report created animated discussions at the time of its presentation and was met with significant resistance on the part of the audience.

Concomitantly and independently of Vasconez' work, Isse began by reevaluating the heritage of knowledge of the basic mechanics of forehead elevation to develop his own technique of brow lifting.[43] The classic studies of Duchenne[44] on the mechanical principles of action of the forehead and periorbital muscles gave Isse a deeper insight into the physiology of age-induced ptosis of these structures, as well as of the relationship between the corrugator–procerus muscle tandem, and the frontal and the depressor superciliary muscles. In 1993 Isse also published the first paper on endoscopic facial rejuvenation, detailing the results obtained in his first series of 61 patients.[45]

Ramirez, inspired by Isse, described his subsequent experience with the above-mentioned technique in subperiosteal lift in 1994. He advocated the endoscopically assisted subperiosteal dissection in treating both the brow and the face.[46,47] The technique of subperiosteal dissection in facelifting was, however, first described by Tessier[48] in 1980. Krastinova-Lolov,[49] Santana,[50] and several others[51,52] contributed further refinements to its application. Fuente del Campo, one of the first strong supporters of the subperiosteal dissection technique in rhytidectomy, considers the endoscopic approach superior to blind dissection in many respects, particularly insofar as the reduction of operative bleeding and of postoperative edema are concerned. These beneficial effects, associated with the endoscopic approach, are due to the improved visualization of the operative field and to the thorough release of the facial muscles afforded by the technique.[53]

Use of the endoscope in conjunction with soft tissue undermining at the subcutaneous level was reported to lead to greater ease and superior performance of the procedure by Aiache in 1993.[54] He describes elevation of the facial skin and subcutaneous tissue, followed by the posterior transfer of the excess facial skin to the hairline, where it is fixed by sutures placed within the hair-bearing scalp. The end result has the effect of displacing the redundant skin to the scalp, where in the short term it is less noticeable and in the long term will be eliminated by contracture.[55]

Toledo described a combined multilayer approach that he used in 22 cases of endoscopically assisted facelift procedures. He reserved the subperiosteal approach for the treatment of the frontal region, using the endoscope for the subcutaneous approach to the mid-third of the face, and combining platysmal suspension and superficial liposculpture for treatment of the cervical region. The latter achieved a restoration of a youthful aspect to the cervicomental angle.[56]

CONCLUSION

The endoscopic modality and its applications are continuing to expand their indications in our specialty. This is attested to by the increasing number of communications reporting on such experience both at scientific meetings and in the form of articles published in peer-reviewed journals. The fast-paced increase in such experience worldwide as well as the growing interest in the endoscopic technique among our entire specialty is unprecedented in any recent development since the advent of the liposuction technique, which also made its debut in a somewhat tentative manner at first and now, only 10 years later, has become one of the most frequently performed techniques in aesthetic plastic surgery. Preliminary conclusions based on the accumulation of individual experience indicate that the endoscopic approach is associated with lower morbidity, decreased postoperative recuperation, improved aesthetic results, and decreased operative time than conventional techniques of open surgery. Long-term results will have to be evaluated in controlled trials and the indications for patient selection will have to be further refined to obtain a clear and detailed comparative analysis of the risks and benefits of endoscopically assisted, minimally invasive procedures versus the traditional open procedures. The very process of accumulating such experience and data is as exciting for those of us engaged in it as is the awareness of being involved in a new and promising advance, which is likely to have a profound impact on the practice of the science and art of aesthetic plastic surgery.

REFERENCES

1. Semm K: In Sanfilippo J, Levine R, editors: *Operative gynecologic endoscopy*, New York, 1989, Springer-Verlag.
2. Bozzini P: *Der Lichtleiter oder Beschreibung einer einfachen Vorrichtung und Anwendung zur Erleuchtung innerer Hohlen und Zwischenraume des lebenden animalischen Korpers*, Weimar, 1807, Landes-Industrie-Comptoir.
3. Stein S: Das Photo-Endoskop, *Berl Klin Wochenschr* Par 3, 1874.
4. Kelling G: Uber Oesophagoskopie, Gastroskopie and Colioskopie, *Munch Med Wochenschr* 49:21, 1901.
5. Jacobaeus HC: Uber die Moglichkeit, die Zystoskopie bei Untersuchung seroser Hohlungen Anzuwenden, *Munch Med Wochenschr* 57:2090, 1910.

5a. Fervers C: Die laparoskopie mit dem Cytoskope. Ein Beitrag zur Vereinfachung der Technik ud zur endoskopischen Strangdurchtrennung in der Bauchole, *Medizinische Klinik* 29:1042.

6. Boesch PF: Laparoskopie, *Schweiz Z Krankenhaus Anstaltsw* 6:62, 1936.
7. Kalk H, Bruhl W, Burgmann W: Leitfaden der Laparoskopie, *Munch Med Wochenschr* 49:21, 1951.
8. Robson MC, Phillips LG, Thomason A, et al: Platelet-derived growth factor BB for the treatment of chronic pressure ulcers, *Lancet* 339:23, 1992.
9. Khouri RK, Upton J, Shaw WW, et al: Prefabrication of composite free flaps through staged microvascular transfer: an experimental and clinical study, *Plast Reconstr Surg* 87:108, 1991.
10. Estes JM, Whitby DJ, Lorenz HP, Longaker MT, Szabo Z, Adzik NS, Harrison MR: Endoscopic creation and repair of fetal cleft lip, *Plast Reconstr Surg* 90(5):743, 1992.
11. Rosenberg P, Lombardo A, Treat M, et al: Laparoscopic harvest of jejunal segments in the dog for esophageal reconstruction. PSEF Symposium on Current Concepts in Microsurgical Tissue Transfer, St Louis, 1992.
12. Rosenberg P, Miller M, Saltz R, et al: Laparoscopic harvest of the jejunum for free tissue transfer. Presented at the 62nd Annual Scientific Meeting of the ASPRS, New Orleans, September 1993.
13. Miller M: Preclinical experience with laparoscopic tissue harvest. Presented at the 72nd Annual Meeting of the American Association of Plastic Surgeons, Philadelphia, 1993.
14. Miller M: Personal communication.
15. Saltz R, Stowers R, Smith M, Gadacz TR: Laparoscopically harvested omental free flap to cover a large soft tissue defect, *Ann Surg* 217:542, 1993.
16. Boss W: Endoscopic omental flap reconstruction of the breast. Presented at the Annual Meeting of the Aesthetic Society, Dallas, April 15, 1994.
17. Miller M, Staley CA, King TJ: Preclinical experience with laparoscopic tissue harvest. Presented at the 72nd Annual Meeting of the American Association of Plastic Surgeons, Philadelphia, 1993.
18. Eaves FF, Price CI, Bostwick J, Nahai F, Jones G, Carlson G, Culbertson J: Subcutaneous endoscopic plastic surgery using a retractor-mounted endoscopic system, *Perspec Plast Surg* 7:1, 1993.
19. Sasaki G: Endoscopic expansion surgery. Presented at the LSNA Forum for Innovative Plastic Surgery, Dallas, April 1994.
20. Anger J, Szego T: Use of videoscopy as an aid in the placement of tissue expanders, *Rev Paul Med* 111(2):363, 1993.
21. Eaves FF, Price CI, Bostwick J, Nahai F, Jones G, Carlson G, Culbertson J: Subcutaneous endoscopic plastic surgery using a retractor-mounted endoscopic system, *Perspec Plast Surg* 7:1, 1993.
22. Teimourian B: Subcutaneous endoscopy in suction lipectomy, *J Plast Reconstr Surg* 74:708, 1984.
23. Gerow F: Personal communication, May, 1991.
24. Dowden R, Anain S: Endoscopic implant inspection. Paper presented at the Annual Meeting of American Society of Aesthetic Plastic Surgery, Los Angeles, May 3, 1992.
25. Dowden R, Anain S: Endoscopic implant evaluation and capsulotomy, *Plast Reconstr Surg* 91:283, 1993.
26. Colon G: Endoscopic examination of intracapsular mophology. Paper presented at the Annual Meeting of American Society of Aesthetic Plastic Surgery, Los Angeles, May 3, 1992.
27. Rosenberg P, Lombardo A, Williams M, Bessler M, Treat M: Endoscopic capsulotomy. Paper presented at the Annual Meeting of the American Society of Aesthetic Plastic Surgery, Los Angeles, May 3, 1992.
28. Rosenberg P, Williams M, Bessler M, et al: Treatment of periprosthetic capsular contracture with endoscopic techniques. Presented at the 62nd Annual Scientific Meeting of the ASPRS, New Orleans, September 1993.
29. Rosenberg P, Williams M, Bessler M, et al: Endoscopic capsulotomy, *Plast Surg Forum* XVI, 128, 1993.
30. Kompatscher P: Endoscopic capsulotomy of capsular contracture after breast augmentation, *Plast Reconstr Surg* 90(6):1125, 1992.
31. Dowden R, Anain S: Endoscopic implant evaluation and capsulotomy, *Plast Reconstr Surg* 91:283, 1993.
32. Rosenberg P: Endoscopic evaluation and grading of silicone breast implant status. LSNA Forum for Innovative Plastic Surgery, Dallas, April 1994.
33. Johnson G, Christ J: The endoscopic breast augmentation: the transumbilical insertion of saline-filled breast implants, *Plast Reconstr Surg* 92:801, 1993.

34. Johnson G: Personal communication, Jan 4, 1994.
35. Ho LC: Endoscopic assisted transaxillary augmentation mammoplasty, *Br J Plast Surg* 46:332, 1993.
36. Johnson G: Personal communication.
37. Faria-Correa M: Videotape presentation. ASPRS Conference, Beverly Hills, CA, March 4, 1993.
38. Mitz V: Endoscopic control during rhinoplasty. Presented at the Fifth Annual Meeting of the European Association of Plastic Surgeons, Geneva, Switzerland, May 14, 1994.
39. Core GB, Vasconez L, Askren C, Yamamoto Y, Gamboa M: Coronal facelift with endoscopic techniques. Presented at the 61st Annual Scientific Meeting of the ASPRS, Washington, DC, September 1992.
40. Core GB, Vasconez L, Askren C, Yamamoto Y, Gamboa M: Coronal facelift with endoscopic techniques, *Plast Surg Forum* XV:227, 1992.
41. Liang M, Narayanan K: Endoscopic ablation of frontalis and corrugator muscles: a clinical report, *Plast Surg Forum* XV:54, 1992.
42. Hamas R: Endoscopic resection of corrugator muscles to reduce glabellar frown lines. Annual Meeting of the American Society for Aesthetic Plastic Surgery, Boston, April 1993.
43. Isse NG: Endoscopic forehead lift, *Plast Surg Forum* XVI 18(1):21, 1993.
44. Duchenne de Boulogne GB: The mechanism of human facial expression, New York, 1990, Cambridge University Press. (Translated and edited by RA Cuthbertson).
45. Isse NG: Endoscopic facial rejuvenation: endoforehead, the functional lift. Case reports, *Aesth Plast Surg* 18:21, 1994.
46. Ramirez OM, Maillard GF, Musolas A: The extended subperiosteal facelift: a definitive soft tissue remodeling for facial rejuvenation, *Plast Reconstr Surg* 88:227, 1991.
47. Ramirez O: Endoscopic full facelift, *Aesth Plast Surg* 18:363-371, 1994.
48. Tessier P: Facelifting and frontal rhytidectomy. Presented at the Seventh International Congress of Plastic and Reconstructive Surgery, Rio de Janeiro, 1979.
49. Krastinova-Lolov, D: Le lifting facial sous-périosté, *Ann Chir Plast Esthet* 34:199, 1989.
50. Santana PM: Metodologia craniomaxilofacial en retidoplastias, *Cirugia Plast Ibero-Latinomer* 10:322, 1984.
51. Psillakis JM: Empleo de tecnicas de cirugia craniofacial en las ritidoplastias del tercio superior de la cara, *Cirugia Plast Ibero-Latinomer* 10:297, 1984.
52. Fuente del Campo A: Facelift without preauricular scars, *Plast Reconstr Surg* 92:642, 1993.
53. Fuente del Campo A: Personal communication, July 7, 1994.
54. Aiache A: Endoscopic facelifting. Poster Presentation at the 62nd Annual Scientific Meeting of the ASPRS, New Orleans, September 1993.
55. Aiache A: Endoscopic face-lifting. ISAPS Meeting, Paris, 1994.
56. Toledo LS: Video-endoscopic facelift, *Aesth Plast Surg* 18:149, 1994.

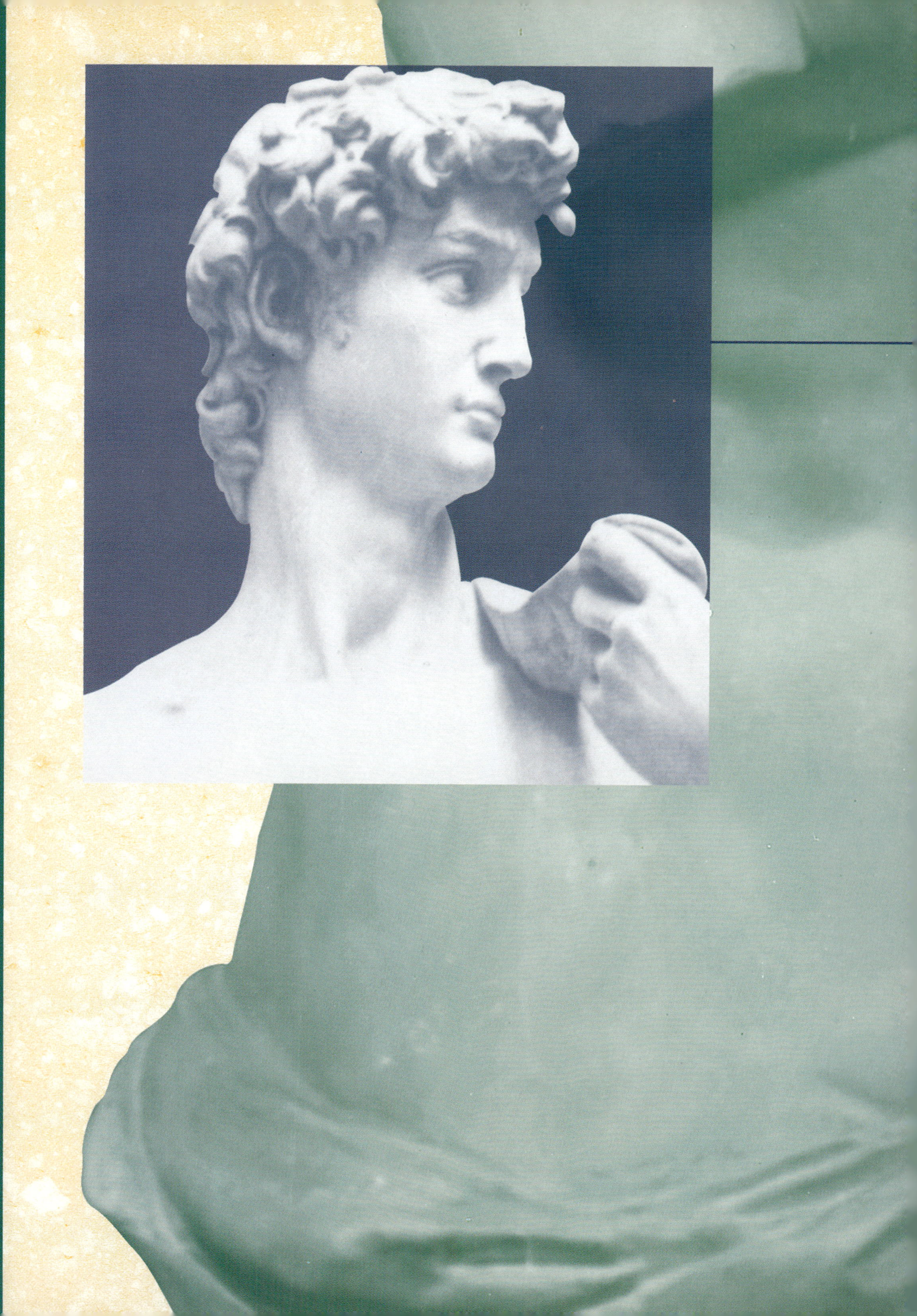

PART I

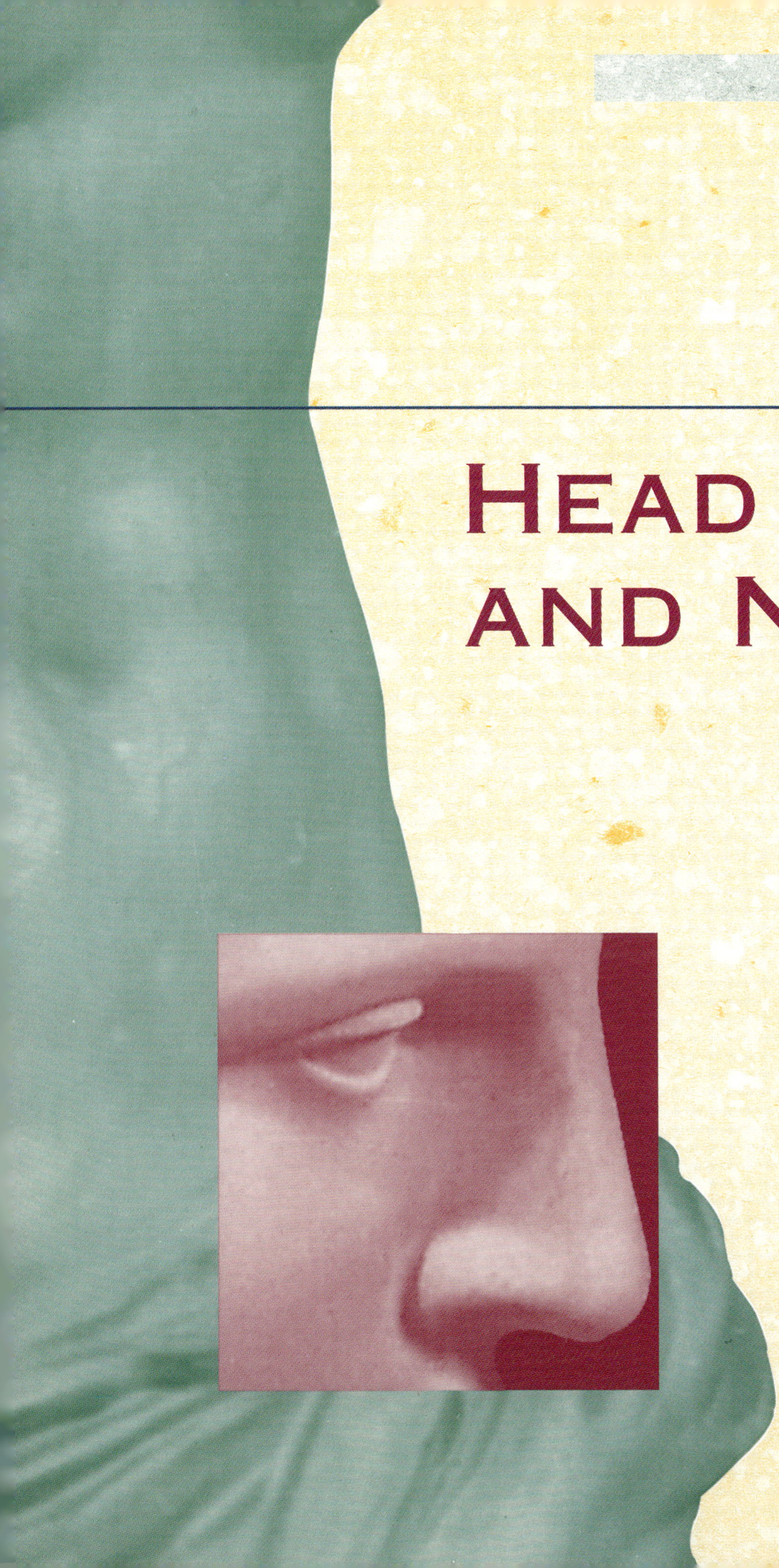

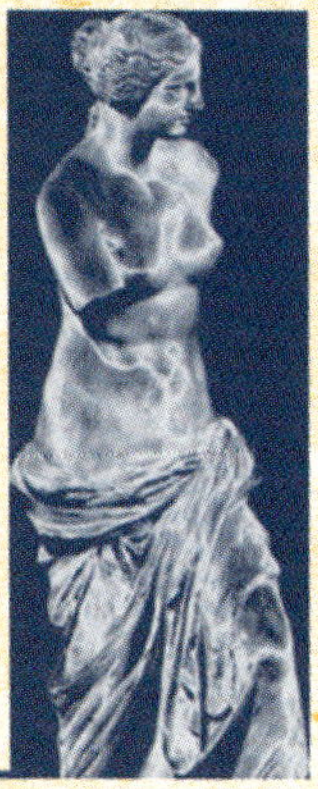

HEAD AND NECK

CHAPTER 1

Anatomic Considerations

Gordon H. Sasaki

The traditional approach to facial anatomy begins at the level of the skin and proceeds in a layered fashion down to bone. For the endoscopic surgeon, however, the view starts from within and extends outward through minimally invasive ports by means of an endoscopic camera. This precise but restrictive window produces a two-dimensional magnified image that may on initial inspection appear to be foreign to the reconstructive surgeon. This chapter identifies landmarks of the deeper structures that are encountered in the journey around specific areas of the face during forehead, periorbital, and midfacial lifts. The deeper anatomy is correlated with the external physical signs of aging.

THE AGING FOREHEAD

Tissue laxity and wrinkle lines characterize the aging forehead. Tissue relaxation occurs primarily in the loose skin that gradually descends and hangs from the superior and lateral orbital rims. During facial relaxation, this redundant tissue creates interbrow fullness, brow ptosis, and lateral hooding of the upper lid (pseudoptosis). These physical findings may become accentuated during certain facial animations, such as frowning or squinting, that actively draw down these ptotic structures. Because facial muscles are inserted into the undersurface of the skin, lines of facial expression become evident during animation. Eventually, these temporary lines become etched into the aging, sun-damaged skin as permanent features. In some patients, significant frontoorbital bony prominences and recessions also develop that accentuate soft tissue ptosis and skin wrinkling during the gradual aging process.

Forehead rejuvenation requires not only a balance between brow elevator and depressor muscles but also repositioning of the ptotic soft tissues, smoothing out of the wrinkle lines, and recontouring of the frontoorbital bony irregularities. A detailed understanding of the static and dynamic (functional) forehead anatomy is essential for the facial aesthetic surgeon.

CLASSIC FOREHEAD ANATOMY

Functional Forehead Anatomy

The sole elevator of the eyebrow-forehead complex is the epicranius, which consists of two frontal-

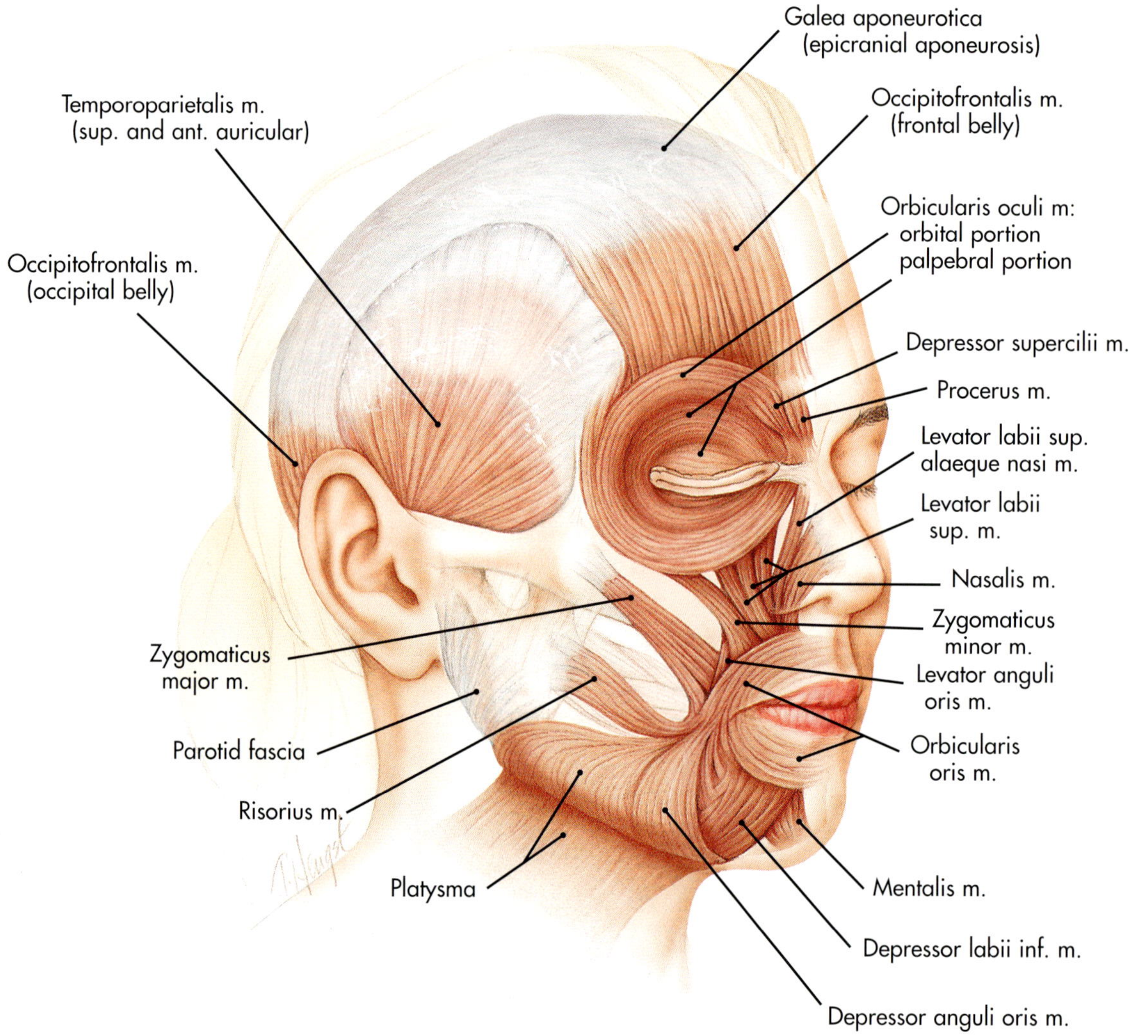

FIGURE 1-1
Muscles of the facial anatomy (front and side views) are shown.

is muscles, interconnecting galea aponeurotica, and two occipitalis muscles (Figure 1-1). The occipital and frontal muscles of the epicranius, acting in concert, draw the scalp back and raise the eyebrows in an expression of surprise. The frontal bellies, acting alone, can raise and produce a pronounced curvature of the eyebrows, making it difficult to assess the contribution from the galea aponeurotica–occipitalis muscle unit. In patients with significant forehead ptosis, compensatory activity of the frontalis muscles develops to counteract the heavy eyebrow–upper lid droop. The constant contraction of the frontalis muscles produces a number of premature horizontal creases across the lateral aspects of the forehead. The antagonist muscles that depress the eyebrows are the central procerus, two corrugator supercilii, two depressor supercilii, and the orbital segments of the orbicularis oculi muscles. Prolonged depressor muscle activity along with the ptotic effects of aging eventually force the forehead-brow complex downward, overpowering the agonist effects of the elevators.

Of the four depressor muscles, the orbital portion of the orbicularis muscle has the most profound effect on lowering the central eyebrow. This muscle is responsible for the many oblique vertical wrinkle lines on the forehead, "crow's feet" area, and upper cheek. The orbicularis oculi is the sphincter muscle of the eyelids. The palpebral portion closes the lids gently, as in blinking or in sleep; the orbital portion is used in more forceful closing, as in winking with one eye. When the entire muscle is brought into action, the skin of the forehead, brow, temple, and cheek is drawn downward and toward the medial angle of the orbit and the eyelids are firmly closed, as in photophobia.

The paired corrugator muscles draw the central part of the eyebrows inward and downward and are considered to be the classic "frown muscles" of suffering. These muscles produce the one to three vertical lines in the glabellar region and in the soft tissue prominence of frowning above the brows. There is an elevation of the medial portion of the brow with corrugator muscle activity that draws the central brow downward and inward but displaces the medial brow upward and inward. The central procerus muscle and the depressor supercilii muscles also displace the eyebrows downward and produce the transverse wrinkle lines across the nasal root and central low forehead.

STATIC FOREHEAD ANATOMY

SKIN

Enriched by closely packed hair follicles, sebaceous glands, and sweat glands, which reach down to the superficial fascia, the skin of the hair-bearing scalp is thicker than in any other area of the body. The enormous number of adnexal structures contributes to the rigidity of the scalp skin and to its adherence to the underlying superficial fascia.

MUSCLES

The facial muscles of expression are cutaneous muscles lying within the layers of the superficial fascia (tela subcutanea). In the head and neck area, the superficial fascia is composed of an outer layer, called the panniculus adiposus, and a thin, inner membranous layer of elastic tissue devoid of fat. In general, facial muscles originate either from the fascia or from the facial bones and are inserted into the undersurface of the skin. An individual muscle seldom remains separate and distinct throughout its length because it merges with neighboring muscles at insertion points. The muscles of facial expression move the skin of the forehead and scalp in defined directions or act as sphincters around the eyes.

ELEVATOR MUSCLES. In the scalp and forehead the frontalis muscles, the galea aponeurotica, and the occipitalis muscles lie between the dense connective layer of the superficial fascia above and the loose connective layer of the superficial fascia below.

Frontalis Muscles (Figure 1-1). Each belly of the frontalis muscle (venter frontalis) is quadrilateral in shape, measuring about 6 cm in width and 7 cm in length. The muscle is wider and longer than the occipitalis muscle and contains fasciculi that are longer, finer, and paler than those of the occipital muscle. The frontalis muscles have no bony attachments: their medial fibers join together for a short distance above the nasal root, comingling at the same level with fibers of the procerus muscle; its intermediate fibers merge with upcoming fibers from the subjacent corrugator muscles, interweaving at the same level with the circling fibers of the orbital portion of the orbicularis oculi muscle; and its lateral fibers blend with the horizontal fibers of the orbital segment of the orbicularis oculi muscle, which lies over the zygomatic process of the frontal bone. From these attachments the frontalis fibers are directed obliquely upward and are encompassed by the galea aponeurotica.

The sensory branches of the supraorbital and supratrochlear nerves course over the frontalis muscles. The supraorbital nerve supplies sensation to the scalp to as far as the crown of the head by dividing into medial and lateral branches. The supratrochlear nerve gives sensation to the forehead in the region of the glabella and the medial part of the upper eyelids. These terminal endings of the larger frontal branch of the ophthalmic division of the trigeminal nerve reach the scalp after passing through the supraorbital and supratrochlear notches of the frontal bones, respectively. The supraorbital notch, or foramen, is located immediately above the upper border of the orbit at the junction of its medial with its lateral two thirds. It harbors the nerve and vessels of the same name. In a small percentage of persons, the main supraorbital nerve or one of its branches may exit about 1 cm above the orbital rim. This anatomic variance can be expected when the familiar notch, or foramen, cannot be palpated on physical examination. The supraorbital nerve can usually be observed, and thus protected, during endoscopic dissection around the supraorbital notch, or foramen. Occasionally, the nerve may be embedded within the corrugator muscle, obscuring its presence until dissection of that muscle is in progress. Blind subperiosteal dissection below the superciliary arch to the superior orbital rim may inadvertently injure a high-exiting branch of the supraorbital nerve. Whereas the supratrochlear nerve runs above the pulley of the superior oblique muscle, exits from its notch, and consistently threads its multiple branches through the corrugator muscles before lying on the frontalis muscles. During endoscopic elevation of the periosteum, the surgeon will not see these thinner branches until the corrugator muscles are dissected.

Galea Aponeurotica (Figures 1-1 and 1-2). The galea aponeurotica (epicranial aponeurosis) covers the cranium between the frontal and occipital bellies of the occipitofrontalis muscles. In addition to its attachment to these muscle bellies, it is firmly attached behind the space between the two occipital muscles to the external occipital protuberance (inion) and the adjacent highest nuchal line of the occipital bone. On either side at the level of the superior temporal line on the parietal bone, the galea merges and receives the superior insertion of the overlying temporoparietalis fascia (often termed the *superficial temporal fascia*). At this point, the galea loses its aponeurotic character and is continuous over the deep temporal fascia, which covers the temporalis muscles. The fusion of the galea aponeurotica, deep temporal fascia, and periosteum at the superior temporal line and the lateral edge of the lateral orbital rim creates a dense and firm attachment of these structures to

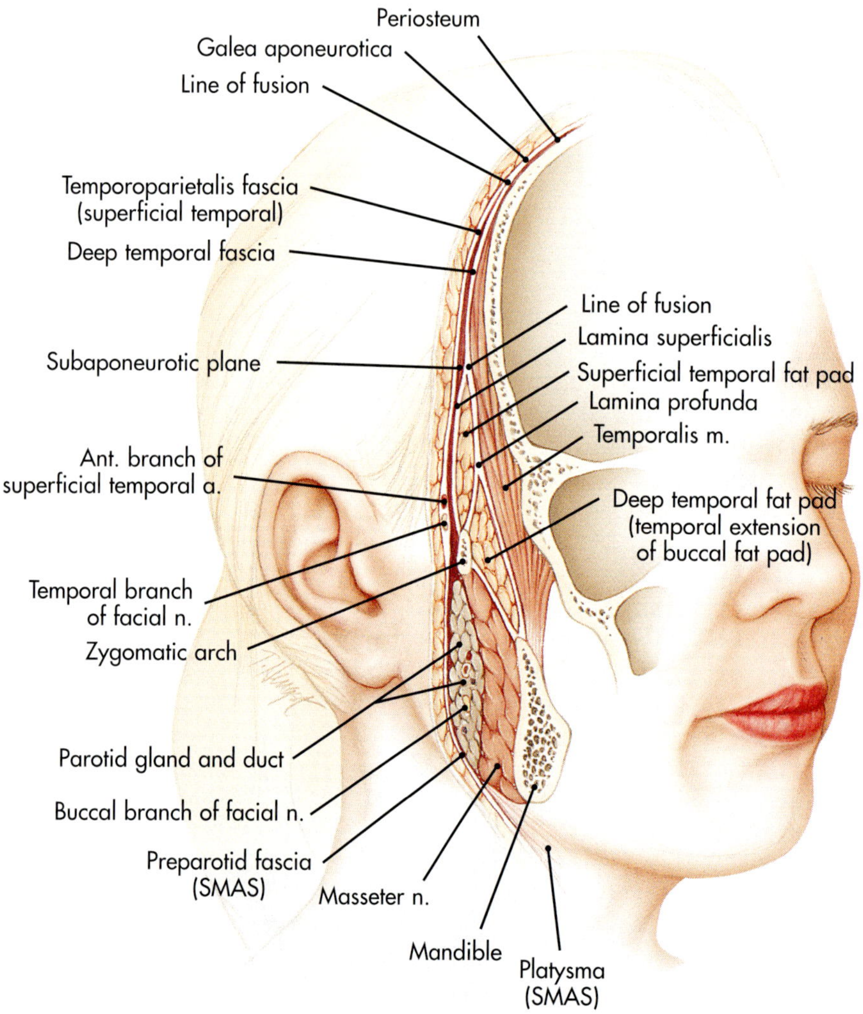

FIGURE 1-2
Coronal section demonstrating the superficial musculo-aponeurotic system (SMAS) is shown.

the underlying bone. These dense thickened attachments to the bone must be sharply divided during the subperiosteal dissection under endoscopic control to release the soft tissue. The galea aponeurosis itself spreads over the loose layer of connective tissue of the superficial fascia, which covers the underlying periosteum.

The temporoparietalis fascia originates from the deep temporal fascia above the ear and spreads out like a fan over the temporal fascia, inserting at the lateral border of the galea at the superior temporal line. The superficial temporal artery (veins), the frontal motor branch to the facial nerve, and the small muscle bellies of the anterior and superior auricularis muscles reside within the temporoparietalis fascia. There is a thin layer of fat between the temporoparietalis fascia and the deep temporal fascia.

Occipitalis Muscles (Figure 1-1). Each belly of the occipitalis muscles (venter occipitalis) is quadrilateral (4 cm wide and 4 cm long) in shape and originates from the lateral two thirds of the superior nuchal line of the occipital bone. The muscle fibers ascend toward the vertex and are inserted into the galea aponeurotica. Between the bellies of the occipitalis muscles is a considerable—although variable—space occupied by a prolongation of the galea aponeurotica.

DEPRESSOR MUSCLES

Corrugator Muscles (Figures 1-1 and 1-3) The corrugator muscle (corrugator supercilii) is small, narrow, and pyramidal in shape, about 1 cm wide and 3 cm long. It is located at the medial end of the eyebrow beneath the frontalis and orbicularis oculi muscles. The corrugator muscle arises from the medial end of the superciliary arch; its fibers pass upward and lateral between the palpebral and orbital portions of the orbicularis oculi muscle and are inserted into the deep surface of the skin above the middle of the brow arch.

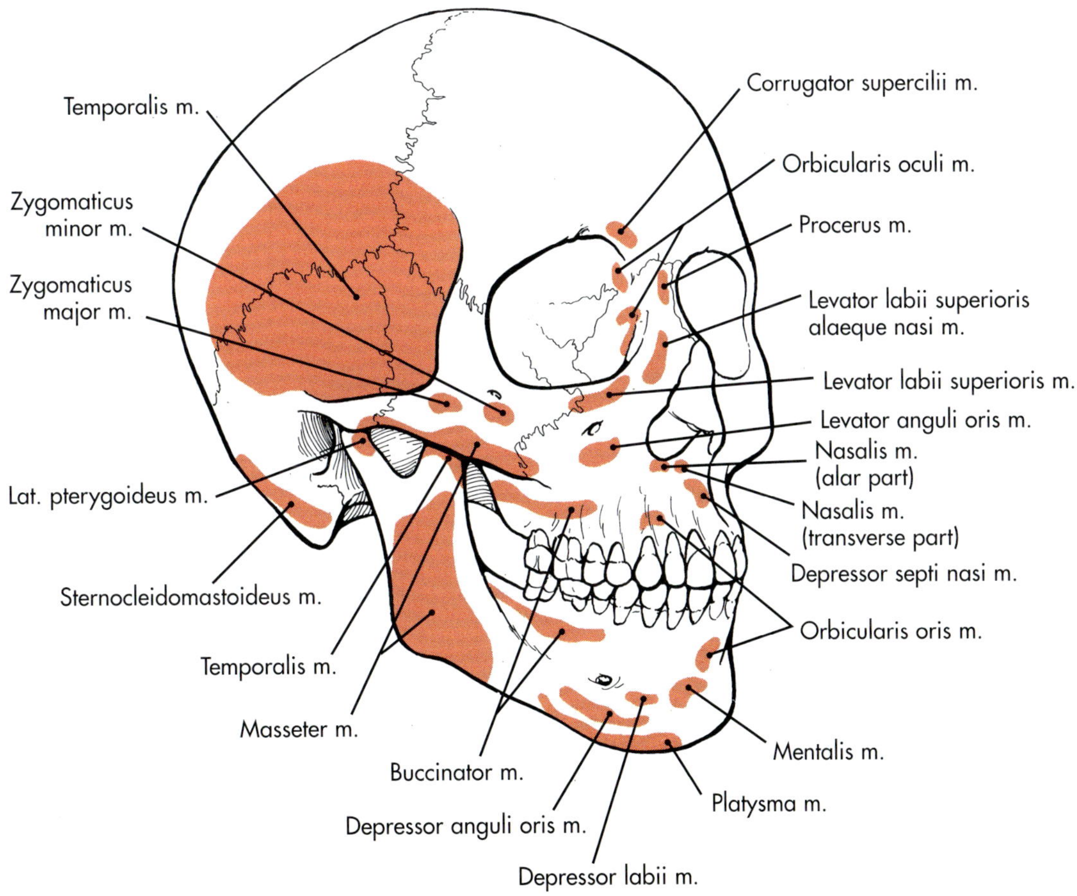

FIGURE 1-3
Attachments of the facial muscles to the skull are shown.

Procerus Muscle (Figures 1-1 and 1-3). The procerus muscle (pyramidalis nasi) is a small pyramidal slip that originates by tendinous fibers from the fascia, covering the lower part of the nasal bones and the adjacent upper portion of the upper lateral nasal cartilages. The muscle decussates with the medial borders of the frontalis muscles and is inserted into the skin over the lower midportion of the forehead, between the two eyebrows. The origin of the procerus muscle is intimately associated with the subjacent nasalis muscle, which plays no significant role in depression of the forehead structures. The nasalis (compressor naris) consists of the transverse and alar parts. The transverse part begins from the maxilla above and runs lateral to the incisive fossae. Its fibers course upward and medially, forming a thin, adherent aponeurotic apron, which is continuous on the nasal bridge with that muscle of the opposite side. The alar portion of the nasalis muscle is attached to the lower alar cartilage and skin at the nasal tip. The nasal muscle depresses the cartilaginous part of the nose and contracts the ala nasi toward the septum.

Depressor Supercilii Muscle (Figure 1-1). The depressor supercilii muscle is located on the medial arc of the orbicularis oculi muscle. It is unclear whether the depressor supercilii muscle is part of the orbicularis oculi muscle or is a separate muscle that aids in pulling down the medial portion of the eyebrows and overlying skin. The depressor muscle arises from the nasal process to the frontal bone and extends upward to interdigitate with fibers of the procerus and frontalis muscles.

Orbicularis Oculi Muscle (Figures 1-1 and 1-3). The orbicularis oculi muscle arises from medial bony origins and is inserted laterally on soft tissues and skin. This large, circular, concentric muscle represents one of the largest facial muscles, extending above the eyebrows and onto the midcheek and lateral temporal zone. It begins from the nasal part of the frontal bone and from the frontal process of the maxilla anterior to the medial palpebral ligament. From this broad origin, its fibers sweep in concentric arcs over the eyelids, the circumference of the orbit, and the temple and cheek.

The orbicularis muscle is arbitrarily divided into orbital, palpebral, and lacrimal portions. The palpebral portion is further subdivided into pretarsal and preseptal sections. The outer orbital portion begins medially from the superomedial orbital margin, the maxillary process of the frontal bone, the medial canthal tendon, the frontal process of the maxilla, and the inferomedial orbital margin. The outer peripheral fibers cross the eyelids in a series of concentric loops, the more central ones forming almost complete rings. In the upper lid, the orbital portion spreads upward onto the forehead, covers and blends with the corrugator and frontalis muscles, and then continues laterally over the temporoparietalis fascia. In the lower lid, the orbital portion covers the origins of the elevator muscles of the upper lip and ala nasi and continues temporally to cover the origin to the masseter. Occasionally, the lower portion may continue downward onto the cheek, as festoons of the aging process. The preseptal portion diverges from its origin on the medial canthal tendon and lacrimal diaphragm and passes across the lid as a series of half ellipses to meet at the lateral canthal raphe. Medially, the orbicularis oculi unites to join the medial canthal tendon, which is inserted on the medial orbital margin and nasal bones. The lacrimal portion of the orbicularis oculi muscle is a thin strip, about 6 mm wide and 12 mm long, situated behind the medial palpebral ligament and lacrimal sac. It arises from the posterior crest and the adjacent part of the orbital surface of the lacrimal bone, passes behind the lacrimal sac, and is inserted by two slips into the superior and inferior tarsus.

NERVES (FIGURE 1-4)

The frontal branch of the facial nerve lies on the periosteum of the proximal one third of the zygomatic arch. This crossing point may be 2.5 cm from the anterior border of the external auditory meatus, but it may vary between 0.8 cm and 3.5 cm from this point. The course of the nerve is within or under the temporoparietalis fascia; it makes an oblique angle 1.5 cm lateral to the brow to enter the frontalis belly on its undersurface, not greater than 2 cm above the eyebrow. The frontal branch also enters the posterior surfaces of the two corrugator and procerus muscles and, occasionally, a portion of the orbicularis oculi muscle. Nerves from the temporal and zygomatic branches of the facial nerve enter the undersurface of the orbicularis oculi and depressor supercilii muscles, while nerves from the buccal branches enter on the undersurface of the procerus and nasalis muscles.

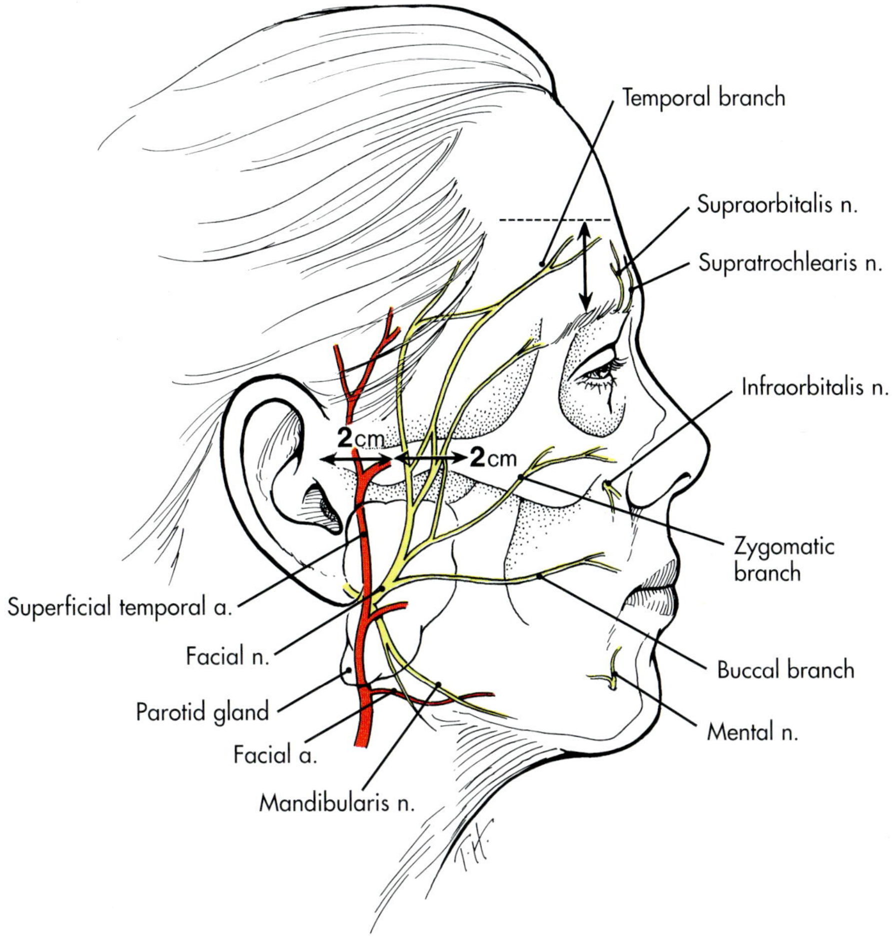

FIGURE 1-4
Landmarks for the temporal branch of the facial nerve are shown.

ENDOSCOPIC ANATOMY OF FOREHEAD AND PERIORBITUM

FOREHEAD AND SCALP POCKETS

Elevation of the forehead and scalp is accomplished both by blind dissection and endoscopically assisted release of more critical areas. Initially, the surgeon elevates—without the assistance of the endoscope—the periosteum from the forehead frontal bone via three 1.5-cm vertical incisions located behind the precapillary hairline, down to the level of the superciliary arches and out laterally to the superior temporal line. This forehead pocket is then connected in continuity with the scalp subperiosteal pocket, which is then blindly elevated with the same dissector. The scalp pocket is defined from the superior temporal lines to the vertex of the scalp. Usually, the right-handed surgeon introduces the endoscope with his left hand through one of the left-sided ports and works with the dissector in his dominant hand through one of the right-sided ports to complete the forehead subperiosteal dissection down to the supraorbital margins, below the nasofrontal suture line in the interbrow space, and laterally along the zygomatic process of the frontal bone past the zygomaticofrontal suture line at the lateral orbital rim. During the endoscopic periorbital dissection, the surgeon views through the small optical window the frontal bone below and the glistening periosteal ceiling above. In the patient with a palpable supraorbital notch, or foramen, the supraorbital nerve and vessels should be observed and endoscopically preserved throughout this dissection. Occasionally, the surgeon may find the main supraorbital nerve exiting from an opening above the rim. Blind dissection may inadvertently injure this nerve and may also produce more bleeding by forced entry through the periosteum at the level of the orbital rim.

Temporal Pocket

The temporal pocket is located over the temporal muscle, bordered above at the superior temporal line, forward along the posterior edges of the zygomatic process of the frontal bone and the frontal process of the zygoma (lateral orbital rim), and below at the cephalic edge of the zygomatic arch. A 1-cm incision in the hair above the ear permits swift access to the temporal pocket by entering through the temporoparietal fascia. When a rhytidectomy is scheduled as part of the facial rejuvenation procedure, the usual temporal incision gives a wider opening for the dissection of the temporal pocket. Blind dissection above the deep temporal fascia gains quick access superiorly into the subperiosteal forehead pocket, after crossing the fusion line at the superior temporal line. Inferior elevation of the temporoparietalis fascia should be conservative because the frontal branch of the facial nerve lies on the undersurface of this fascia, above the zygomatic arch. Sharp dissection with scissors of the fascia and periosteum along the posterior edge of the orbital rim is necessary to further connect these two pockets. This dissection is safely accomplished by passing the endoscope through the midforehead precapillary scalp port and cutting through the lateral precapillary scalp opening. Endoscopic isolation and cauterization of a solitary sentinel vein may be necessary during this portion of the endodissection. The sentinel vein is predictably located 5 mm lateral to the frontozygomatic suture line and marks the most inferior level of dissection of the forehead and temporal pockets.

When a periorbital release is planned to elevate the lateral commissure, a 5-mm incision at the lateral canthus through the periosteum covering the lateral orbital rim permits a blind dissection cephalad along the frontal process of the zygoma. A safer breakthrough of the dissector from the periorbital pocket into the frontal pocket is facilitated by an optical view, with the endoscope positioned through the lateral precapillary port of the scalp. Further endodissection of the tough attachments of periosteum along the posterior edge of the zygoma that have not yet been released during development of the temporal pocket is now completed. If the surgeon plans to release more of the subperiosteal pocket under the zygoma over the zygomatic arch and infraorbital rim, a great part of it can be done through this lateral canthal incision.

Release of Arcus Marginalis and Depressor Muscles

The surgeon returns to the frontal pocket to complete an endoscopic release of the periosteum at the level of the arcus marginalis, above the level of the superior orbital rim and across the interbrow area to the lateral bare area of the anterior superior temporal line behind the upper lateral orbital rim. An effective, complete periosteal release will elevate the forehead-brow complex by 1 to 2 cm without upward traction. The origin and insertion of the corrugator muscles may be marked transcutaneously with methylene blue dye injected with a needle. Endoscopic avulsion, myotomy, or myectomy of the red, fleshy corrugator muscle may be performed precisely. Identification and preservation of the supraorbital neurovascular bundles from the notch, or foramen, can be easily done during release of the corrugator muscles. The finer intramuscular fibers of the supratrochlear nerve within the corrugator muscles can be teased away from the muscle. Further dissection of fleshy muscle lateral to the supraorbital nerve represents the orbital portion of the orbicularis oculi muscle. Endoscopic release of a paler muscle within the interbrow area represents the procerus muscle. Blind release with long scissors of the medial portion of the orbicularis muscle at the level of the medial brow represents release of the depressor supercilii muscle.

THE AGING MIDFACE

Changes in the midface during the aging process are believed to be due primarily to skin laxity as it drapes from the malar cheekbone down to the mandible and into the neck proper. Midface skin is adherent to the deeper structures between the cheek and ear, tethered by the zygomatic ligament and the anteriorly located mandibular ligament. In the lateral neck proper, below the lobule of the ear and behind the ear posterior to the sternocleido-

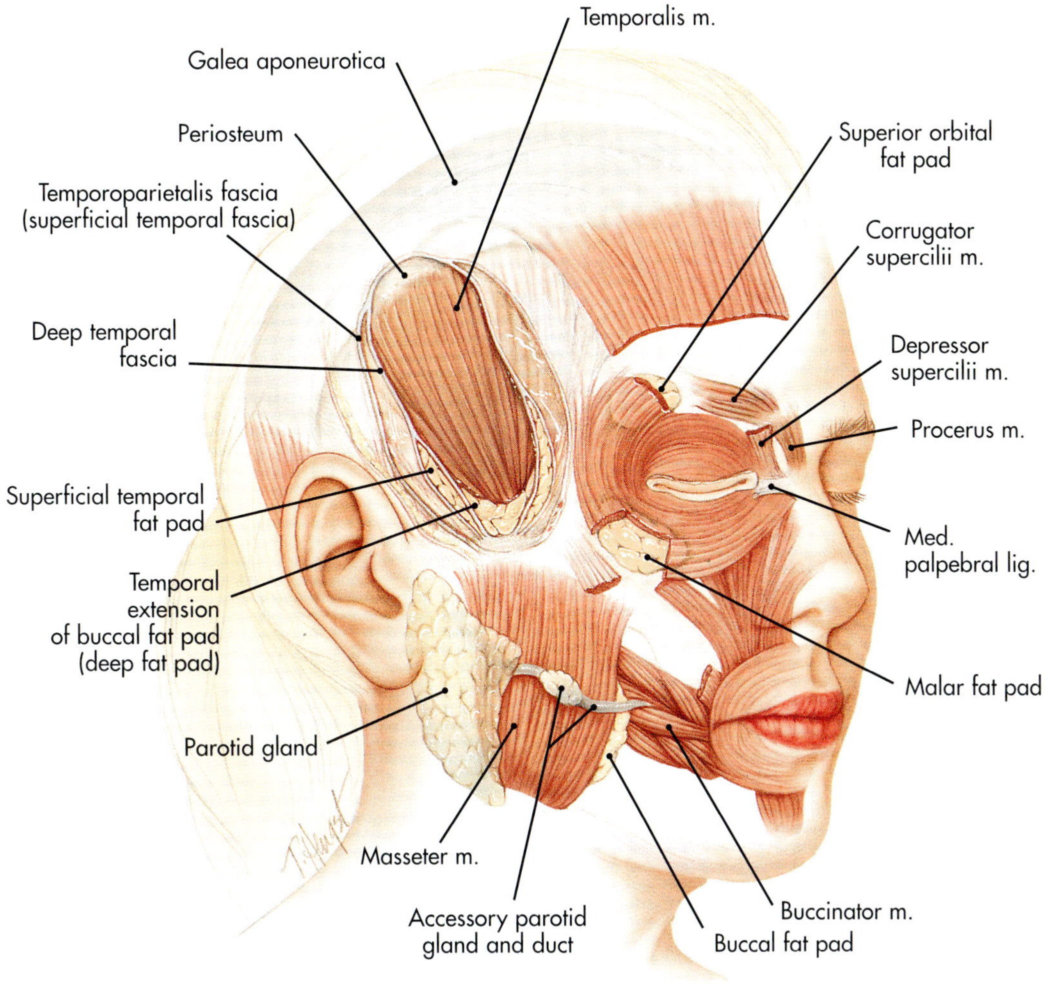

FIGURE 1-5
Head and upper cervical region from the left side are shown.

mastoid muscle, neck skin is also adherent to the deeper fascial coverings. The stigmata of the aging midface is thus located in the anterior half, between the cheek and naso-oral structures, referred to as the nasolabial folds, labiomandibular folds (marionette lines), and jowls. In the complex area of the nasolabial folds, activity of the lip elevators and zygomatic major and minor muscles accentuate the formation of the folds during animation. With aging, the folds remain due to lax skin and ptosis of the cheek fat along the lateral edge of the nasolabial line. The marionette lines are produced primarily by skin sagging and laxity of the underlying anterior border of the platysma. The jowls above the inferior border of the mandible are created by lax skin and the loose platysma muscle that has no bony attachments in the midface region.

CLASSIC MIDFACE ANATOMY

FUNCTIONAL MIDFACE ANATOMY (FIGURE 1-5)

The levator labii superioris muscle is the proper elevator of the upper lip and, at the same time, carries it a little forward. The levator labii superioris alaeque nasi muscle also dilates the naris and forms with the levator labii superioris and the zygomaticus minor muscles the nasolabial furrow, which is deepened in expressions of sadness. When these three muscles act in conjunction with the levator anguli oris, the furrow is deepened into an expression of contempt or disdain. The zygomaticus major draws the angle of the mouth upward and backward, as in laughing.

The risorius muscle retracts the angle of the mouth. The depressor labii inferioris draws the lower lip directly downward and laterally, as in the expression of irony. Being the antagonist of the levator anguli oris and zygomaticus major, the depressor anguli oris depresses the angle of the mouth and, acting with the levator, draws the angle of the mouth medially. The mentalis raises and protrudes the lower lip and, at the same time, wrinkles the skin of the chin, expressing doubt or disdain. Retracting and depressing the angle of the mouth, the platysma acts with this group.

The orbicularis oris effects the direct closure of the lips by its deep fibers, assisted by its oblique fibers; it closely applies the lips to the alveolar arch. The superficial part brings together the lips and also allows them to protrude forward.

The buccinator muscle compresses the cheek and is an important accessory muscle of mastication, holding the food under the immediate pressure of the teeth. When the cheeks have been distended with air, the buccinators compress them and tend to force the cheeks out between the lips, as in blowing a trumpet.

STATIC MIDFACE ANATOMY

MUSCLES AND FASCIA

LEVATOR LABII SUPERIORIS (FIGURES 1-3 AND 1-5). The levator labii superioris muscle has a rather broad origin from the lower margin of the orbit immediately above the infraorbital foramen, with some of its fibers attaching to the maxilla and others to the zygomatic bone. Its fibers converge and insert into the muscular substance of the upper lip between the levator anguli oris and the levator labii superioris alaeque nasi and are overlapped by the orbicularis oculi.

LEVATOR LABII SUPERIORIS ALAEQUE NASI (FIGURES 1-3 AND 1-5). The levator labii superioris alaeque nasi muscle arises by a pointed extremity from the upper part of the frontal process of the maxilla and passes obliquely downward and laterally, dividing into two slips. One of these is inserted into the greater alar cartilage and skin of the nose, and the other is prolonged into the upper lip, blending with the levator labii superioris.

ZYGOMATICUS MAJOR AND MINOR (FIGURES 1-3 AND 1-5). The zygomaticus major muscle, which arises from the zygomatic bone in front of the zygomaticotemporal suture and descends obliquely with a medial inclination, is inserted into the angle of the mouth where the muscle blends with the fibers of the levator, depressor anguli oris, and orbicularis oris. The zygomaticus major is both longer and thicker than the minor and is referred to as the "smiling muscle." The zygomaticus minor arises from the malar surface of the zygomatic bone immediately behind the zygomaticomaxillary suture and passes downward and medially as a narrow slip to be inserted into the upper lip between the levator labii superioris and the zygomaticus major.

LEVATOR ANGULI ORIS (FIGURES 1-3 AND 1-5). The levator anguli oris muscle arises from the canine fossa immediately below the infraorbital foramen. Its fibers are inserted into the angle of the mouth, intermingling with those of the zygomaticus major, depressor anguli oris, and orbicularis oris.

RISORIUS (FIGURE 1-5). The risorius muscle arises in the fascia over the masseter muscle, passes horizontally forward superficial to the platysma, and is inserted into the skin at the angle of the mouth. By drawing the angle of the mouth in a lateral direction, the muscle plays a large part in the production of a smile and has been referred to as the "grinning muscle."

DEPRESSOR LABII INFERIORIS (FIGURE 1-5). The depressor labii inferioris muscle is a small quadrilateral muscle. It arises from the oblique line of the mandible between the symphysis and the mental foramen and passes upward and medially to be inserted into the integument of the lower lip. Its fibers blend with the orbicularis oris and with those of the opposite side. At its origin it is continuous with the fibers of the platysma, and a significant amount of yellow fat is intermingled with the fibers of this muscle.

DEPRESSOR ANGULI ORIS (FIGURES 1-3 AND 1-5). The depressor anguli oris muscle arises from the oblique line of the mandible, where its fibers converge and are inserted by a narrow fasciculus into the angle of the mouth. At its origin it is continuous with those fibers of the levator anguli oris.

MENTALIS (FIGURES 1-3 AND 1-5). The mentalis muscle is a small conical muscle situated at the side of the frenulum of the lower lip. It arises from the incisive fossa of the mandible and is inserted into the integument of the chin.

ORBICULARIS ORIS (FIGURES 1-3 AND 1-5). The orbicularis oris is not a simple sphincter muscle as is the orbicularis oculi. It consists of numerous strata of muscular fibers surrounding the orifice of the mouth in different directions and partly of fibers derived from the other facial muscles that are inserted into the lips and lip proper. A considerable number of fibers are derived from the buccinator and form the deeper stratum of the orbicularis. Some of the buccinator fibers, namely, those arising from the maxilla, pass to the lower lip and those from the mandible to the upper lip. The uppermost and lowermost fibers of the buccinator pass across the lips from side to side without decussation. Formed on either side by the levator anguli oris and depressor anguli oris and superficial to this stratum is a second layer of fibers that cross each other at the angle of the mouth. The fibers from the levator anguli oris pass to the lower lip and those from the depressor anguli oris to the upper lip, along which they run, and are inserted into the skin near the median line. In addition to these, there are fibers from the quadratus labii superioris, the zygomaticus, and quadratus labii inferioris muscles that intermingle with the transverse fibers described above. The proper fibers of the lips are oblique and pass from the undersurface of the skin to the mucous membrane, through the thickness of the lip. Finally, there are fibers by which the muscle is connected with the maxillae and the septum of the nose above and with the mandible below. In the upper lip, these consist of two bands, lateral and medial, on either side of the midline. The lateral band arises from the alveolar border of the maxilla opposite the lateral incisor tooth, and it arches laterally and continuously with the other muscles at the angle of the mouth. The medial band connects the upper lip to the back of the septum, to the nose. The interval between the two medial bands, called the philtrum, corresponds with the depression and is seen on the lip beneath the septum of the nose. The additional fibers for the lower lip constitute a slip on either side of the midline, which arises from the mandible, lateral to the mentalis, and intermingles with the other muscles at the angle of the mouth.

BUCCINATOR (FIGURES 1-3 AND 1-5). The buccinator is the principal muscle of the cheek and forms the lateral wall of the oral cavity. It lies deeper than the other facial muscles, is quadrilateral in form, and occupies the interval between the maxilla and mandible lateral to the teeth. It arises from the outer surfaces of the alveolar processes of the maxilla above and mandible below, alongside three molar teeth and from the pterygomandibular raphe. A tendinous inscription gives origin to both the buccinator and the superior constrictor muscle of the pharynx. The fibers of the upper and lower portions follow a slightly converging course forward and are inserted by blending with the deeper stratum of muscle fibers in the lips. The fibers of the center portion converge toward the angle of the mouth and decussate those fibers above from becoming continuous with the orbicularis oris of the lower lip and those from below with that of the upper lip. The superficial surface of the buccinator is covered by the buccopharyngeal fascia and the buccal fat pad. The deep surface is in relation to the buccal glands and the mucous membrane of the mouth, and it is pierced by the duct of the parotid gland opposite the upper second molar tooth.

NERVES

Branches from the temporal, zygomatic, buccal, and mandibular sections of the facial nerves innervate these muscles on their undersurfaces.

DEEP TEMPORAL FASCIA
(FIGURES 1-2 AND 1-5)

The deep temporal fascia is a strong, fibrous, aponeurotic sheet that covers the temporalis muscle and is used by it for the attachment of its fibers. The deep temporal fascia is the most cranial extension of the deep fascia. Above it, the deep fascia is represented only by the pericranium. The deep temporal fascia is covered by the superficial temporal fascia (temporoparietalis fascia) and the orbicularis oculi muscle anteriorly, and in front of the ear it is crossed by the superficial temporal vessels and the auriculotemporal nerve. Its uppermost portion is a thin, single sheet that is attached to the entire extent of the superior temporal line. Its lower portion, which is 1 to 2 cm above or near the attachment of the zygomatic arch, is thickened and laminated. The inner leaf (lamina profunda) ends by attaching to the medial border of the arch; the outer leaf (lamina superficialis), after attaching to the lateral border, continues downward below the arch as the masseteric fascia. Between the leaves is a small quantity of fat (superficial temporal fat) that sits on the superior surface of the zygomatic arch. The middle temporal artery, which arises from the superficial temporal artery at the level of the zygomatic arch, enters the deep temporal fascia immediately above the zygomatic arch, supplies the fascia and the superficial temporal fat pad, and gives off branches to the temporalis muscle itself. A filament from the zygomatic branch of the maxillary nerve also travels within the interlamellar fat pad.

The superficial temporal fascia, which lies immediately deep to the dermis, is continuous with the galea aponeurotica above and the superficial musculo-aponeurotic system (SMAS) of the face below. The superficial temporal artery and its anterior and posterior branches lie within the fascia, and the accompanying veins are located immediately superficial to it. On its superficial surface, the superficial temporal fascia is attached to the subdermal tissue; whereas on its deep aspect, there is an avascular plane separating it from the deeper structures. The temporal branch of the facial nerve lies on the deep aspect of the fascia, 1 to 2 cm posterior to the lateral orbital rim. A surgical approach that goes deep to the superficial layer of the deep temporalis fascia inferior to the line of fusion will avoid injury to this nerve.

ENDOSCOPIC ANATOMY OF THE MIDFACE

Endoscopic midface procedures are currently in the early stages of development; thus, long-term results are still lacking. The benefits and complications of open subperiosteal midface approaches have begun to be documented. It remains to be seen whether endoscopic releases will contribute significantly, other than allowing smaller incisions, to procedures that commonly involve skin removal. Technically, endoscopic midface subperiosteal dissections can be performed safely when certain areas of dissection are approached with an awareness of anatomic concerns.

Zygomatic Pocket

Dissection under the periosteum of the zygomatic arch and its release is critical to the entry into the midface. Although there are a number of favored surgical approaches to freeing this tight area, a simple and safe method involves a dissection over the zygoma through the lateral canthal incision, coupled with a small incision along the preauricular crease line down to the zygomatic arch. Careful and gentle elevation of the periosteum off the complete arch will not transect the frontal branch as it crosses abruptly over the proximal third of the bone, heading toward the undersurface of the frontalis muscle on the undersurface of the temporoparietalis fascia. However, this subperiosteal dissection can result in temporary nerve palsy from traction injury to the nerve.

A 2-cm transverse incision is then made below the fusion line of the superficial and deep laminae of the deep temporal fascia. Endodissection under the superficial lamina down to and over the arch into the zygomatic pocket allows entry into the midface. This is accomplished by elevating the masseteric fascia as a continuation of the superficial lamina below the zygomatic arch for a short distance over the masseter muscle.

Maxillary Pocket

The periosteum over the maxilla and zygoma can be quickly and safely elevated through the Caldwell-Luc operation. Endoscopic preservation of the infraorbital nerve ensures its function in the postoperative period. The maxillary pocket is connected with the periorbital and zygomatic pockets for a complete subperiosteal release of the midface. The midface muscles are not usually observed during this extensive dissection.

CONCLUSION

The endoscopic surgeon has a unique opportunity to observe and dissect soft tissue structures of the forehead and midface through small optical windows using an endoscope. This anatomic view is from within; therefore, it must be understood for an effective and safe dissection and release of deep structures prior to their elevation for correction of ptosis in the aging face. It is hoped that this detailed review of the dynamic functions and static anatomy of the face will aid the endoscopic surgeon when using this new and exciting technique.

Suggested Readings

Anderson J: *Grant's atlas of anatomy,* Baltimore, 1983, Williams & Wilkins.

Duchenne GB: In Cuthbertson RA, editor: *The mechanism of human facial expression,* Cambridge, 1990, Cambridge University Press.

Larrabee WF Jr, Makielski KH: *Surgical anatomy of the face,* New York, 1993, Raven Press.

Thorek P: *Anatomy in surgery,* Philadelphia, 1962, JB Lippincott.

Zide BM, Jelks GW: *Surgical anatomy of the orbit,* New York, 1985, Raven Press.

CHAPTER 2

Scalp Tissue Expansion for Treatment of Male-Pattern Baldness

Gordon H. Sasaki

Endoscopy has represented a standard procedure in most surgical specialties for the past 10 years.[1] In plastic surgery, endoscopy was first introduced for carpal tunnel release[2,3] and endodiagnosis and management of ruptured breast implants.[4] As the benefits of this new technique were realized in the field of reconstructive plastic surgery, it was inevitable that endoscopic assistance became available for forehead lifts,[5-7] augmentation mammoplasty,[8] and abdominoplasty.[9]

Endoscopic assistance has also been useful in certain steps during tissue expansion procedures for alopecia that require placement of expanders under the periosteum.[10] In these cases, the optical window is enhanced by the presence of a bloodless, intact periosteal ceiling and shiny bony floor. In other soft tissue areas of the body, endodissection is more difficult due to soft tissue collapse around the endoscope in a field frequently stained with blood and body fluids. Another benefit is the creation of miniincisions, which are placed distant from the expansion pocket, permitting earlier, safer expansion. In addition, the use of endoscopy allows precise visualization of important structures through small optical windows and produces minimal trauma during endoinsertion of expanders. After expansion is begun, endocorrection of implant or capsular problems permits the expansion process to continue with minimal interruption. At the final stage, endoscopic capsulotomy and dissection create a larger defined pocket for more effective intraoperative expansion. The disadvantages of this technique, however, include indirect contact with the tissue, a two-dimensional image with altered depth perception, restricted mobility and visual field, a need for new instruments and video equipment, and time and effort to learn a new technique. This chapter reviews the author's early experience with endoscopy in the surgical management of male-pattern baldness.

CHRONIC TISSUE EXPANSION FOR MALE-PATTERN BALDNESS

Chronic tissue expansion of flaps for correction of alopecia and male-pattern baldness has improved results over those previously obtained with punch grafts, serial reductions, and rotation-advancement and transposition flaps. The goal of expansion procedures is to provide even, dense coverage across the frontal hairline and occipital vertex, while minimizing scars and producing a natural direction of hair flow. Chronic expansion requires a two-staged approach. First, the introduction of the balloons (800 ml, smooth rectangle, 8 × 20 cm) is made in the subgaleal pocket; second, advancement of the stretched flaps is done. Thus, the use of chronic expansion is best indicated for the highly motivated patient who can cope with the physical deformity, social incapacity, withdrawal from the workplace, and the number of office visits throughout the 3- to 4-month expansion period. In addition, there may be another expansion period to complete areas of inadequate coverage from the first advancement. Furthermore, the presence of tissue expanders increases the risk of infection because of exposure of the foreign body through healing incision lines. Infection of the prostheses can also occur from inadvertent contamination during filling of the expanders with percutaneous needle sticks into the valve systems.

INSTRUMENTS AND VIDEO EQUIPMENT

Endoscopy requires the acquisition of a limited assortment of minidissectors, scissors, graspers, and knives. Many of these instruments are available from the instrument packs currently in use for endoscopy in other areas of the body. Specific instruments can be obtained from a number of plastic surgery instrument companies that are actively involved in the field of endoscopy.

The video endoscopic system consists of a light source, monitor, recording and duplication system, and most importantly, a camera and lens on the endoscope. There are a number of reliable video systems on the market for office, surgical-center, and hospital use. An extension hood inserted around the tip of the endoscope is useful to elevate tissue away from the lens. An intraoperative balloon (2.5 to 10 ml) is helpful to act as an umbrella to open the visual field so that endodissection can be performed with safety and efficiency.

SURGICAL TECHNIQUE FOR ENDOINSERTION

After preparing and draping the operative site, the area is infiltrated with 1% lidocaine (Xylocaine) with epinephrine (1:200,000 dilution). Two 1.5- to 2.5-cm incision ports are strategically placed about 5 cm apart for insertion of a 4-mm, 30-degree-angled endoscope in one opening (left-sided port for right-handed surgeon) and the dissecting instruments in the other one (right-sided port for the right-handed surgeon). The incisions may be selected, for example, either along each of the postauricular precapillary line or within the central area of male-pattern baldness so that a relative distance exists from the small incisions to the eventual temporoparietooccipital subperiosteal or subgaleal pockets for the expanders. Blind dissection with a periosteal elevator establishes a 3- to 5-cm, fan-shaped working space from each port in order to connect the two spaces. To minimize the collection of tissue fluid on the lens, a trocar within the cannula is first introduced into one of the ports and withdrawn to allow passage of the endoscope into the cannula. The cannula may be mounted with a hood extension to facilitate the opening of the optical window. An irrigation tube, attached to a saline-filled syringe, is connected to the cannula and flushed intermittently to cleanse the lens of moisture and debris. The endodissector is positioned into the other port and viewed through the endoscope as elevation of the appropriate-sized pocket is developed with this instrument. At times, a small intraoperative expander (5 to 10 ml round, smooth-walled) may also be inserted through one of the ports and inflated to open the collapsing soft tissue envelope, until endodissection is completed. Relaxing incisions in the galea aponeurotica do not contribute significantly to a smoother or faster expansion period. A smooth-walled tissue expander is then inserted with a cotton swab and positioned during partial filling with saline into the remote microvalve. After the expander is located in its optimal position, the remote valve is inserted into its own pocket. Trial filling and withdrawal of saline percutaneously from the buried remote valve should be done to ensure a competent expander system.

ENDOCORRECTION

During serial expansion a defective expander system and its environment may not allow effective inflation to continue. This problem may involve malposition of the balloon, tubing, or valve. The balloon may have settled away from its original location, thus not efficiently expanding the donor tissue. The tubing may be located too close to the skin's surface or curled upon itself, thus partially obstructing flow. The valve may have migrated too near the balloon or overturned in the original location. These occurrences may be diagnosed and corrected by endoscopic evaluation and management.

A defective expander system may also involve leakage from the balloon, tubing, or valve. Introduction of an endoscope will document and confirm the site of leakage, determining which portion of the expander system requires replacement. A leak within the balloon proper or tubing is corrected with a new expander and tubing. However, valve leakage requires only valve replacement.

The development of a capsular septum between adjacent expanders prevents full effective expansion of the soft tissue. Endoscopic capsulotomy or capsulectomy removes this barrier and permits expansion to continue. In these cases, the balloons are deflated and pushed aside to prevent inadvertent injury to them during the procedure.

ENDOSCOPICALLY ASSISTED INTRAOPERATIVE EXPANSION

When expansion is completed, endoscopy can still be of benefit to maximize tissue recruitment by intraoperative expansion prior to flap advancement. Intraoperative expansion is most effective when stretch is applied in a closed cavity. Suboptimal chronic expansion may have occurred because the expander migrated away from a leading edge of donor tissue. To correct this situation, first endoscopic capsulotomy is performed followed by intraoperative expansion.

At surgery, the balloon is deflated and temporarily removed from its pocket through a slight enlargement of one of the ports previously used for endoinsertion of the expander. The endoscope is inserted through this port to visualize the capsular cavity. The endoknife and scissors may be passed through the previously made second port to open the capsule distally for a partial capsulotomy. After reinsertion of the uninjured expander into its pocket, intraoperative expansion of the modified pocket is done serially to recruit additional flap tissue most efficiently. After the defect is excised and the expander removed, further capsulotomy and capsulectomy unfurl the domed flap, which is advanced into its final position.

CASE 1

SINGLE-STAGE EXPANSION FOR MALE-PATTERN BALDNESS

This 45-year-old man selected surgical correction for male-pattern baldness by expansion techniques after previous consultations for hairpieces, hairplug transplantation, transposition scalp flaps, and serial reduction procedures (Figure 2-1). The advantages of tissue expansion of his bitemporoparietooccipital donor sites included minimizing crossing scars, retention of scalp sensation, provision of a relatively dense and uniform amount of hair, growing in a natural direction. Some of the disadvantages of the expansion technique were the unnatural appearance of the scalp during expansion, possible episodes of infection, and eventual provision of sufficient forward advancement after 3 to 4 months of expansion for a natural frontal hairline (widow's peak and anterior temporal recession). The patient was informed about a possible second expansion period (at the earliest, 4 months after his first advancement) to minimize any significant midsagittal scar alopecia from stretchback and to advance forward his scalp for a more natural frontal hairline.

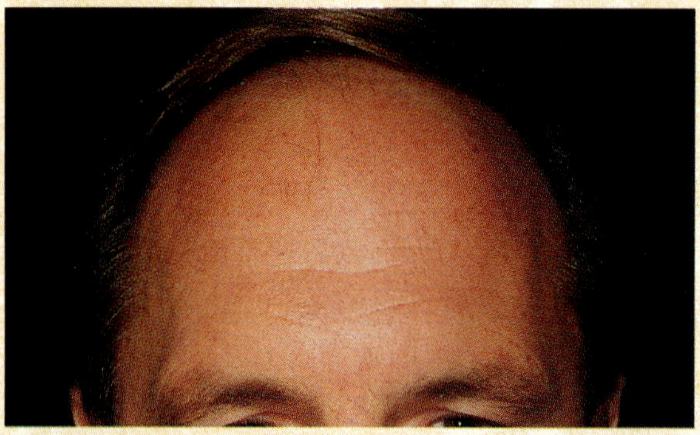

FIGURE 2-1
This 45-year-old man developed type 4 male-pattern baldness with bitemporal and occipital donor sites. The patient relies on brushing his long hair from the left side of his scalp to cover the alopecia and create an artificial frontal hairline.

On preoperative examination (Figure 2-2), the central area of alopecia measured 12 cm across at the anteriotemporal hairline, 10 cm across at the midscalp, and 8 cm across at the vertex. The sagittal length of the bald spot measured about 15 cm. The forehead height from the lateral brow to the recessed precapillary line at the anterior temporal juncture was 12 cm on each side. On October 25, 1993, endoscopic insertion of two 700-ml rectangular expanders (7 X 20 cm) was performed through two 1.5-cm ports about 4 cm apart in a bald spot on the scalp's vertex. Filling of the expanders through the microvalves was begun 6 days after surgery (Figure 2-3). After 5 months of gradual expansion up to 650 ml into each expander, the bald area was excised with a sagittal line closure and frontal advancement with a forehead height of 12 cm (Figure 2-4).

The patient has plans for a second expansion of his midscalp after 4 months to diminish the area of hair thinness adjacent to the slightly widened sagittal scar and to further advance the frontal hairline to 7 cm from the brows.

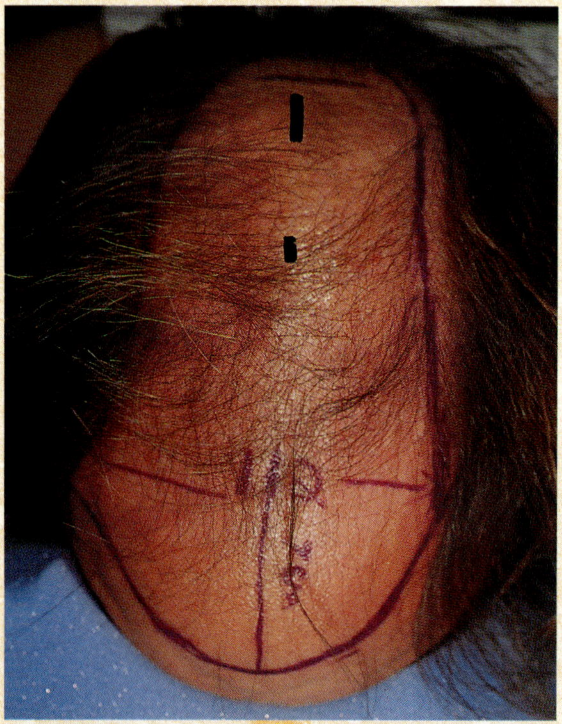

FIGURE 2-2
Shown here is, on preoperative examination the width of the bald spot across the anteriotemporal hairline measured 12 cm. A 7-cm midfrontal advancement from the anteriotemporal level was necessary to produce an optimal forelock brow height of 7 cm. The two 1.5-cm incisions are marked 4 cm apart, with the bald area for endodissection on either side for insertion of the tissue expanders.

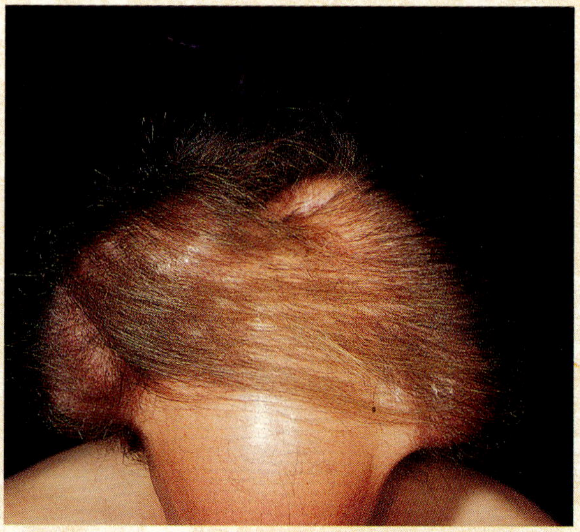

FIGURE 2-3
Serial filling of expanders began less than 1 week after endoinsertion through two remote microvalves located under the anterior half of the bald scalp. After 5 months of gradual expansion—about 20 to 30 ml every 2 weeks—the final volume achieved within each expander was 650 ml.

A

B

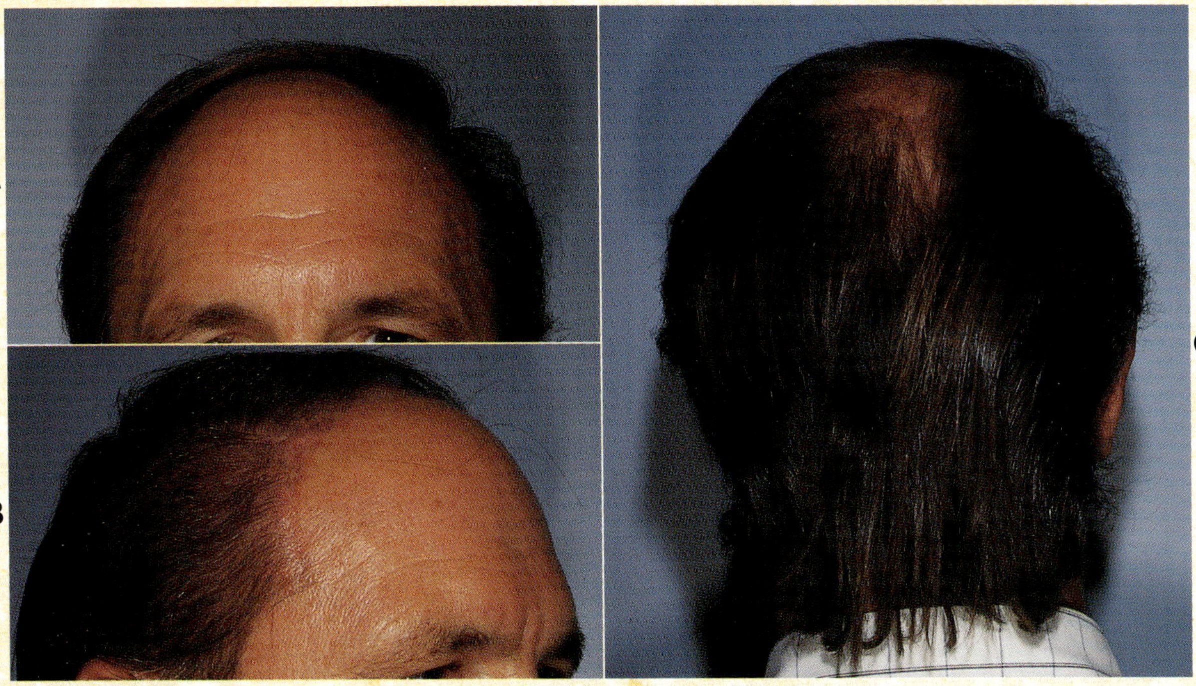

C

FIGURE 2-4
The patient is shown 6 weeks after advancement of flaps toward the midsagittal line (**A** through **C**). The distance of midfrontal advancement from the anteriotemporal level was only 2 to 3 cm (**B**). There still remains a 2 to 3 cm area of sparse hair to frank alopecia at the sagittal line of closure (**C**). The patient is scheduled for another endoinsertion of expanders placed in the midscalp area adjacent to the temporary frontal hairline to complete the reconstruction.

CASE 2

EXPANSION OF TRANSFERRED JURI FREE FLAP AND SCALP FOR CORRECTION OF MALE-PATTERN BALDNESS

This 49-year-old man underwent successful microsurgical transfer of a right Juri flap to the left superficial temporal artery and vein in 1984 (Figure 2-5, *A*). Later, multiple punch grafts from the occipital area were able to partially fill the vertex of the scalp and areas behind the Juri flap (Figure 2-5, *B*). On the preoperative examination, the forehead height was 11 cm long from the precapillary line to the midbrow (Figure 2-6, *A*). Also, there was a 2 X 10 cm wide scar along the right temporoparietooccipital area above the ear (Figure 2-6, *B*), a 2 X 7 cm scar alopecia along the left temporoparietal scalp (Figure 2-6, *C*), a 2 X 7 cm area of alopecia from the occipital donor site, two 3 X 5 cm areas of sparsely filled hairplug transplants behind the Juri flap, and a 4 X 7 cm area of thin hairplug transplants in the vertex of the scalp (Figures 2-6, *C* and *D*).

On March 1, 1994, endoscopically assisted insertion of two 1120-ml smooth-walled expanders (8 X 20 cm) were positioned under the periosteum of the Juri flap anteriorly and the temporoparietooccipital areas through a 3.5-cm incision along each postauricular hairline (Figure 2-7). The remote valves were positioned on each side of the posteriolateral neck. After 9 weeks of expansion with about 600 ml into each expander (Figure 2-8), reconstruction of the anterior hairline was accomplished by a 4.5-cm advancement to produce a widow's peak and frontolateral recessions (Figure 2-8, *D*). The forehead height was measured at 6.5 cm from the midbrow. In addition, the areas of alopecia along the temporoparietal scalp and occipital scalp were excised. The thinly covered areas of hair transplantation behind the transposed Juri flap and scalp vertex were also removed. The patient also underwent endoscopic release of the corrugator and procerus muscles (Figure 2-9).

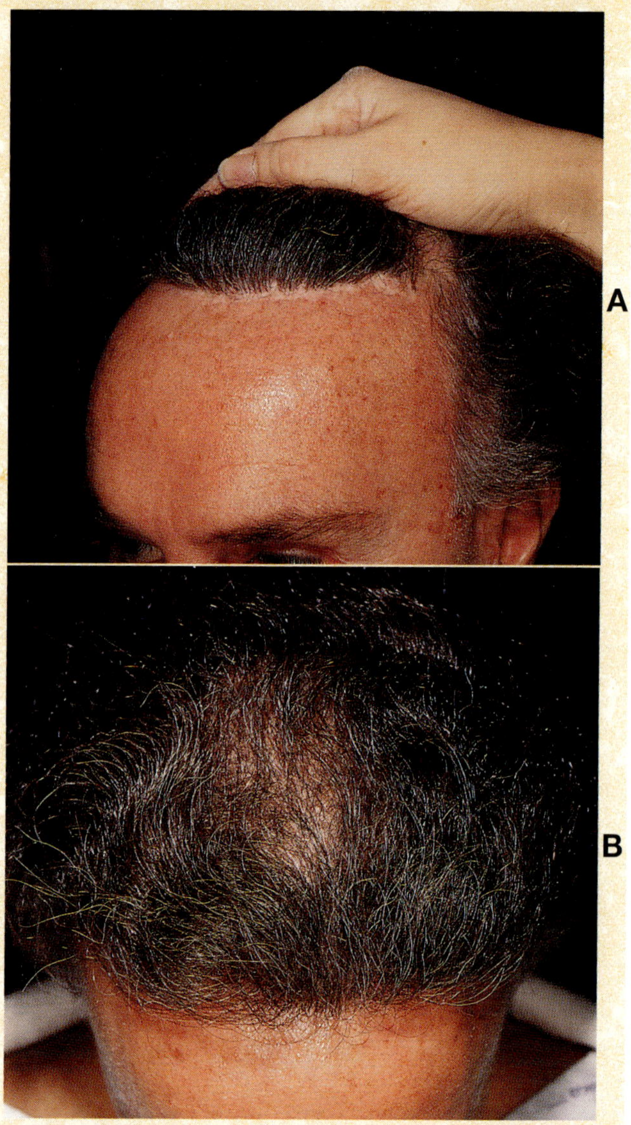

FIGURE 2-5
A, This 49-year-old patient underwent a successful microvascular transfer of a right Juri flap to the left superficial temporal vessels. **B,** Later, multiple punch grafts were transplanted from the occipital site to fill in the bald areas of the scalp vertex and posterior to the Juri flap.

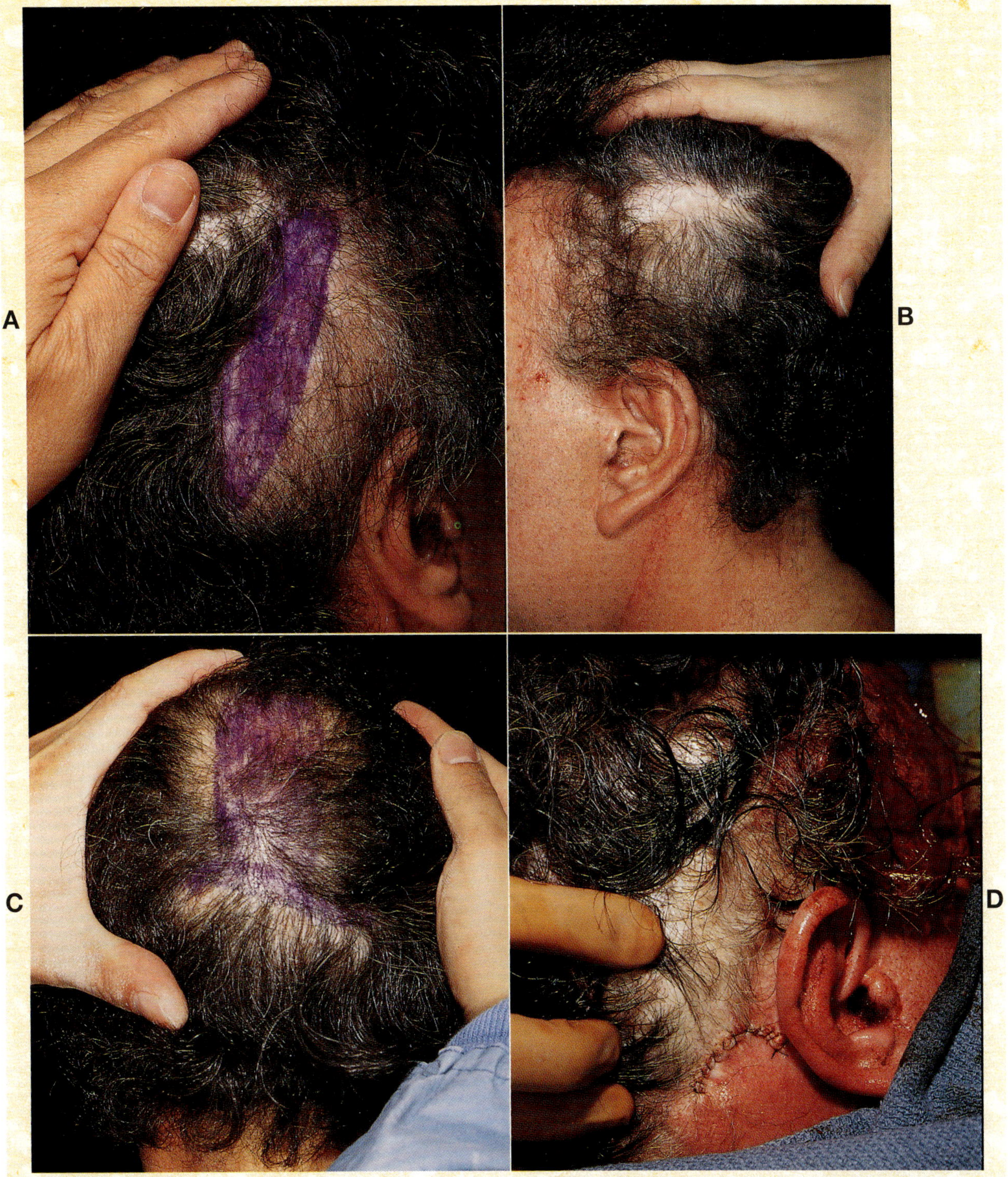

FIGURE 2-6
As shown here, on preoperative examination the forehead height from the forelock to brow measured 11 cm. The excellent results with microsurgical transfer and punch grafts left areas of surgical alopecia or incomplete coverage at the occiput, vertex, and bitemporal areas. **A,** There was a 2 × 10 cm strip of surgical alopecia from the Juri flap donor site on the right scalp. **B,** and **C,** There was a 2 × 7 cm strip of scar alopecia at both the left temporal area and the occipital donor site. **D,** In addition, the sparse areas of hairplug transplants at the scalp vertex and behind the Juri flap produced spot alopecia.

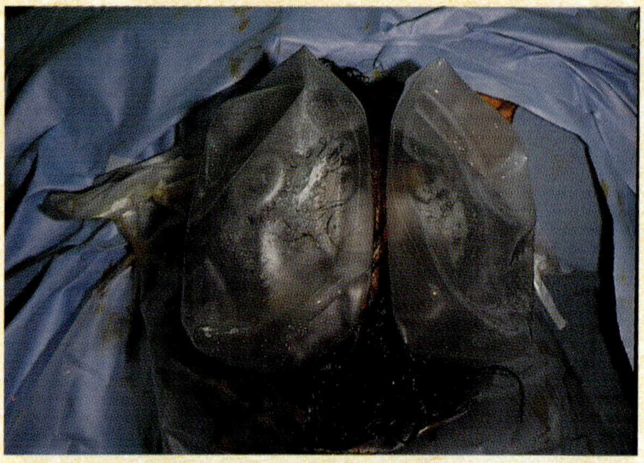

FIGURE 2-7
Endoinsertion of two 1120-ml, smooth-walled expanders (8 × 20 cm) was accomplished through 3.5-cm postauricular incisions. The remote valves were positioned at the posterior lateral neck.

A

B

C

D

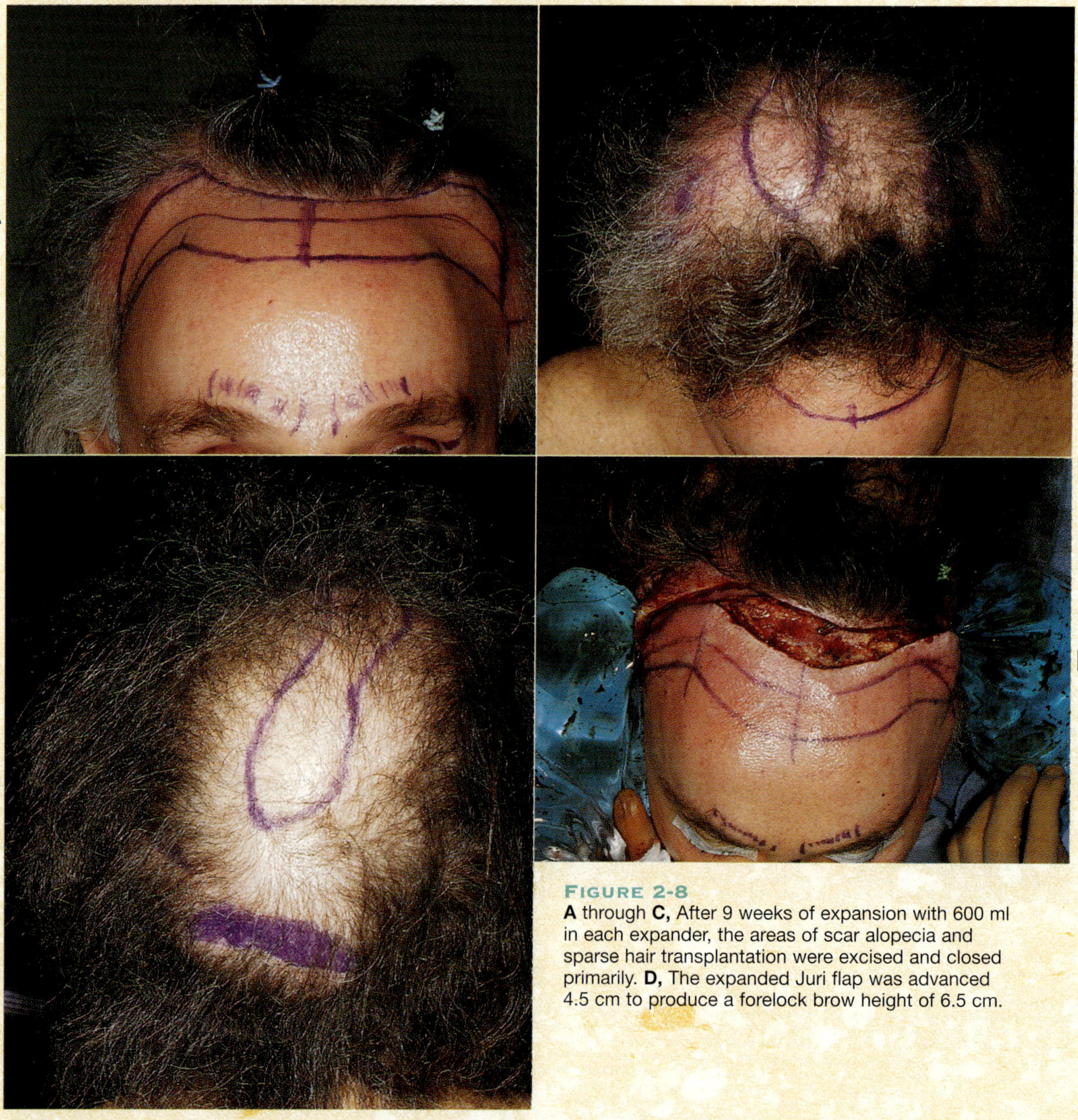

FIGURE 2-8
A through **C,** After 9 weeks of expansion with 600 ml in each expander, the areas of scar alopecia and sparse hair transplantation were excised and closed primarily. **D,** The expanded Juri flap was advanced 4.5 cm to produce a forelock brow height of 6.5 cm.

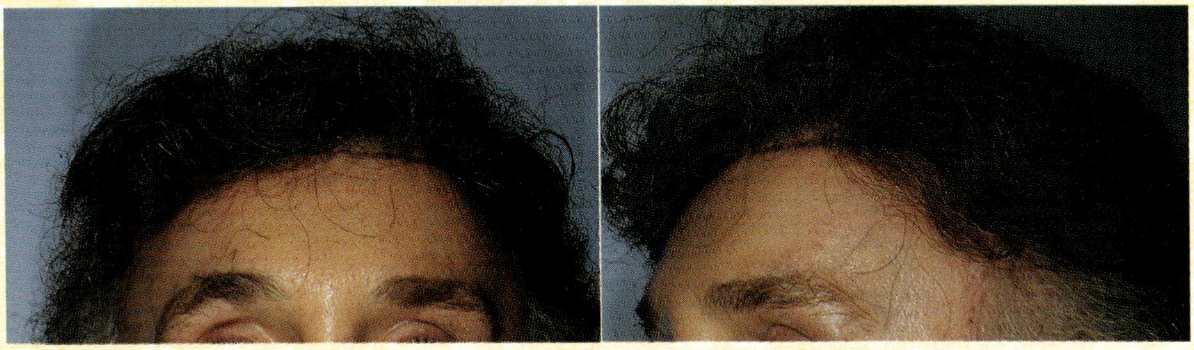

FIGURE 2-9
The patient is shown 2 weeks after surgery, with a significant reduction in the areas of alopecia. The forelock brow relationship has been improved with a height of 6.5 cm and a reduction in procerus muscle and corrugator muscle activity.

COMBINED EXPERIENCE

ENDOINSERTION

The author's early experience with endoinsertion of expanders, in addition to these two cases of male-pattern baldness, includes 34 patients with scars, skin grafts, and congenital large nevi (Table 2-1). A total of 51 expanders were used. Each expander was inserted via a 1.0- to 2.5-cm port after the pockets were endoscopically dissected. Minimal trauma with distant miniincisions permitted by endoscopy results in earlier, safer expansion. Endovisualization during dissection was enhanced by the use of small intraoperative balloons to open the optical windows. It was the author's impression that less ecchymosis and pain were observed postoperatively.

TABLE 2-1 ENDOINSERTION OF 51 EXPANDERS

LOCATION	NO. OF CASES	REASON FOR PROCEDURE
Scalp	11	Baldness, scars, large nevi
Forehead	4	Scars, large nevi
Face	12	Skin grafts, scars, large nevi
Neck	2	Scars, large nevi
Breast	5	Delayed reconstruction
Trunk	6	Skin grafts, scars, large nevi
Upper extremity	7	Skin grafts, scars, large nevi
Lower extremity	4	Skin grafts, scars, large nevi

ENDODIAGNOSIS AND CORRECTION

In five cases, endoscopic evaluation of problems that developed after the expanders were inserted were accurately diagnosed and corrected (Table 2-2). The malpositioned expander balloon was relocated adjacent to the defect by opening the capsule endoscopically. The two valves that required repositioning had either overturned or moved under the expander balloon. The periorbital balloon was observed endoscopically, requiring replacement of the expander. A capsulotomy between adjacent expanders permitted more effective expansion of the donor site. Because surgical management was relatively atraumatic through miniincisions, expansion was not significantly delayed. This enabled the expansion process to be completed with minimal complications.

TABLE 2-2 ENDODIAGNOSIS AND CORRECTION IN FIVE CASES

PROBLEM	NO. OF CASES
Malposition of balloon	1
Malposition of valve	2
Leakage of balloon	1
Septum between balloons	1

COMPLICATIONS

Only one complication was observed with endoscopically assisted expansion surgery, involving an injury to the balloon during capsulotomy. This complication can be avoided by removal of the expander from its pocket before endodissection or manipulation is begun.

CONCLUSION

Endoscopy has been of assistance during tissue expansion surgery. In scalp expansion, endoinsertion is facilitated by the subperiosteal window. In other areas of the body, the optical window can be established with the use of small intraoperative expanders. Miniincisions and precise dissection reduce the complication rate and postoperative morbidity. Endodiagnosis and correction of expander-related problems can be managed effectively with the use of an endoscope. The overall complication rate appears to be low enough to consider endoscopy as an adjunctive procedure in specific aspects of expansion surgery. Further experience is required to evaluate its potential use in reconstructive and aesthetic surgery.

REFERENCES

1. Grimes D: Frontiers of the operative laparoscopy: a review and critique of the evidence, *Am J Obstet Gynecol* 166:1062, 1992.
2. Chow JC: Endoscopic release of the carpal ligament: a new technique for carpal tunnel syndrome, *Arthroscopy* 5:19, 1989.
3. Okutsu I, Niromiya S, Takatori Y, et al: Endoscopic management of the carpal tunnel syndrome, *Arthroscopy* 5:11, 1989.
4. Dowden R, Arian S: Endoscopic implant evaluation and capsulotomy, *Plast Reconstr Surg* 91:283, 1993.
5. Core GB, Vasconez LO, Askren C, et al: Coronal facelift with endoscopic techniques, *Plast Surg Forum* XV:227, 1992.
6. Ramirez OM, Oneal R: First International Workshop on Facial Rejuvenation: The Subperiosteal and Other Deep Plane Techniques, Baltimore, April 1992.
7. Isse NG: Endoscopic facial rejuvenation: endoforehead, the functional lift. Case reports, *Aesth Plast Surg* 18:21, 1994.
8. Johnson GW, Christ JE: The endoscopic breast augmentation: the transumbilical insertion of saline-filled breast implants, *Plast Reconstr Surg* 92:801, 1993.
9. Johnson GW: The Johnson endoscopic abdominoplasty. Endoscopic Plastic Surgery Seminar, University of California, Los Angeles, March 1994.
10. Anger J, Szego T: Use of videoscopy as an aid in the placement of tissue expanders, *Rev Paul Med* 111(2), 1993.
11. Elliot RA: The lateral scalp flap for anterior hairline reconstruction, *Clin Plast Surg* 9:241, 1982.

CHAPTER 3

Forehead Rejuvenation

Nicanor G. Isse
Peter Bela Fodor

The use of endoscopically assisted surgical techniques for diagnostic and surgical endeavors is now routine. The use of the endoscope in plastic surgery, however, especially its reconstructive aspects, is a much more recent development. Within the last 2 years surgeons in the United States, Europe, and South America have made exciting and important contributions to this exploding new field.

The authors believe that endoscopically assisted surgical procedures will be an extremely significant addition to the art and science of facial rejuvenation. We believe, in fact, that "the impact of endoscopic plastic surgery (EPS) on the reconstructive and cosmetic aspects of our specialty will soon be compared in magnitude to microvascular, craniofacial, and tissue expansion techniques."[1]

This chapter discusses our current philosophy and approach to the endoscopically assisted treatment of the aging face. Because most of the experience to date has been in the management of the upper third of the face, emphasis is placed on the endoforehead and endomidface rejuvenation procedures.

THE AGING PROCESS

In the aging process a series of forces and anatomic characteristics act in concert to produce changes in the face. Some of the forces pull downward, while other muscle actions pull the soft tissues upward. The bony architecture of the face is the platform on which this action takes place. Other elements, such as genetics, the environment, and nutrition, also play an important role in the way we look as we age. This discussion focuses on those elements that can be modified with endoscopically assisted facial rejuvenation procedures.

The forces that affect the face in the downward direction are both static and dynamic, that is, gravity and the action of the depressor muscles, respec-

The authors would like to extend sincere thanks to Stryker Endoscopy and Wells Endoscopy Company for their invaluable assistance in developing the techniques described in these pages.

tively. The dynamic force exerted by the depressor muscles is present primarily in the periorbital glabellar area and the perioral–mental regions of the face. The activity of these muscles produces depression of the upper portion of the face, the corners of the mouth, the jaw, and the mental areas.

The dynamic forces exercising an upward pull are the elevator muscles, such as the frontalis-galea-occipitalis complex, the function of which is counteracting the action of the depressor muscles. This dynamic but opposing muscle activity eventually produces hypertrophy and a series of wrinkles and folds in the glabellar, orbital, perioral, and mental areas. Gravitational forces, in the meantime, produce malposition of the facial skin and the fat pads in each of these areas.

The other major factor that influences the outcome of aging is the underlying bony architecture of the face: the "bone structure" of the individual. This bony topography consists of both depressions and prominences in the glabellar area, the radix of the nose, the mental area, and the malar area. Such relative facial bony depressions can result from hypoplasia of the malar bone or from underdevelopment of the mentum. Prominences include bossing of the supraorbital ridge of the frontal bone, isolated bossing of the glabellar region, or bossing of the supraorbital rim, with relative depression in the midforehead area.

If such prominences and depressions are not appreciated and dealt with in the course of facial rejuvenative procedures, the ultimate result will be compromised because, in time, the soft tissues will tend to slide back down into these bony depressions. Grafting, adding implant material, and bone shaving are some of the techniques that can be added to endoscopically assisted techniques to alter the surface architecture of the facial skeleton.

SURGICAL RATIONALE FOR THE ENDOFOREHEAD PROCEDURE

Traditional approaches to rejuvenate the aging forehead involve coronal, hairline, midforehead, and eyebrow incisions. Direct excision of the corrugator muscles is an integral part of these procedures. One of the authors (Dr. Isse) pioneered a new surgical intervention that incorporates the use of endoscopic techniques through small, inconspicuous access incisions. This procedure allows "physiologic" brow elevation to occur by the release of the depressor muscles and the soft tissue attachments at the level of the supraorbital rim, without direct forehead excision and without removal of the corrugator muscles, thus avoiding the creation of a depression over the center of the forehead. Direct skin excision is not necessary with this procedure.

Through small incisions within the hair-bearing scalp, an endoscope and appropriate instruments are introduced. With this approach, wide undermining and release of the soft tissues of the forehead are accomplished. As a result, the muscle balance described above is offset, in favor of the elevation of the eyebrows and the forehead skin.[2,3]

FUNCTIONAL ANATOMY OF THE MUSCLES OF EXPRESSION OF THE UPPER FACE

There are two sets of muscles (Table 3-1 and Figures 3-1, *A* and *B*) that control upper facial expression. They can be grouped into elevator muscles and depressor muscles of the forehead. Their individual contracture is reflected in the facial expressions of attention, pain, reflection, and aggression.

The orbicularis oculi muscle is a very strong sphincteric muscle. Its main function is to draw the tissue around the eye inferiorly and centrally toward the longitudinal axis of the orbit. In other words, the orbicularis draws the forehead soft tissues downward, in the direction of the globe.

The orbicularis has three portions: the orbital portion covering the superciliary arch, the preseptal portion located between the lower border of the

TABLE 3-1 MUSCLES OF HUMAN FACIAL EXPRESSION

MUSCLE	CLASSIFICATION	TYPE OF FACIAL EXPRESSION[4]
Frontalis m.	Elevator	Attention
Corrugator m.	Elevator (of head of brow)	Pain
Orbicularis oculi m.	Depressor	Reflection
Procerus m.	Depressor	Aggression
Corrugator m.	Depressor (of tail of brow)	Pain
Depressor supercilii m.	Depressor	Reflection

A

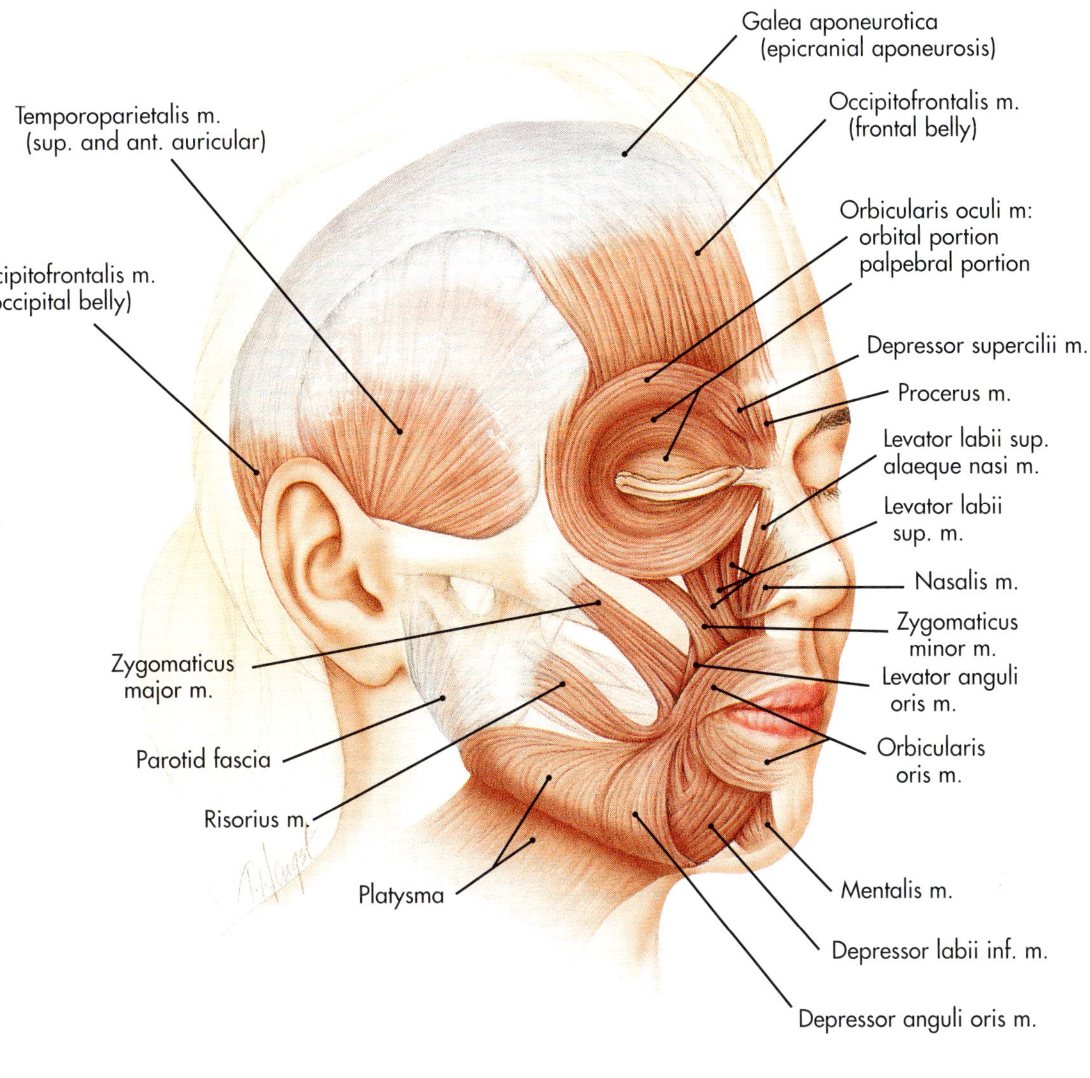

FIGURE 3-1
A, The muscles of human facial expression are shown: the occipitofrontalis muscles, the orbicularis oculi muscle, with the palpebral and orbital portions, the depressor supercilii muscle, and the procerus muscle.

Continued.

eyebrow and the upper margin of the tarsal plate, and the pretarsal portion covering the tarsus. The preseptal and pretarsal portions are also known as the palpebral portion.

These three portions have different actions. The orbital portion mainly depresses the eyebrow. For example, when we squint tightly, the eyebrow moves down and toward the center of the eye because of the strong sphincteric action of the orbicularis. The preseptal portion functions primarily to close the upper eyelid. The pretarsal portion is responsible for blinking. Its function is almost entirely involuntary in nature. The same portions and division of functions of the orbicularis are also present in the lower eyelid. The medial superior portion of the upper lid orbicularis has developed into a small but functionally strong muscle called the depressor supercilii. This muscle is a forceful depressor of the head of the brow.

The innervation of the upper lid orbicularis oculi muscle is derived from the temporal and zygomatic branches of the facial nerve for the preorbital portion, and from the zygomatic branch of

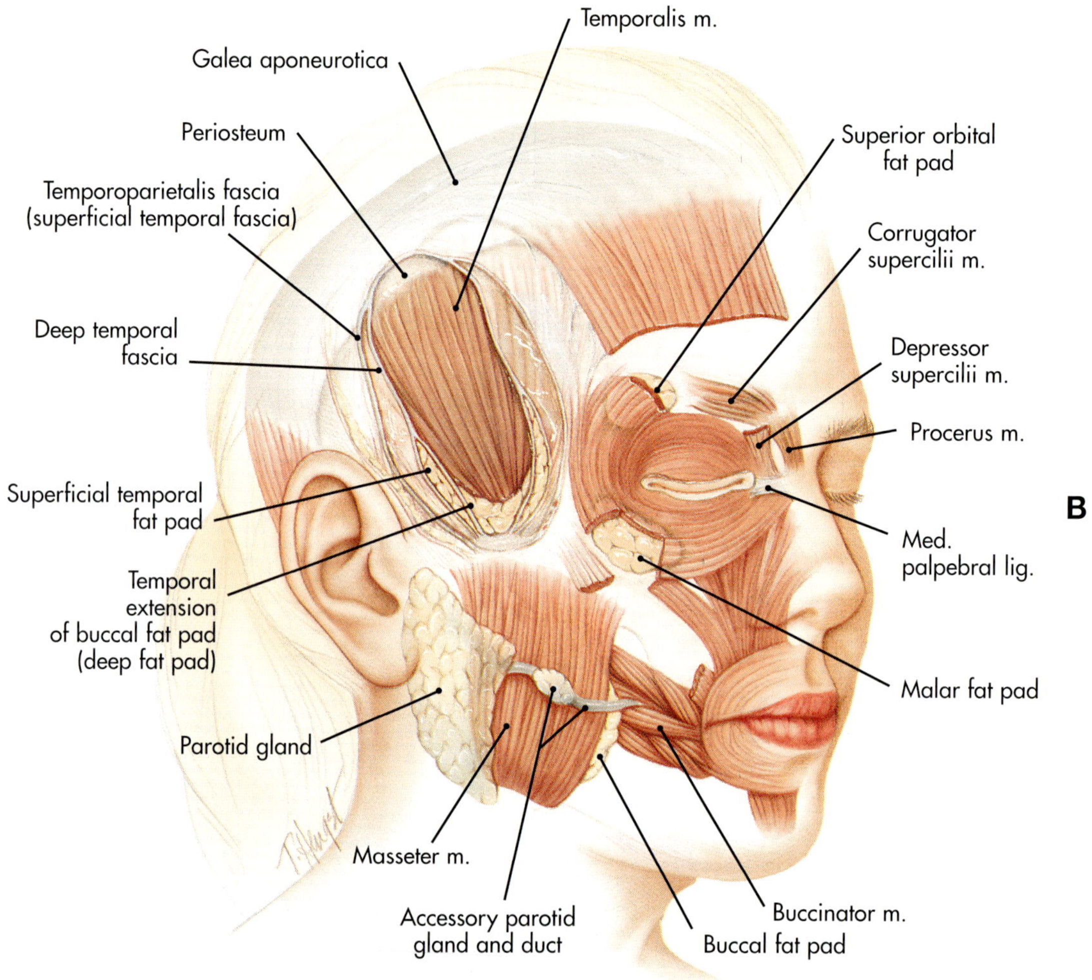

FIGURE 3-1, CONT'D.
B, A window was created through the frontalis muscle, the orbital portion of the orbicularis muscle, and the depressor supercilii muscle to see deep inside to the origin and trajectory of the corrugator supercilii muscle.

the facial nerve for the rest of the upper lid. The inferior portion corresponding to the inferior eyelid is supplied by the buccal branch of the facial nerve and the zygomatic branch.

The corrugator is a beef-colored, long, meaty, fleshy muscle the orientation of which is generally from the superior to the inferior direction. It originates in the supraorbital arch and in the glabellar area and is inserted into the skin (Figure 3-2). The muscle belly has a head portion and a tail portion and is slightly horizontal, bowing underneath the eyebrow (Figures 3-3, *A* and *B*). When the head of the corrugator muscle contracts, the head of the brow is displaced upward, and the whole eyebrow becomes slightly sinuous, taking on a lazy S-like shape. On the other hand, the lateral portion of the corrugator muscle—or the tail—that is intermingled with the orbicularis produces depression of the tail of the brow when it contracts. As a result, the tail is drawn medially toward the center of the eye.

The corrugator muscle, because of this activity, has produced a very strong imprint on the glabellar and medial supraorbital arch of the frontal bone. The "corrugator facets" usually have the shape of the "Roman Empire eagle" (Figure 3-2).

According to classic teaching *(Gray's Anatomy)* the corrugator muscle's innervation comes mainly from the temporal branch of the facial nerve and, occasionally, from the zygomatic branch. Recent studies confirm that most of the innervation of the corrugator muscle comes only from the temporal

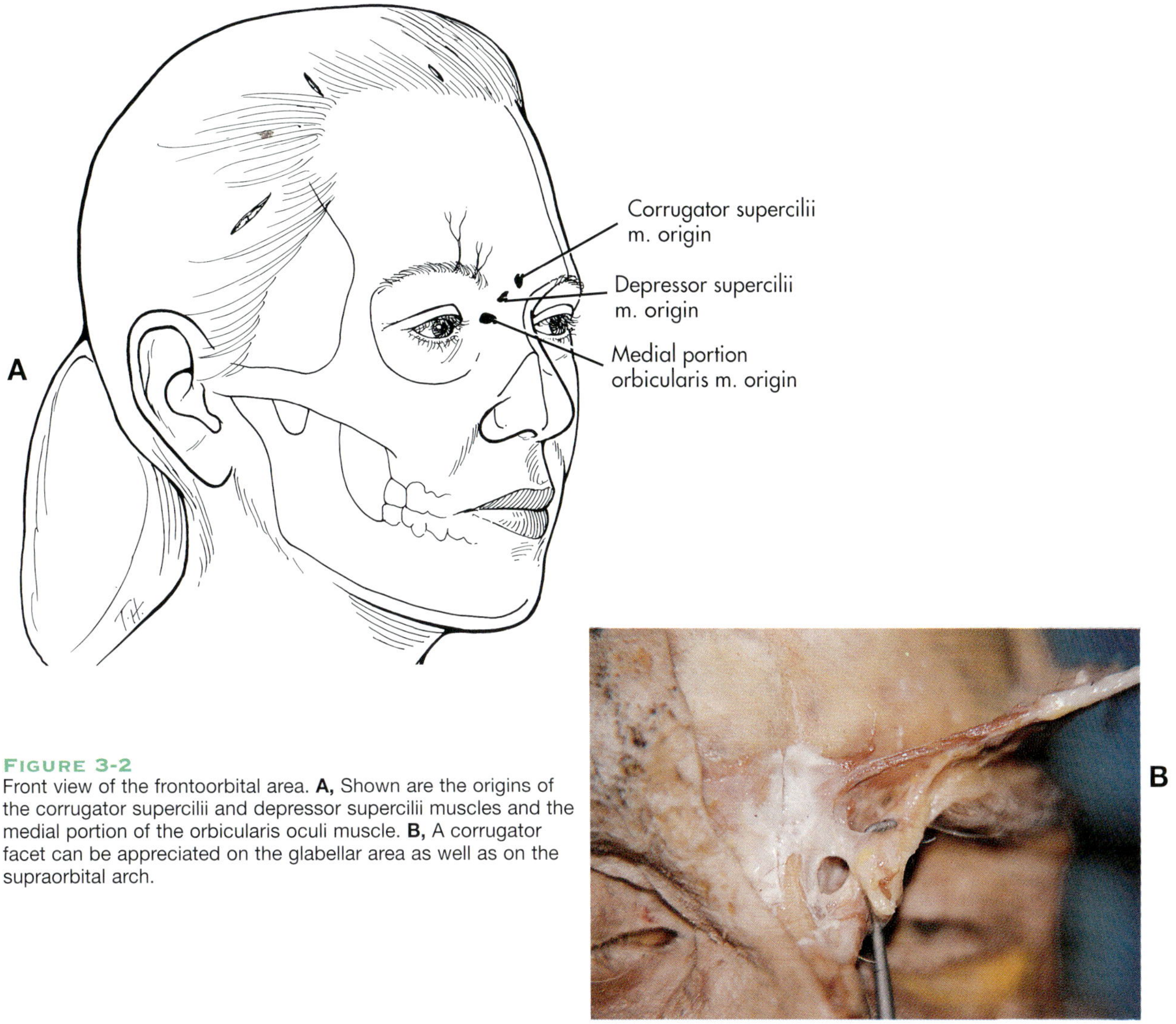

Figure 3-2
Front view of the frontoorbital area. **A,** Shown are the origins of the corrugator supercilii and depressor supercilii muscles and the medial portion of the orbicularis oculi muscle. **B,** A corrugator facet can be appreciated on the glabellar area as well as on the supraorbital arch.

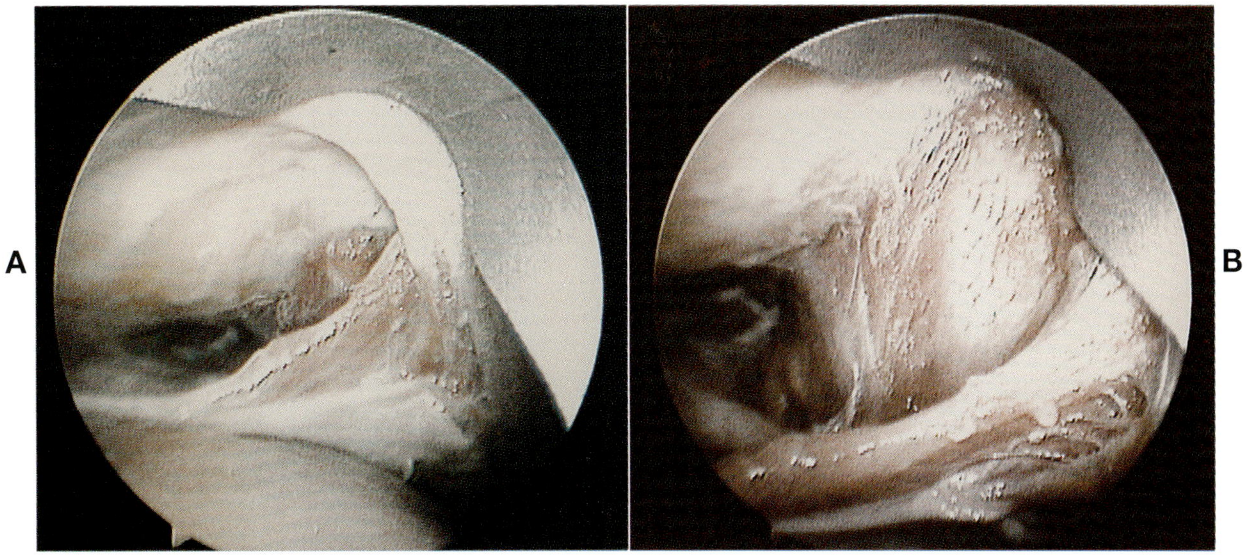

Figure 3-3
A, Endoscopic view of the glabellar origin of the corrugator supercilii muscle is shown; the picture was taken from the medial hairline incision, midway into the frontal area of the forehead. Anterior to the corrugator supercilii muscle are the vertical fibers of the depressor supercilii muscle, which originate from the nasal process of the frontal bone. **B,** Endoscopic view of the depressor supercilii muscle as the scope passes over the glabellar origin of the corrugator supercilii muscle. The superior flaps contain the procerus muscle. The floor of this tunnel is made up of the nasal bones.

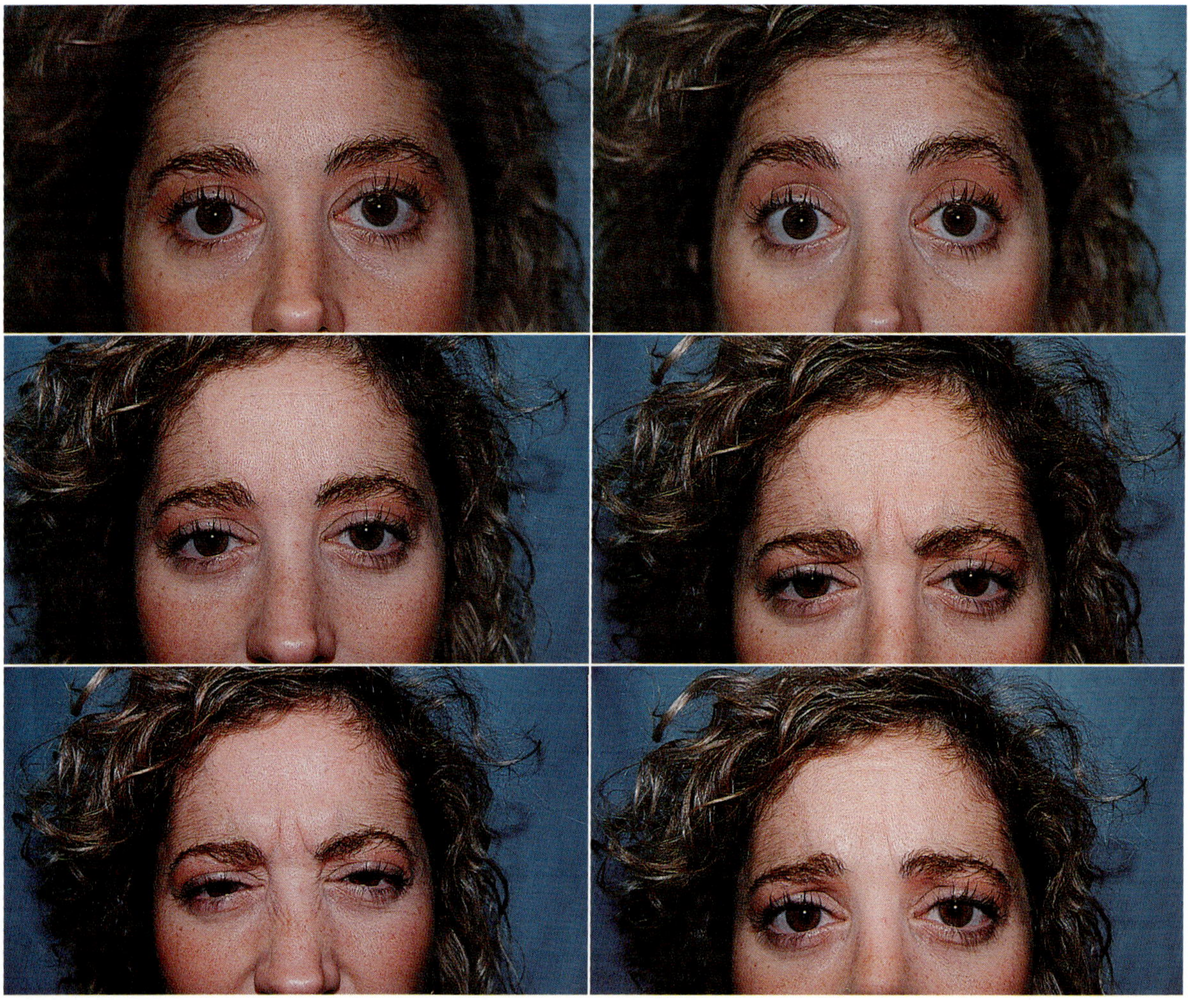

FIGURE 3-4
A, Shown is the face at rest. **B,** Attention: frontalis muscle action elevates the brow and produces horizontal wrinkles of the forehead. **C,** Reflection: orbicularis muscle action causes total depression of the brow. **D,** Anger: depressor supercilii muscle action causes depression of the head of the brow and vertical wrinkles in the glabellar area (frowning). **E,** Aggression: procerus muscle action lowers the head of the brow and produces horizontal wrinkles at the root of the nose. **F,** Pain and suffering: corrugator muscle action elevates the head of the brow, depresses the tail of the brow, and shortens the brows, producing a corrugation laterally to medially.

branch of the facial nerve, to a branch that courses under the preorbital portion of the orbicularis muscle and penetrates the corrugator muscle at a point slightly medial to the supraorbital nerve.

Table 3-2 summarizes the functions of the muscles of the forehead. Figure 3-4, *A*, shows the face at rest.

An understanding of the functional classification of the muscles of expression of the forehead provides the basic rationale for our endoscopic forehead procedure. To produce the desired elevation, first the soft tissues are dissected from the frontal area in a subperiosteal plane. Next soft tissue modification consisting of (1) periosteal release, (2) muscle modifications (mainly myotomies); and (3) neurotomies is performed. Consequently, the frontalis-galea-occipitalis muscle sling, now unopposed, will elevate the brow. In addition to muscle modification and neurotomies, the periosteal release will facilitate the action of the elevator muscles of the forehead.

The surgical procedures can be custom tailored for each patient. In general terms, based on the extent of the dissection, the endoscopic facial rejuvenation procedures can be classified into the following groups: (1) endoscopic forehead lift (standard, extended, limited); (2) endoscopic midface lift; (3) endoscopic temporal lift; (4) endoscopic full facelift; (5) endoscopic cervicoplasty; and (6) endoscopic facial rejuvenation combined with other procedures, such as superficial musculo-aponeurotic system (SMAS) modification, facial implants, open facelift, and open cervicoplasty.

TABLE 3-2 FUNCTION OF THE FOREHEAD MUSCLES

MUSCLE	CLASSIFICATION	FUNCTION
Frontalis m.	Elevator	Produces total elevation of the eyebrow (Figure 3-4, *B*)
Corrugator m. (medial part)	Elevator	Produces partial elevation of the head of the eyebrow (Figure 3-4, *F*)
Orbicularis oculi m.	Depressor	Orbital portion produces total depression of the brow (Figure 3-4, *C*)
Depressor supercilii m.	Depressor	Produces depression of the medial portion of the brow (Figure 3-4, *D*)
Procerus m.	Depressor	Depresses the medial portion of the brow and the glabellar region (Figure 3-4, *E*)
Corrugator m. (lateral part)	Depressor	Depresses the tail of the brow (Figure 3-4, *F*)

EQUIPMENT AND INSTRUMENTS

Endoscopic facial rejuvenation procedures require a complete endoscopic unit, which includes a medical videocamera, a camera control unit, a light source, a monitor, fiberoptic cables, a documentation device (such as a photographic camera), a VCR, and a printer, all mounted on moveable stands.

In our experience, compact endoscopic units (Figure 3-5) designed for use in the office are less costly and often more convenient for plastic surgeons to use than the larger ones used in hospitals. The wattage of the smaller lamps (150 W) is more than adequate for endoscopic facial rejuvenation procedures because the white bony surfaces of the facial skeleton reflect light. In addition, because these surgeries are performed in a small cavity, the compact endoscopic unit can be moved very close to the object.

One-chip cameras generally are sufficient for surgeries in the facial area. If crisp documentation of specific cases is needed for publication or teaching purposes, the surgeon may wish to use a three-chip camera because it provides superior resolution, more detail, and better definition.

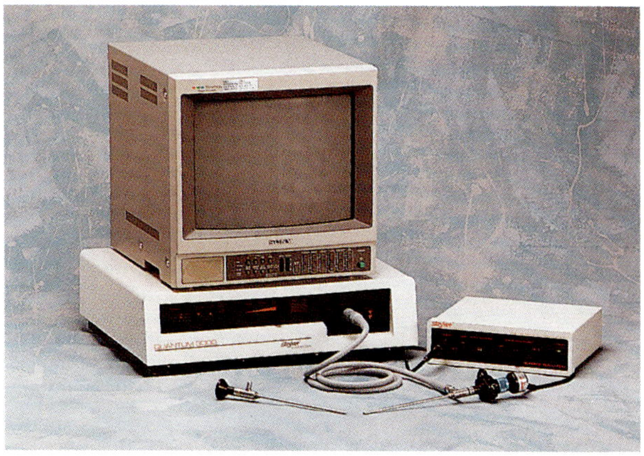

FIGURE 3-5
Endoscopic equipment: monitor, camera, and light source, with 30-degree angle scope attached are shown.

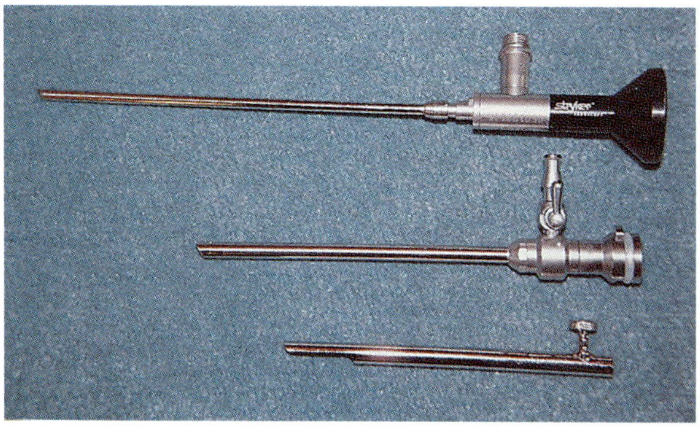

FIGURE 3-6
Endoscopic equipment: 4-mm diameter, 30-degree angle scope, irrigating cannula, and moveable soft tissue retractor sleeve are shown.

The surgical instruments used in facial rejuvenation procedures are designed to help the surgeon visualize, dissect, or suspend tissue. The *visualizing instruments* include the following: (1) a 30-degree angle arthroscope, 4 mm in diameter; (2) an irrigating cannula (saline is often mixed with adrenalin or epinephrine solution to control bleeding and reduce oozing); and (3) a retractor cannula for the endoscope (Figure 3-6). *Dissecting instruments* fall into two categories: tissue dissectors (Figure 3-7) and neurovascular dissectors (Figure 3-8). The most common types of dissectors for endoscopic facial rejuvenation are summarized in Table 3-3. For *suspension and fixation,* different types of equipment are needed. For suspension of soft tissue, a Reverdin needle or suture passer is used. For suspension to bone, a tiny drill; microscrews, 1×2.5 mm (also called miniscrews); and a locking screwdriver are among the devices available to surgeons (Figure 3-9).

TABLE 3-3 BASIC DISSECTORS USED IN ENDOSCOPIC FACIAL REJUVENATION

TYPE	DESCRIPTION	PURPOSE
Tissue	Soft tissue dissector (diameter, 1.0 cm)	For dissecting the temporal area
Tissue	Sharp 0.5 or 0.8 cm periosteum dissector	For dissecting the glabellar area, lateral orbital rim, zygomatic arch, and frontal bone
Tissue	Sharp, small endoscopy scissors, or sharp Cottle mucoperichondrium elevator	For periosteal release at the orbital ridge
Tissue	Small endoscopic grasper	To aid in dissection and control bleeding
Neurovascular	Narrow, spoon-shaped instrument	To isolate the nerves and blood vessels
Neurovascular	Thin, 90-degree angled instrument	To skeletonize the nerves and blood vessels

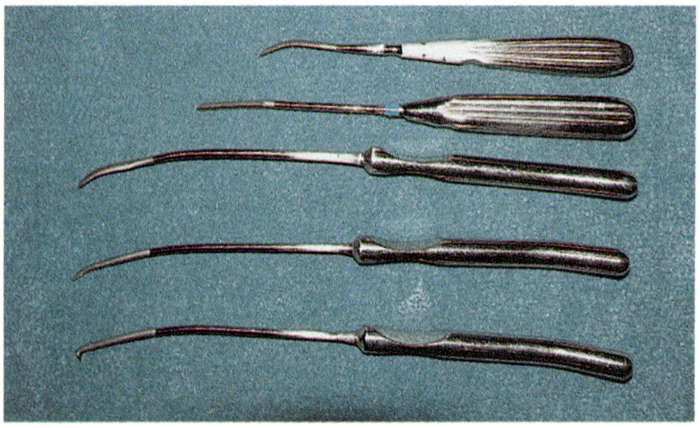

FIGURE 3-7
Tissue dissectors: frontal periosteum dissector, glabellar and nasal dissector, temporal soft tissue dissector, and two supraorbital rim dissectors are shown.

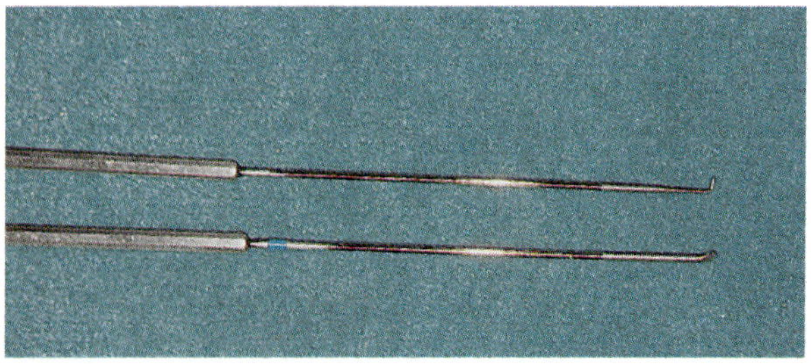

FIGURE 3-8
Neurovascular dissectors are shown.

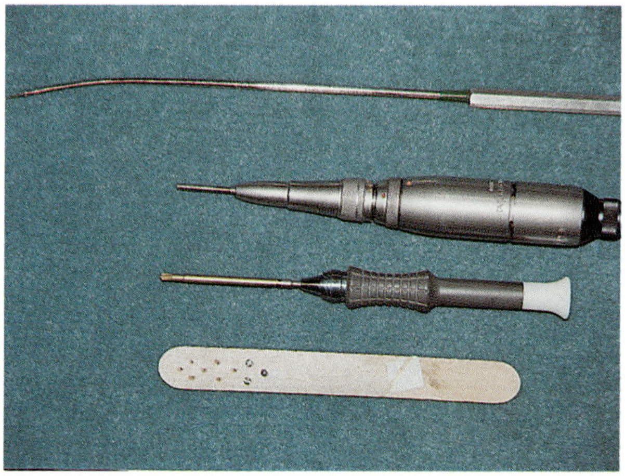

FIGURE 3-9
Fixation instruments: suture passer (Reverdin needle), a drill machine, a 2.5-mm drill tip, a 1-mm microscrew, and corresponding screwdriver are shown.

ENDOFOREHEAD LIFT

In general terms, the endoforehead lift is performed to improve the following conditions: ptosis of the eyebrows; pseudoptosis of the upper eyelids; lateral pulling and fullness of the upper eyelid; glabellar wrinkles; horizontal wrinkles of the forehead and root of the nose; "sunken" eyes; and "crow's feet" of the upper eyelid. Contraindication for the procedure is the absence of the above-mentioned conditions. The presence of tight forehead skin, as often seen in persons of Latino, Asian, and Native American descent, might require a more superficial (supraperiosteal or subcutaneous) dissection. For patients with tight forehead skin, it also appears that selected myotomies and neurotomies are more important than the actual skin suspension in the frontal area.

In the *standard endoscopic forehead lift* the entire forehead, including the temporal area, is freed up laterally to the level of the supraorbital rim and medially in the glabella, down to the radix of the nose, and at times over the bony nasal pyramid. Dissection continues in the temporal area medially to the sentinel vein (Figure 3-10).

In the *extended endoscopic forehead lift*, dissection is similar to the standard endoscopic forehead lift, except that the temporal dissection is carried out on top of the lateral orbital rim, all the way to the insertion of the lateral canthal ligament medially, and inferiorly to the junction of the orbital rim and the body of the malar bone laterally. This more extended dissection allows for further elevation of the tail of the brow and, at same time, for elevation of the lateral raphe of the lateral canthal ligament and for improving crow's feet. Based on work done using the open approach by de la Plaza and others,[5] we currently perform this lateral orbital dissection in most patients in the supraperiosteal plane (Figure 3-11).

In the *limited endoscopic forehead lift* the dissection can be limited to either the glabellar and nasal areas or to the lateral supraorbital rim. To dissect the glabellar and nasal areas, the approach could be made through a forehead, upper eyelid, or nasal incision, in order to dissect the depressor supercilii and the procerus muscles, and occasionally the head of the corrugator.

The lateral supraorbital rim is approached through a blepharoplasty incision to modify the periosteum and the retroorbicularis fat pad and to perform myotomies and neurotomies of the orbicularis and corrugator muscles. This is done to improve or elevate the tail of the brow, to modify the shape of the brow, and to improve crow's feet (Figure 3-12).

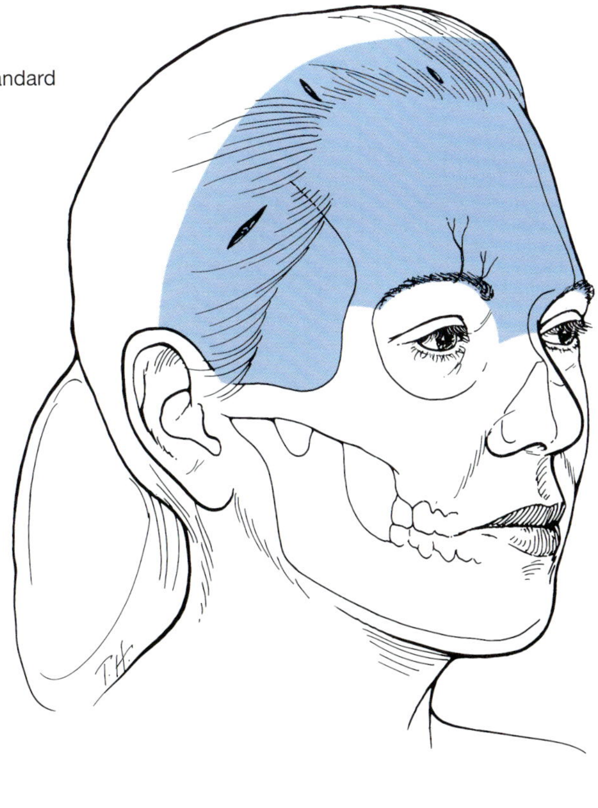

FIGURE 3-10
Endoforehead classification: extent of dissection in standard endoforehead is shown.

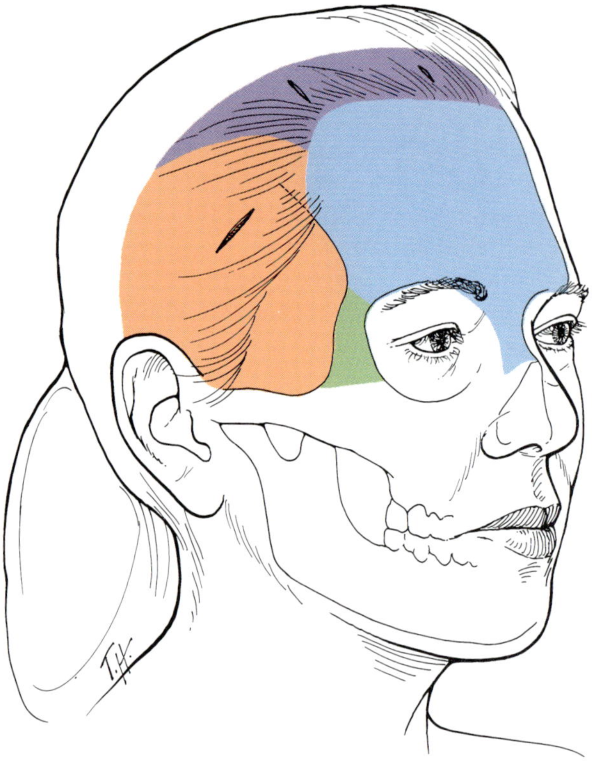

FIGURE 3-11
Endoforehead classification: extent of dissection in extended endoforehead is shown.

FIGURE 3-12
Endoforehead classification: extent of dissection in limited endoforehead with two variations, limited glabellar and limited lateral supraorbital, is shown.

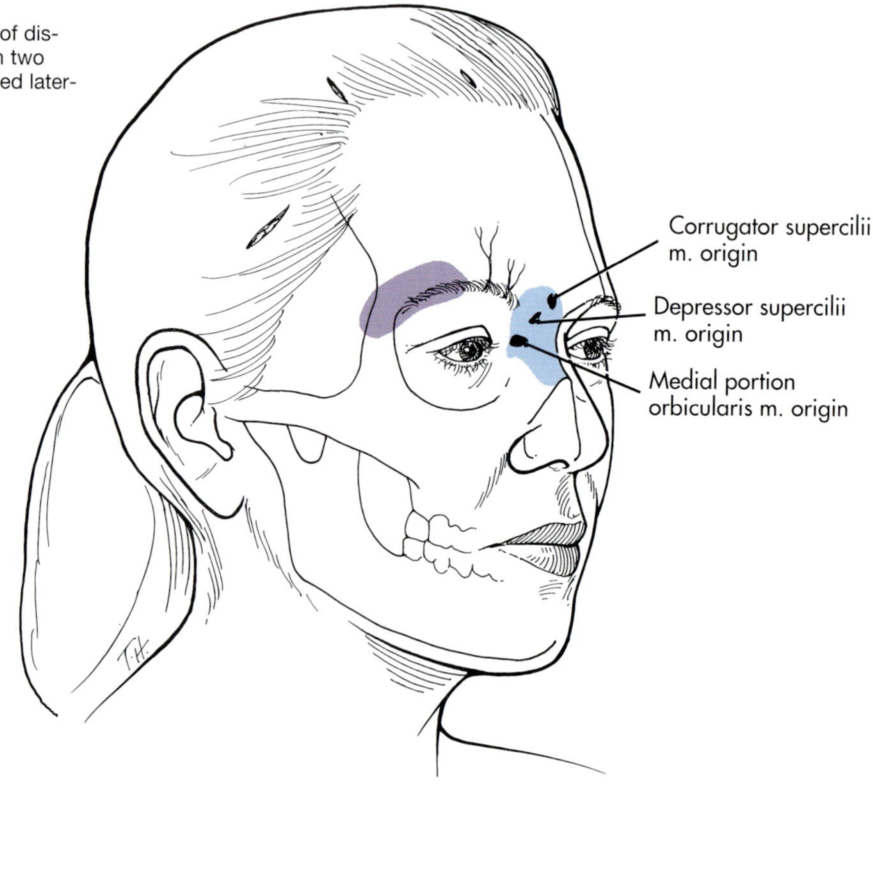

For the temporal endoforehead dissection is in the temporal area down to the lateral orbital rim and medially over the frontal bone to the supraorbital nerve. This technique is indicated for elevation of the lateral brow, crow's feet, and pseudoptosis of the upper eyelid (Figure 3-13).

ENDOFOREHEAD SURGICAL TECHNIQUE

As mentioned previously, the surgical technique used for the endoforehead lift is described in detail.

ANESTHESIA

For anesthesia, general or intravenous (IV) sedation with local anesthetic can be adequately used. For local anesthesia, nerve blocks are carried out with 1% lidocaine (Xylocaine) with epinephrine (1:100,000). In addition, the soft tissues of the scalp and forehead are infiltrated with 0.25% Xylocaine with epinephrine (1:400,000).

SKIN MARKINGS

Several skin markings are made (Figures 3-14, *A* and *B*). First, the trajectory of temporal, buccal, and zygomatic divisions of the facial nerve are outlined. The temporal branch begins at the point just inferior to the tragus where it rises obliquely, ending at a point about 1.5 cm above the eyebrow. The course of the buccal branch is from the ear lobe to the base of the nose. The zygomatic division generally follows the line that bisects the triangle formed by the trajectories of the temporal and buccal divisions.

The next landmark is the trajectory of the supraorbital nerve. The location of the supraorbital notch, or foramen, is palpable in most patients. This point is usually 2.7 cm lateral to the midline of the forehead. Over 60% of the time the nerve emerges from inside the orbit through a notch in the supraorbital rim. About 32% of the time, it comes out from a foramen in the supraorbital rim. About 8% of the time, the supraorbital nerve has supernumerary branches that arise approximately 1.5 cm superior to the orbital rim. We find that this normal variant occurs more commonly over the right side of the forehead. The supratrocheal nerve is located approximately 1 cm medially from the supraorbital nerve.

In addition, we usually mark the site of the incisions and the areas to be dissected. In so doing we differentiate between the areas where we will use the endoscope and the areas where dissection can be performed in a "blind" manner.

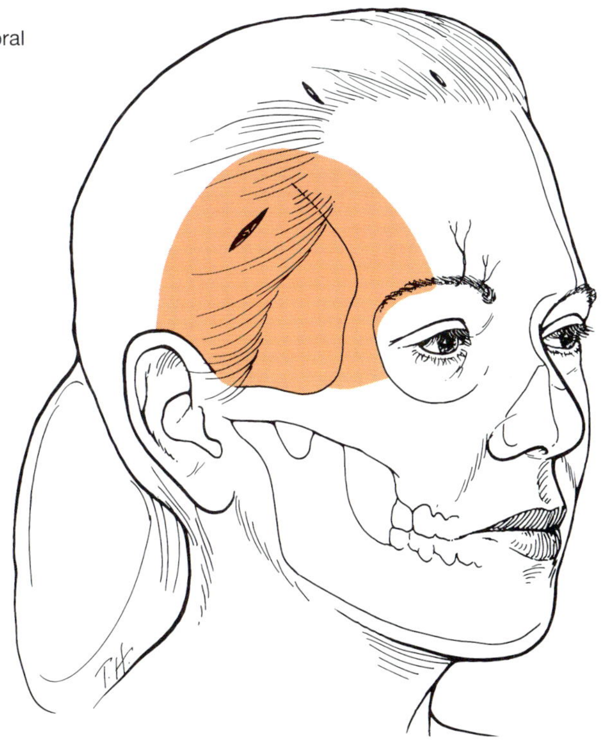

FIGURE 3-13
Endoforehead classification: extent of dissection in temporal endoforehead is shown.

FIGURE 3-14
A, Landmarks are given. Trajectories of branches of the facial nerve and supraorbital and supratrochlear nerves. The frontal branch of the facial nerve runs from the lower portion of the tragus to 1.5 cm above the eyebrow. The buccal branch of the facial nerve runs from the tragus to the columella labial angle. The zygomatic branch of the facial nerve runs at a 45-degree angle from the previous branches. The supraorbital nerve can be located 2.5 to 3.0 cm from the midglabellar line laterally; a notch can usually be felt at that level. The supratrochlear nerve is located 1 cm medial and 0.8 cm inferior to the supraorbital nerve. About 8% of the time the lateralmost branch of the supraorbital nerve rises 1 to 2 cm above the supraorbital rim, and in some instances leaves an imprint on the frontal bone as a "nerve groove." **B,** The anatomic trajectory of different branches of the facial nerve and its relationship with the zygomatic arch and the eyebrow are shown.

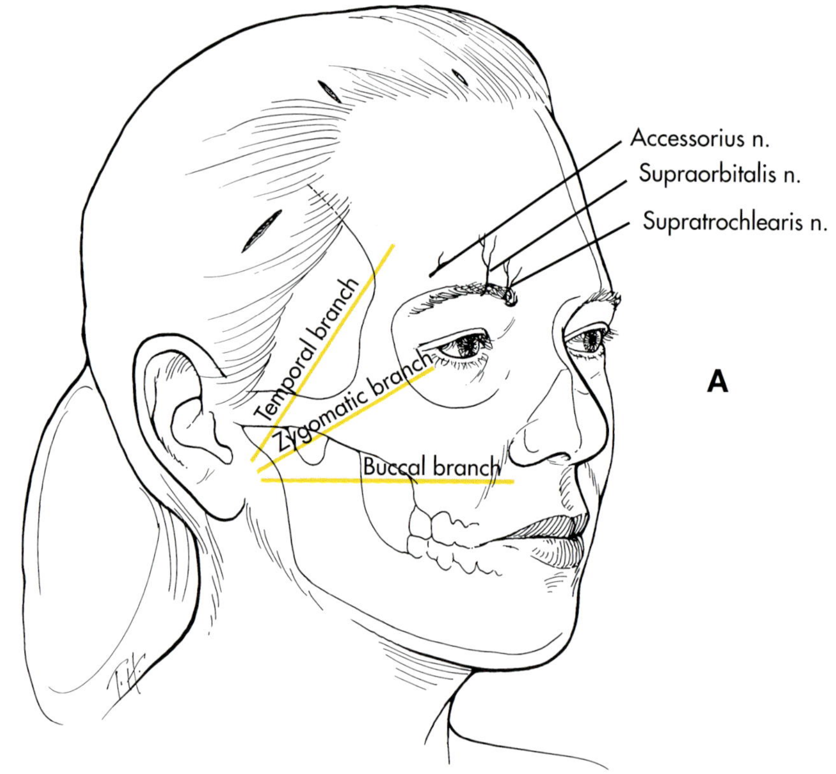

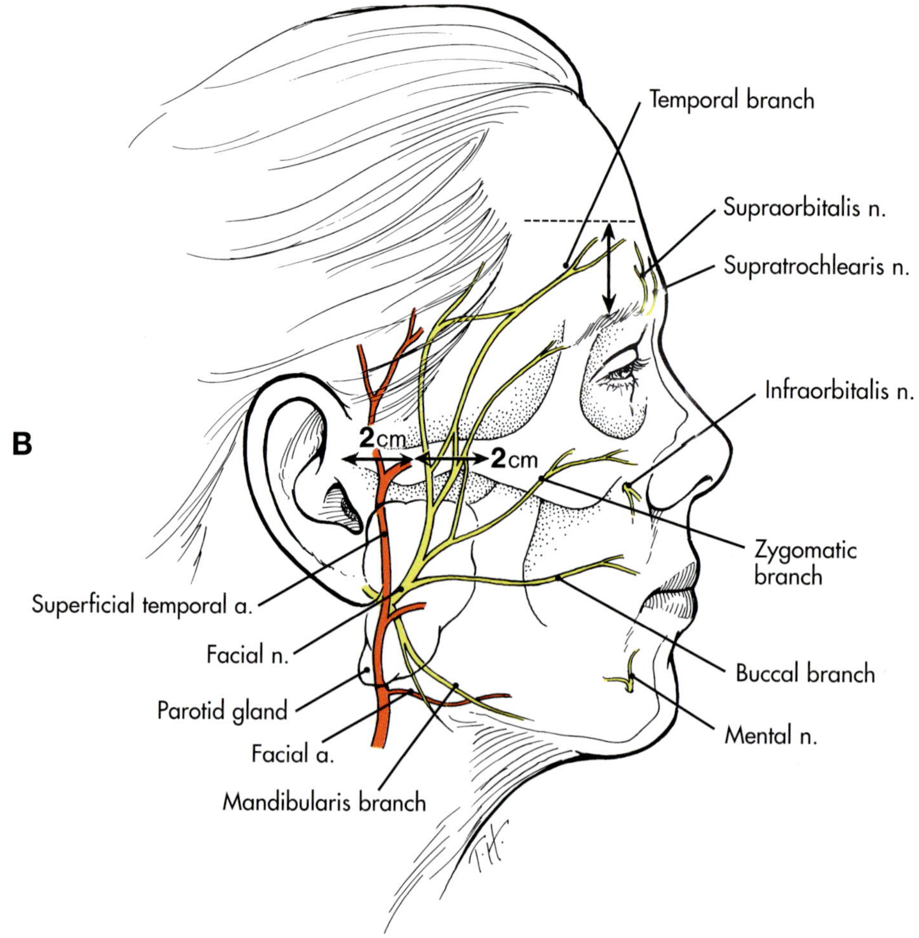

INCISIONS

For the endoforehead, usually five incisions are made. The first is in the *midline*, 1 cm long, vertical in direction, and just behind the hairline. The next two, similar in length and direction, are the *paramedian* incisions, approximately 5 cm on either side of the midline incision. Two other incisions, one in each *temporal* area, approximately 2 cm long and running behind the temple hairline, are also marked.

The central and paramedian incisions are made all the way down through the periosteum. The temporal incisions are made into the superficial dermis. This incision is carefully deepened, usually with a blunt instrument, such as a hemostat, to the level of the superficial layer of the deep temporal fascia. Care is taken not to injure the superficial temporal vessels because this can cause premature bleeding, which could obscure the view, prolong the procedure, and even produce a hematoma (Figure 3-15).

DISSECTION

After making the incisions, dissection without the use of the endoscope proceeds in the temporal, frontal, and posterior scalp areas, creating pockets in each of these areas (Figure 3-16). *Temporal dissection* is usually performed first, in a blind fashion,

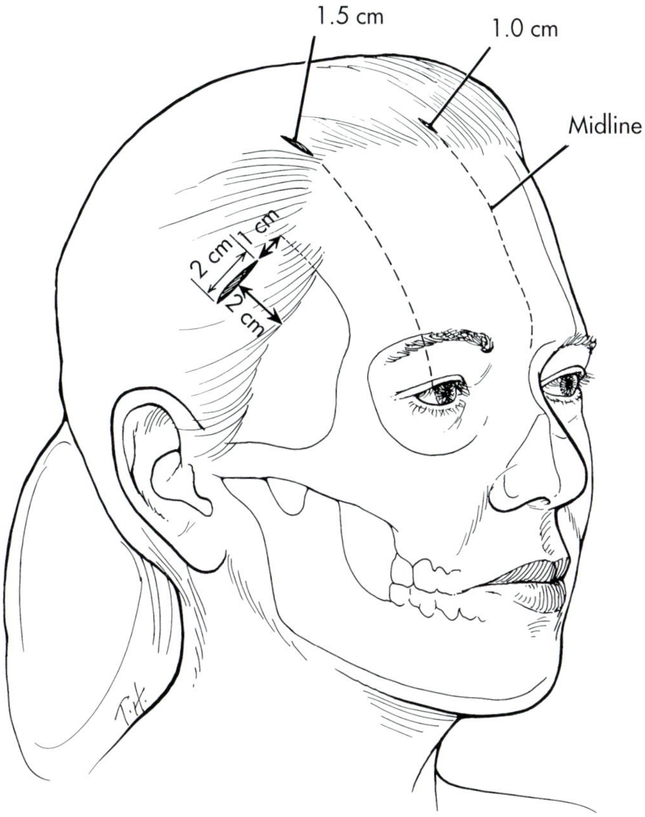

FIGURE 3-15
Marking the incisions is shown. The midline incision is the upward projection of the midforehead line. Paramedian incisions are 5 cm lateral to the midline incision. Temporal incisions are in the medial portion of the temporal area 1 cm lateral from the temporal crest.

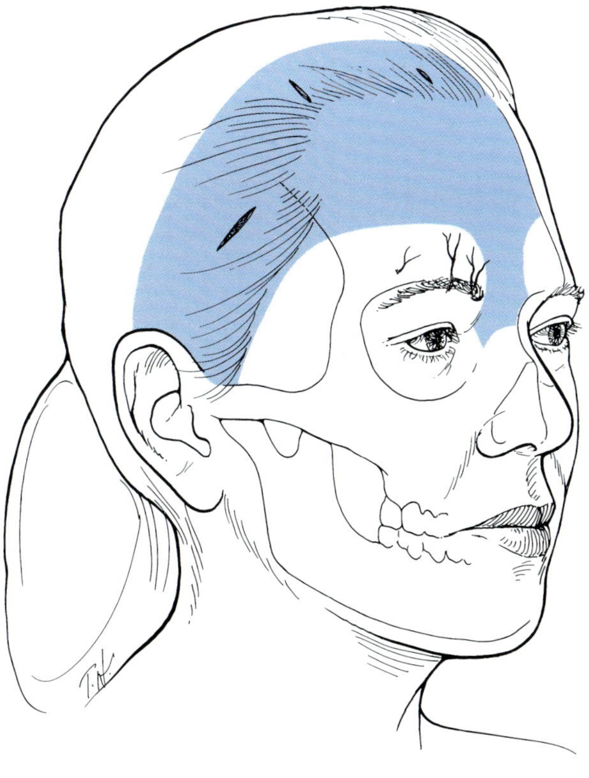

FIGURE 3-16
Extent of the "blind" dissection is shown. Without the use of the endoscope this is carried out to 3 cm above the supraorbital rim to prevent injuring branches of the supraorbital nerve that might exit the frontal bone above the superior orbital rim.

between the temporoparietal fascia and the superficial layer of the deep temporal fascia. This undermining is carried posteriorly into the postauricular area, inferiorly and anteriorly, to about 1 cm superior to the premarked course of the temporal branch of the facial nerve. Medially, the dissection of the pocket is carried to the level of the temporal crest.

In the *posterior scalp* (coronal area), we prefer to use a subgaleal plane of dissection, although it can be done subperiosteally as well. Subgaleal dissection allows for better contraction or redraping of the posterior scalp flap.

Frontal pocket dissection also begins in a blind fashion. Its plane is subperiosteal. It is usually carried out with a sharp periosteal elevator. If the periosteum is loose and flimsy, a soft tissue elevator can be used as well.

In the *center over the glabella* the dissection is carried blindly all the way to the radix of the nose. Laterally, the dissection is stopped at a level approximately 2 cm superior to the superior orbital rim. Next, the endoscope is inserted and dissection under endoscopic visualization is continued in the subperiosteal plane until the superior orbital rim is reached.

Once these pockets are developed (subperiosteal in the frontal area and subgaleal in the temporal area), they are joined between the paramedian and temporal incisions, dissecting from a lateral to a medial direction. Once the pockets are joined at this level, still blindly, a lateral sweep with a periosteal elevator is carried out. This detaches the junction of the periosteum and the galea at the superior portion of the temporal crest.

ENDOSCOPIC DISSECTION

Next with the aid of the endoscope (Figure 3-17, *A*) the dissection of the temporal pocket is continued inferiorly to the level of the zygomatic arch, and anteriorly to the lateral orbital rim until the sentinel vein (so named by de la Plaza)[6] is reached (Figure 3-17, *B*). This vein is a tributary of the internal maxillary vein. For a standard endoscopic forehead lift, this vein is preserved. If an extended forehead lift or an endoscopic midface lift is carried out, this small vein will sometimes be sacrificed.

Next the fibrous tissue present at the junction of the frontal and temporal pockets over the temporal crest is divided as dissection continues all the way down to the beginning of the lateral orbital rim. Here, commonly, other small vessels that also need to be controlled are encountered. Following this the dissection is returned to the frontal region, where at the level of the superior orbital rim the periosteum is usually found to be very tightly attached. Here a sharp, narrow periosteal elevator usually is used. If the dissection needs to be carried into the orbit, then a similar sharp elevator with a 75- to 90-degree angle is used. During this surgical step care is taken to preserve the supraorbital and supratrocheal nerves (Figure 3-17, *C*).

Once the periosteum is dissected away from the superior orbital rim the dissection is continued medially into the glabellar area. Additional subperiosteal dissection using a sharp, wider instrument is used to detach the tight periosteal attachments. In addition to dissecting the superior portion of the radix of the nose, the dissection also continues laterally to the level of the medial canthal ligament. In this way the soft tissues are detached from the prominences and depressions of the glabellar region (Figure 3-17, *D*).

As previously mentioned, based on the patient's individual anatomy, the glabellar bony structures may include depressions in the center of the glabella or protrusions of bone immediately lateral to the glabella toward the superior orbital rim. The radix of the nose may be high, somewhat depressed, or very acutely depressed. Each of these bony configurations should be addressed properly, and all of the soft tissue should be elevated from the underlying bone, in order to deal with the bony anatomy. For example, if a patient is presenting with a protruding glabellar area and a very acute depression over the radix of the nose, the results of surgery will be minimal if we only address the soft tissues. This is because, in time, the tissues will tend to slide back into the bony depression. To prevent this, the bony configuration can be modified as needed by rasping, by shaving the protuberant bone, or by grafting the radix of the nose.

FIGURE 3-17
A, The extent of endoscopic dissection is shown. Direct visualization is mandatory at this level to prevent injury to motor and sensory branches of cranial nerves and blood vessels, which may lead to premature bleeding and hematoma. **B,** Endoscopic view of the temporal area showing the temporoparietalis fascia above and the temporal aponeurosis (deep temporal fascia) below. **C,** The sentinel vein near the lateral orbital rim. The temporal crest with the "temporal septum" (fusion of periosteum, temporoparietalis fascia, and temporal aponeurosis). **D,** Endoscopic view of the supraorbital area showing the supraorbital nerve, superior orbital rim, the corrugator muscle, and some branches of the supratrochlear nerve. **E,** Endoscopic view of the glabella area showing the origin of the corrugator muscle, the depressor supercilii muscle anterior to the corrugator muscle, the procerus muscle and the nasal bone, the periosteum as a superior flap, and the frontal bone as the floor of the dissected pocket.

A

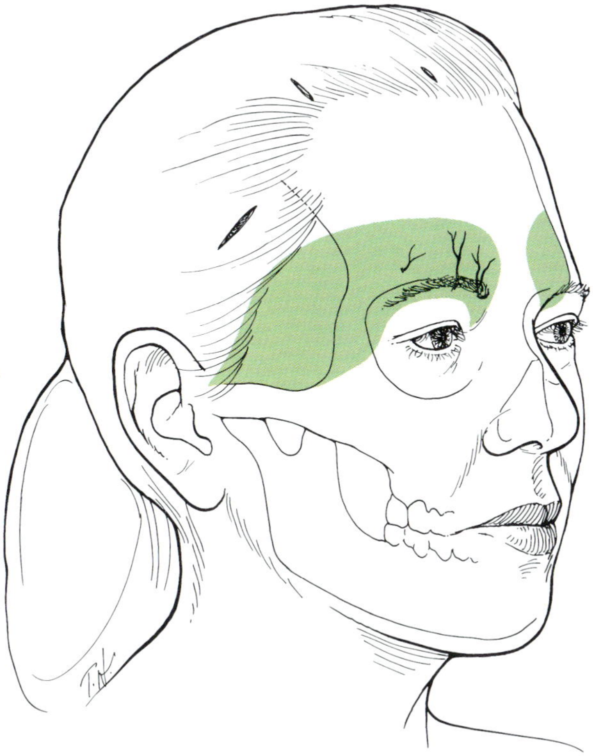

B C D E

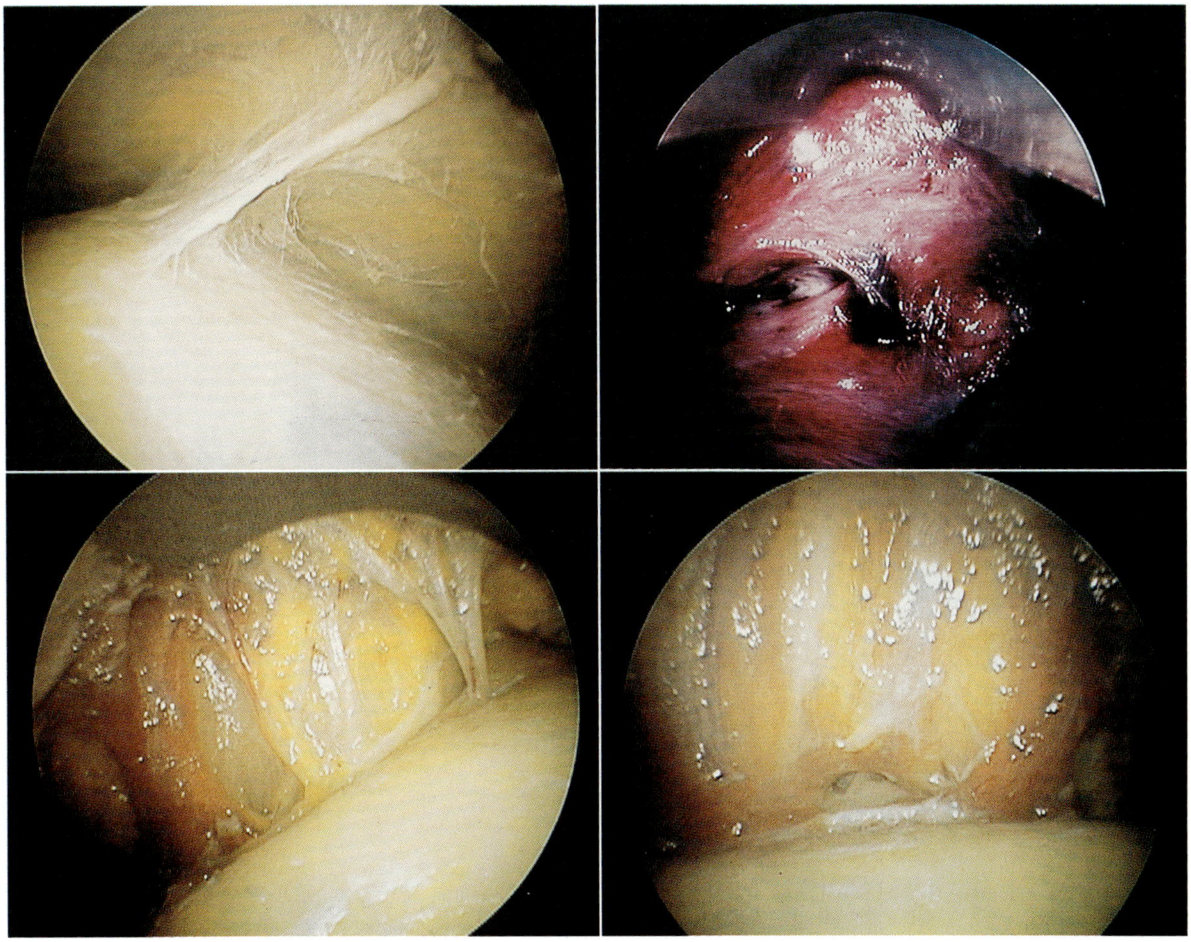

SOFT TISSUE MODIFICATION (FIGURE 3-18)

Periosteal release: the periosteum is released both horizontally and vertically. *Horizontal release* (Figure 3-19, *A*) consists of division of the periosteum across the superior orbital rim from the uppermost part of orbital process of the frontal bone laterally, all the way into the glabellar area medially. This release is done only after the supraorbital nerves are identified. Generally, in order to identify these nerves, one can look for an apparent transparency of the neurovascular bundle, a convex image coming from the supraorbital notch, or foramen, and a bluish tinge of discoloration. Once the location of the neurovascular bundle is identified, a long-handled no. 15 blade is introduced, and an incision is made lateral to the nerve, exactly at the level of the superior orbital rim.

Next, this incision is extended laterally and, eventually, medially. The *medial periosteal release* is sometimes easier to accomplish using only the periosteal elevator. Additional spreading of the edges of the periosteum is carried out to a point where a gap of approximately 1 to 1.5 cm in width exists between the periosteal edges. Preperiosteal fibrous tissue is often encountered at this point, which also needs to be released from the periosteum until one can clearly see either the orbicularis oculi muscle fibers or the subjacent fat pad.

As the medial periosteal release is performed, another vessel that joins the supraorbital vascular bundle and the corrugator muscle is encountered. The corrugator is beefy red in color and is usually extremely friable. Release of the periosteum continues next over the glabella. Here, again, although the periosteum tends to tear at different points, a complete release should be performed.

The previously mentioned *vertical release* (Figure 3-19, *B*) of an approximately 0.5-cm-wide gap should be completed throughout the length of the horizontal release. This vertical release of the periosteum allows the eyebrow to stretch out and relax horizontally. This maneuver also helps to elevate the tail of the brow. This vertical release in the glabellar region allows the skin to stretch out, thus improving the glabellar wrinkling.

MYOTOMIES (FIGURE 3-20, *A*)

Next the myotomies are carried out. Essentially, these are incisions of the muscles without myec-

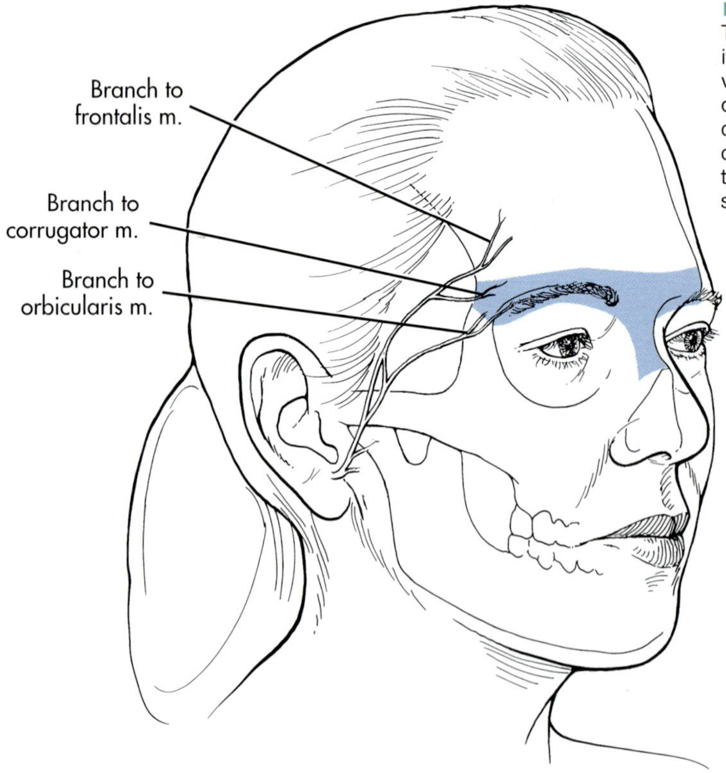

FIGURE 3-18
The shaded area shows where the soft tissue modification is done: periosteum release (horizontal and vertical), myotomies of the orbital portion of the orbicularis oculi muscle and the corrugator and depressor supercilii muscles. Release of the retro-orbicularis oculi fat pad (ROOF). Neurotomies of the orbital portion of the orbicularis, depressor supercilii, and corrugator muscles.

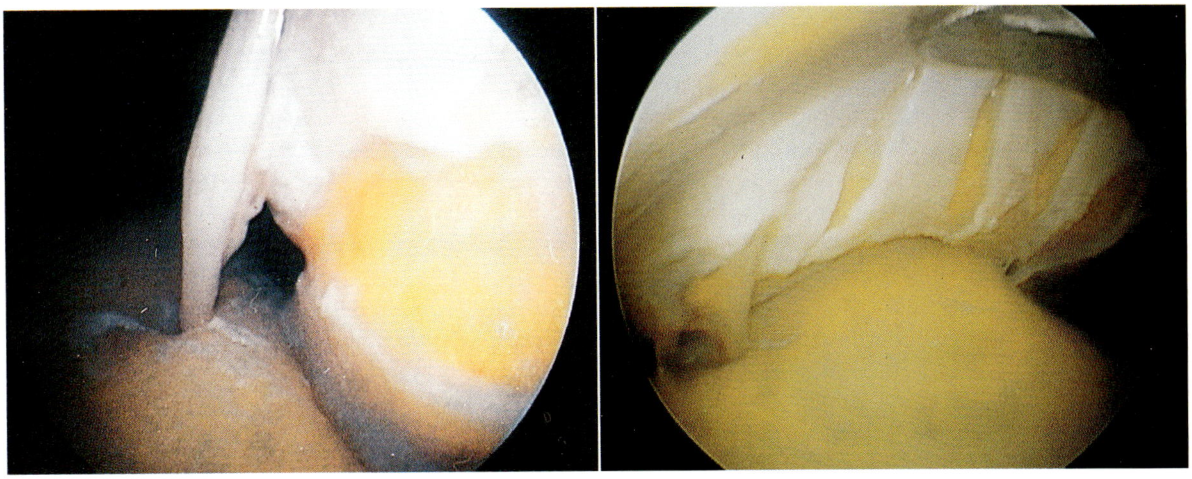

FIGURE 3-19
A, Horizontal periosteotomy: in this particular picture is shown a periosteotomy lateral to the supraorbital nerve. **B,** Vertical periosteotomy: serial vertical release of the periosteum, approximately 3 to 5 mm apart. Anterior to the periosteum can be seen the retro-orbicularis oculi fat pad (ROOF).

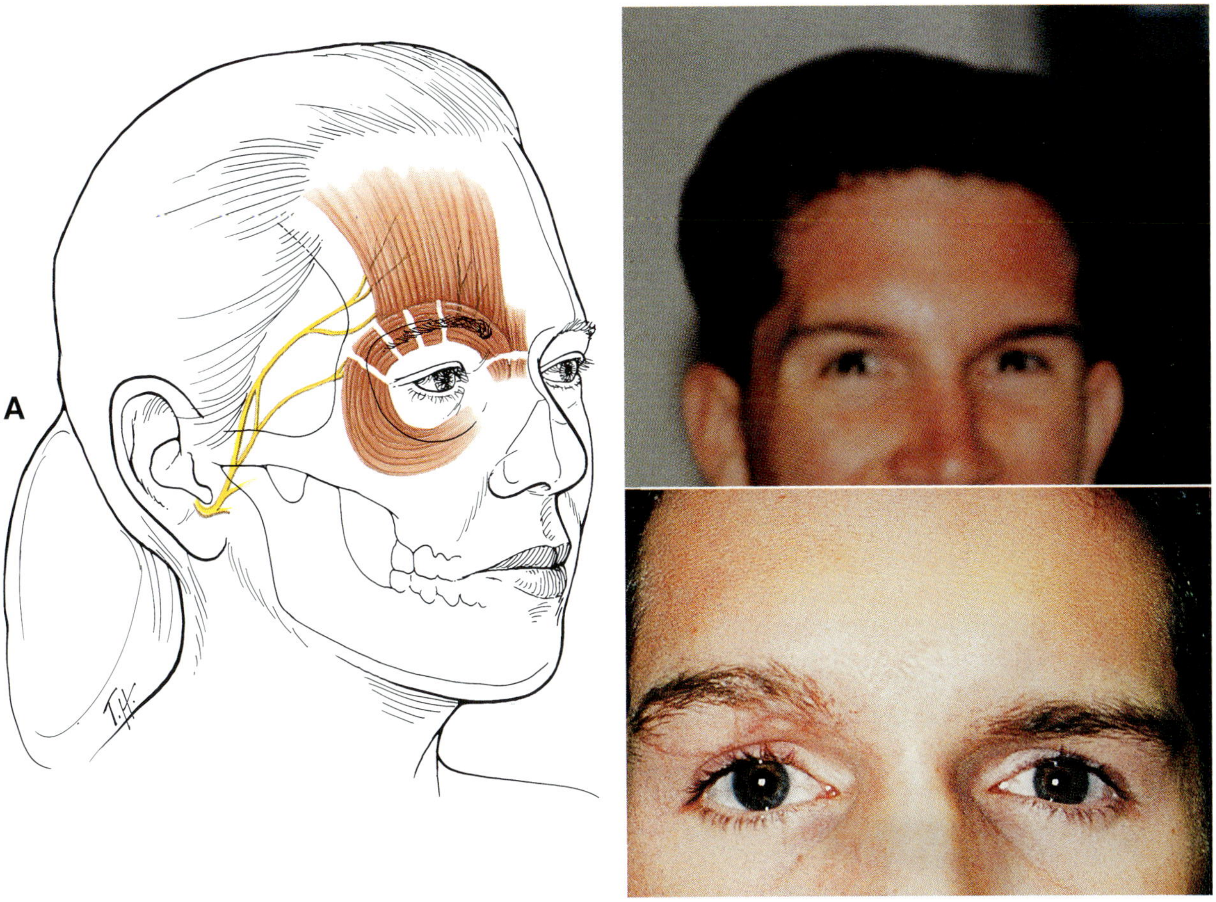

FIGURE 3-20
A, Myotomies and neurotomies: shown are the myotomies of the orbital portion of the orbicularis, lateral to the supraorbital nerve, and the myotomies of the depressor supercilii and procerus muscles at the level of the nasoglabellar area. **B,** A 21-year-old man before he was involved in a car accident. Photograph reproduced from family album shows eyebrows to be at a symmetric level. **C,** Appearance a year and a half after patient sustained a traumatic transection of the orbital portion of the orbicularis, depressor supercilii, and corrugator muscles and the corresponding neurotomies. This patient is an example of the changes that can occur after myotomies and neurotomies even in the absence of any tissue undermining and fixation.

tomies (muscle excisions). The effect of these myotomies is well demonstrated in this 21-year-old man (Figure 3-20, *B*). He was involved in a motor vehicle accident approximately 2 years prior, resulting in traumatic unilateral superior periorbital myotomies and neurotomies.

Rarely in patients with severe hypertrophy, muscle excision may be indicated to debulk the soft tissues and ensure a smooth contour.

We do myotomies of four facial muscles: the depressor supercilii, the procerus, the lateral portion of the corrugator, and the orbital portion of the orbicularis oculi.

Myotomy of the *orbicularis muscle* (Figure 3-20, *C*), which we believe to be the most important myotomy, is done lateral to the supraorbital nerve in the vertical fashion to weaken the orbital portion of this muscle. The myotomies, each about 1 cm in height, are performed every 3 to 5 mm apart, over the area subjacent to the eyebrow. The most lateral myotomy is done at the point where the orbicularis dives down, that is, at the superior orbital portion of the frontal bone, at the tail of the brow. This last myotomy is done roughly at a 30-degree angle from the superior orbital rim.

More medially, we also weaken the *depressor supercilii muscle*. This can be done either directly through the lateral glabellar area, transnasally, or through a window created in the medial portion of the corrugator muscle. As blunt dissection passes through the friable medial portion of the corrugator muscle, the supratrocheal nerve, which is usually sandwiched between the corrugator and the depressor supercilii muscles, comes into vision. Deep to this nerve, we find the depressor supercilii, which we then transect. This myotomy is done in a horizontal direction to allow the head of the brow to move upward.

Myotomy of the *procerus muscle* is also horizontal and is generally performed at the level of the radix of the nose. We usually prefer to do this at the level of the lowermost horizontal skin wrinkle. Sometimes, however, as recommended by Connell,[7,8] the procerus can be myotomized at a little higher level, so that when the residual procerus contracts downward, it will fill the radix of the nose. This can improve the nasal profile of patients with a low radix.

NEUROTOMIES

In the course of performing these myotomies, neurotomies are performed simultaneously by division of the tiny branches that course within the orbital portion of the orbicularis and the corrugator muscles. If we wish to do selective neurotomies to the corrugator muscle without affecting the lateral (orbital) portion of the orbicularis muscle, we can make a vertical incision medial to the supraorbital nerve and lateral to the supratrocheal nerve, in the uppermost portion of the corrugator muscle where the nerve pierces it, or above the superior margin of the eyebrow by approximately 5 to 7 mm.

Once the soft tissue release is complete, the frontalis-galea-occipitalis muscle sling will pull the brow posteriorly, producing a functional elevation (Figure 3-21).

FIXATION

Fixation is performed next to keep the tissues elevated, especially in the first few weeks when edema is intense and the tissues are heavy and might counteract the elevation produced by the frontalis muscle. The need for fixation is only temporary; usually 2 or 3 months are sufficient. We stress that in the endoforehead approach, fixation is used only to **stabilize** the tissues and **not** for the purpose of pulling and elevating.

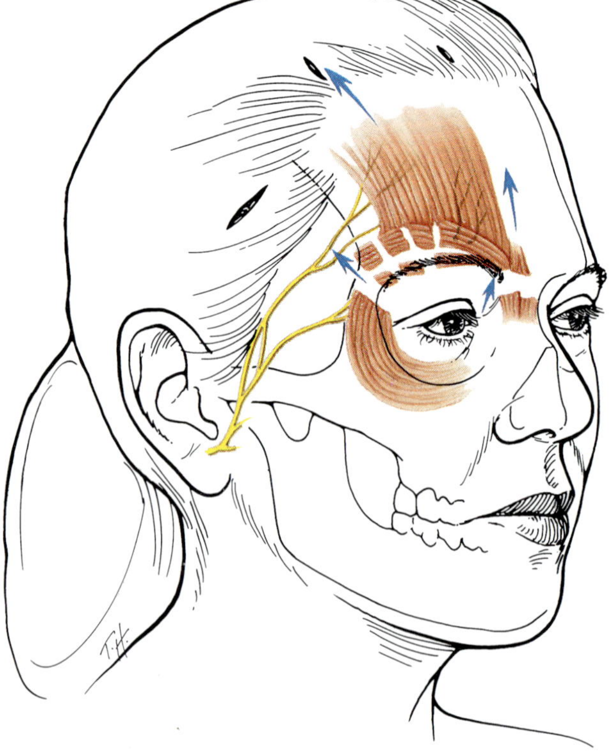

FIGURE 3-21
Functional elevation of the eyebrow by the frontalis muscle after release of the soft tissue and depressor muscles is shown.

Fixation in the temporal area is performed routinely by advancing the temporoparietalis fascia posteriorly and fixing it to the temporal aponeurosis. Nylon sutures or 2.0 or 3.0 polydioxanone sutures (PDS) are used. The anterior part of the suture is either placed into the temporoparietalis fascia or a portion of the dermis. This then is advanced posteriorly and sutured to the temporal fascia (Figures 3-22 and 3-23).

In the frontal area, fixation is done at the level of the paramedial incisions. Different types of fixation using miniplates, miniscrews, cortical tunnels (Figure 3-24), and other suturing techniques can be used.

For bandages, micropore, paper, or foam tape can be used to help control swelling and to act as an external splint or suspension device. After 4 or 5 days, the bandages are removed and replaced by more tape, or by a headband. Skin sutures are removed in approximately 7 days. Ecchymosis may last a week or so, depending on the patient.

In addition, intraoperatively, the administration of dexamethasone (Decadron), 8 or 10 mg, in conjunction with 50 mg diphenhydramine (Benadryl), is used. Dilute solution of Decadron and bupivacaine (Marcaine) is sprayed under the flaps. Postoperatively, dexamethasone is administered for 2 or 3 days in decreasing amounts. These measures appear to help with postoperative edema. Patients are asked to return in 1 year for additional postoperative evaluation.

SELECTED CLINICAL CASES: ENDOFOREHEAD

See Figures 3-25 through 3-28.

COMPLICATIONS

The results of the endoforehead lift are similar to those provided by conventional coronal forehead lift operations. Complications are minimal. In our patients, complications ranged from itching, bleeding, nerve injury, and insufficient release of

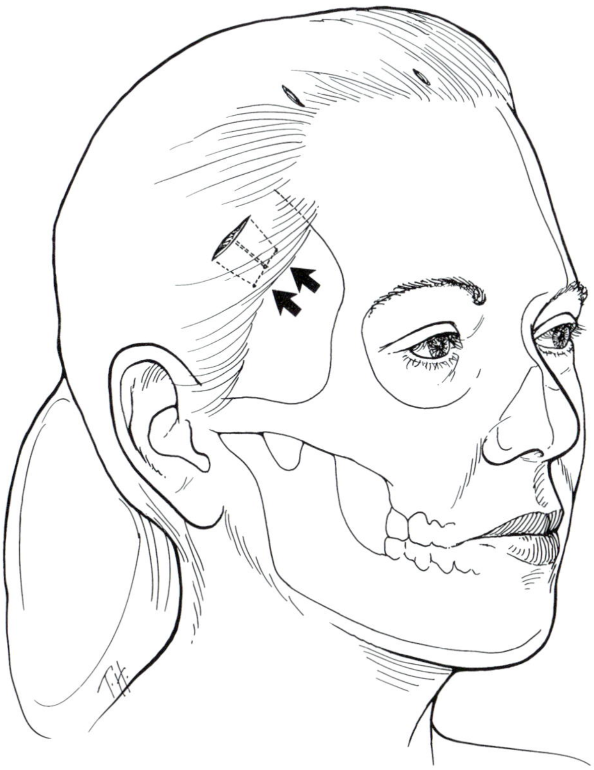

FIGURE 3-22
The temporal fixation between temporoparietalis fascia and the temporal aponeurosis is shown.

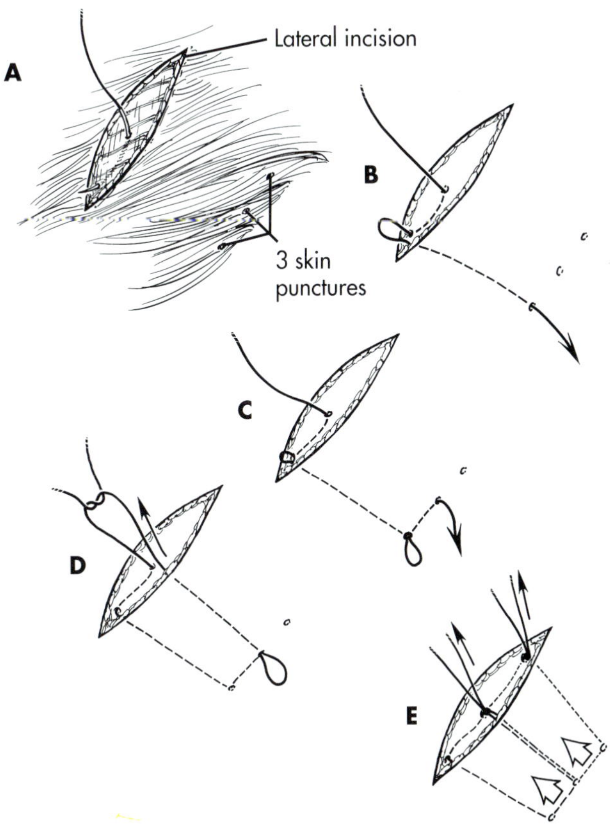

FIGURE 3-23
Different steps for placement of stitches for temporal fixation are shown. **A,** Suture under temporal aponeurosis posterior to the temporal incision. **B,** Suture passing from inside out through a temporoparietalis fascia of skin, puncture wound. **C,** Suture going outside through same puncture wound as **(B),** then traveling under the dermis to the next puncture wound, then coming out. **D,** Suture going from outside in through puncture wound **(C),** attaching dermis to temporoparietalis fascia. **E,** Two sutures are suspending the temporoparietalis fascia to the temporal aponeurosis.

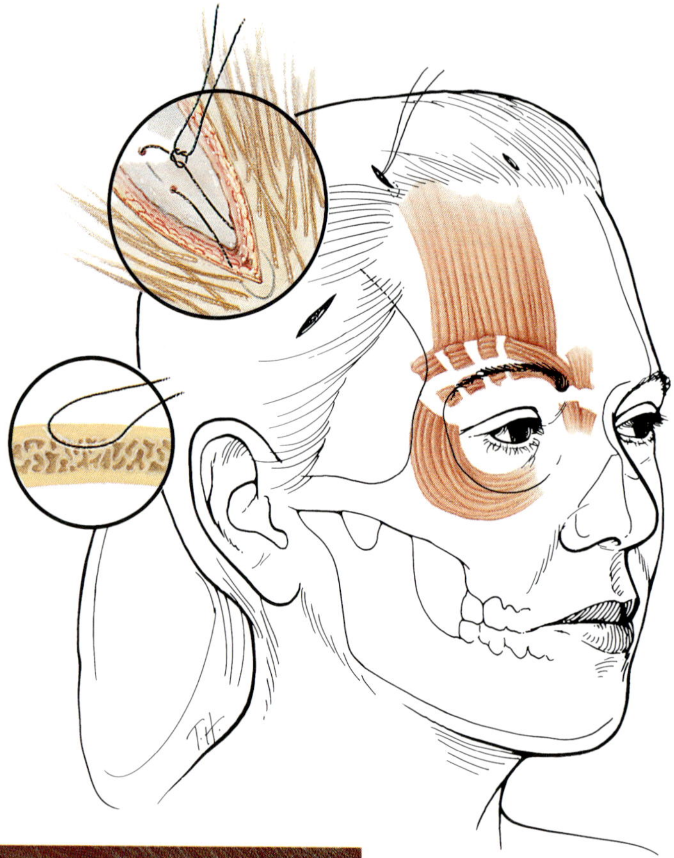

FIGURE 3-24
Frontal fixation by means of the cortical tunnel is shown.

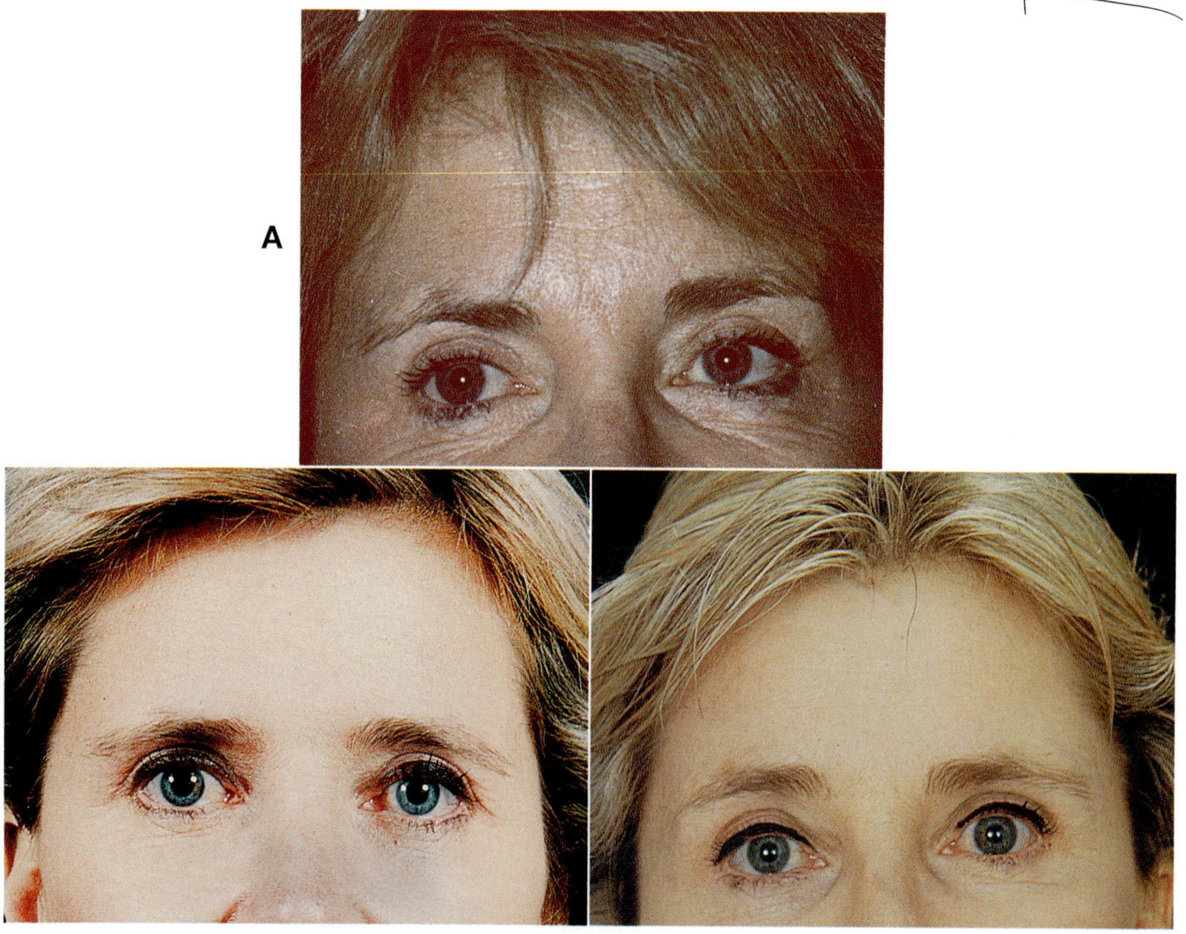

FIGURE 3-25
Case study 1. **A,** A 48-year-old woman before conventional "open" approach forehead plasty and blepharoplasty performed by another surgeon is shown. **B,** Patient at 4 months after the first operation. **C,** Patient at 10 months after endoscopic forehead plasty. A repeat blepharoplasty was not performed.

A

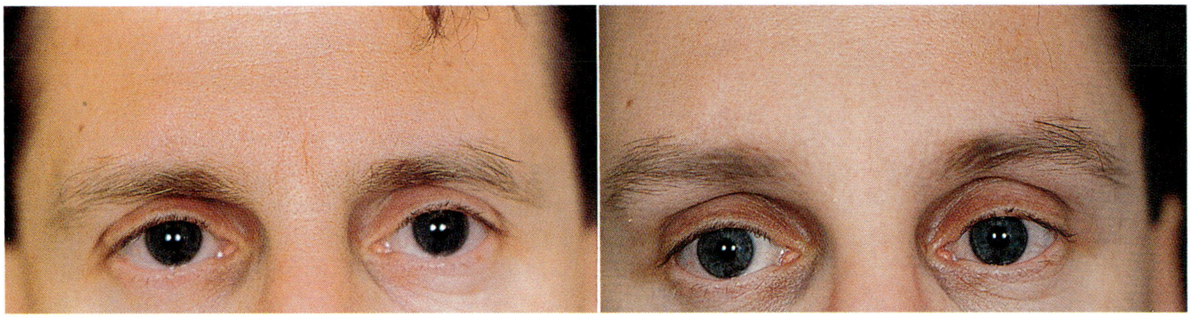

B

FIGURE 3-26
Case study 2. **A,** A 36-year-old man is shown before, and **B,** 7 months after endoscopic forehead plasty. A blepharoplasty was not performed.

A

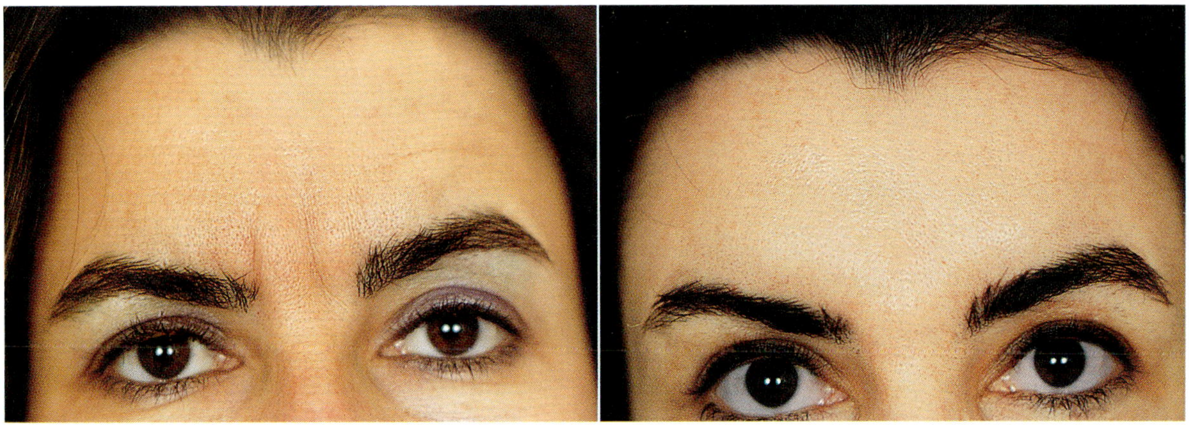

B

FIGURE 3-27
Case study 3. **A,** A 39-year-old woman is shown before, and **B,** 8 months after endoscopic forehead plasty. A blepharoplasty was not performed. Note on the preoperative photograph the bulges caused by the hypertrophic depressor supercilii muscles. Also note that our attempt to correct the asymmetry in the height of the eyebrows was not successful.

A

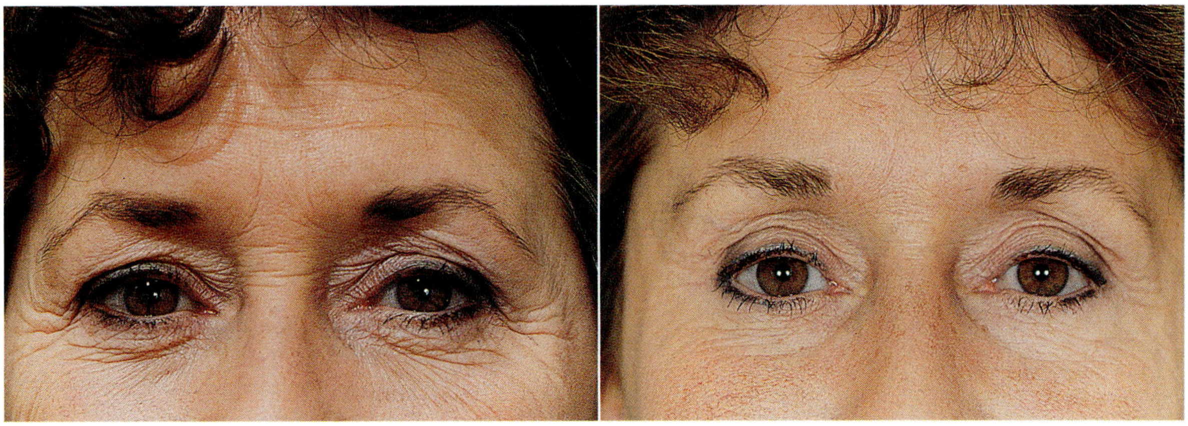

B

FIGURE 3-28
Case study 4. **A,** A 55-year-old woman is shown before, and **B,** 16 months after endoscopic forehead lift. An upper lid blepharoplasty was not performed.

the periosteum, to asymmetry which is caused mainly by uneven dissection. Table 3-4 shows the complications that occurred in our series of endo-forehead lifts (most performed by Dr. Isse) over a 2-year period.[3,9]

In the cases of seroma, we drained the excess fluid. The stitch abscesses were rather minor and occurred only when silk sutures were used for fixation. Once the suture material was removed, the stitch abscess resolved. Subsequently, we switched from silk to PDS suture material, and we have not observed another case of stitch abscess. The rest of the complications resolved with time.

Although at first glance the rate of complications appears to be high, in actuality most of them have been minor in nature and required minimal, if any, intervention for their treatment. One male patient with significant forehead bossing experienced complete relapse of the eyebrow ptosis at 3 months postoperatively and represented the only entirely unsatisfactory result. Five additional patients demonstrated partial recurrence of the eyebrow ptosis. Despite this, these patients remained content with the results obtained.

By far, most of the complications and less-than-satisfactory results occurred early on. As we gained experience in preoperative patient selection, and as our technique evolved, complications have been practically eliminated and patient satisfaction has been uniformly high. In general, our experience with endoscopic forehead rejuvenation procedures has been very satisfactory. We remain enthused and are looking forward to future developments in endoscopically assisted plastic surgery.

TABLE 3-4 POSTOPERATIVE COMPLICATIONS IN 110 CASES OF ENDOFOREHEAD LIFT

COMPLICATION	NO. OF CASES	COMMENT
Seroma	4	Located on top of scalp
Ecchymosis (2 weeks' duration)	5	Located in periorbital area
Numbness (4 weeks' duration)	2	Located on scalp
Paresis (6 weeks' duration)	1	Located in frontal branch of facial nerve on right side
Stitch abcess	4	Located at temporal fixation point
Complete relapse of brow ptosis	1	Occurred 3 months post-operatively in a male patient with severe forehead bossing
Partial relapse of brow ptosis	5	Occurred 6 months post-operatively; these female patients were of Latino and Asian descent

REFERENCES

1. Fodor PB: Endoscopic plastic surgery, a new milestone in plastic surgery, (Editorial), *Aesth Plast Surg* 18:31, 1994.
2. Isse NG: Endoscopic facial rejuvenation: endoforehead, the functional lift. Presented at the Los Angeles Society of Plastic Surgery Conference, Los Angeles, November 17, 1992; also presented at the XII Congress of the International Society of Aesthetic Plastic Surgery (ISAPS), Paris, September 7, 1993.
3. Isse NG: Endoscopic facial rejuvenation: endoforehead, the functional lift, *Aesth Plast Surg* 18:21, 1994.
4. Duchenne de Boulogne GB: *The mechanism of facial expression*, New York, 1990, Cambridge University Press.
5. de la Plaza R: Supraperiosteal lifting of the upper two-thirds of the face, *Br J Plast Surg* 44:325, 1991.
6. Connell BF: Finesse in rhytidectomy, *Rec Adv Plast Surg* 3:137, 1985.
7. Connell BF, Lambros VS, Neurohr GH: The forehead lift: techniques to avoid complications and produce optimal results, *Aesth Plast Surg* 13:217, 1989.
8. Isse NG: Unpublished data, 1994.

SUGGESTED READINGS

Artz JS, Dinner MI, Foglietti MA: Planning the aesthetic forehead plasty, *Ann Plast Surg* 225:1, 1990.

Aston SJ, Thorne CHM: *Aesthetic surgery of the aging face.* In Smith JW, Aston SG, editors: *Plastic surgery*, Boston, 1991, Little, Brown.

Baker TJ, Gordon HL: *Surgical rejuvenation of the face*, St Louis, 1986, Mosby–Year Book.

Bames HO: Frown disfigurement and ptosis, *Plast Reconstr Surg* 19:337, 1957.

Castanares S: Forehead wrinkles, glabellar frown and ptosis of the eyebrows, *Plast Reconstr Surg* 34:406, 1964.

Connell BF: *Eyebrow and forehead lifts.* In Courtiss EH, editor: *Male aesthetic surgery*, St Louis, 1981, Mosby–Year Book.

Connell BF: Eyebrow, face, and neck lifts for males, *Clin Plast Surg* 5(1):15, 1978.

Connell BF: Finesse in rhytidectomy, *Recent Adv Plast Surg* 3:137, 1985.

Connell BF, Lambros VS, Neurohr GH: The forehead lift: techniques to avoid complications and produce optimal results, *Aesth Plast Surg* 13:217, 1989.

Correia P de C, Zani R: Surgical anatomy of the facial nerve as related to ancillary operations in rhytidoplasty, *Plast Reconstr Surg* 52:549, 1973.
Duchenne de Boulogne GB: *The mechanism of facial expression*, New York, 1990, Cambridge University Press.
Farkas LC, Kolar JC: Anthropometrics and art in the aesthetics of women's faces, *Clin Plast Surg* 14:599, 1987.
Fomon S: *Cosmetic surgery principles and practice*, Philadelphia, 1960, JB Lippincott.
Forrest CR, Phillips JH, Bell AB, Gruss JS, Chir B: The biomechanical effects of deep tissue support as related to brow and facelift procedures, *Plast Reconstr Surg* 88:427, 1991.
Furnas DW: Landmarks for the trunk and the temporofacial division of the facial nerve, *Br J Surg* 52:694, 1965.
Gleason M: *Forehead lift*. In Fisher J, editor: *Manual of aesthetic surgery*, New York, 1985, Springer-Verlag.
Gonzalez-Ulloa M: Facial wrinkles, integral elimination, *Plast Reconstr Surg* 29:658, 1962.
Griffiths CO: A new approach to the operative management of forehead, brow, and frown rhytidectomies, *Int Micro Aesth Plast Surg* 1974B.
Guyuron B, Davies B: Subcutaneous anterior hairline forehead rhytidectomy, *Aesth Plast Surg* 12:77, 1988.
Hinderer UT: Blepharocanthoplasty with eyebrow lift, *Plast Reconstr Surg* 56:402, 1972.
Isse, NG: Endoscopic facial rejuvenation: endoforehead, the functional lift. Presented at the Los Angeles Society of Plastic Surgery Conference, Los Angeles, November 17, 1992; also presented at the XII Congress of the International Society of Aesthetic Plastic Surgery (ISAPS), Paris, September 7, 1993.
Isse, NG: Endoscopic facial rejuvenation: endoforehead, the functional lift, *Aesth Plast Surg* 18:21, 1994.
Kaye BC: *Forehead and brow*. In Rees TD, editor: *Aesthetic plastic surgery*, Philadelphia, 1980, WB Saunders.
Kaye BL: The forehead lift: a useful adjunct to facelift and blepharoplasty, *Plast Reconstr Surg* 60:161, 1977.
LeRoux P, Johes SH: Total permanent removal of wrinkles from the forehead, *Br J Plast Surg* 27:359, 1974.
Liang M, Narayanan K: Endoscopic ablation of frontalis and corrugator muscles: a clinical study, *Plast Surg Forum* XV:54, Washington, DC, 1992.
Marino H: Treatment of wrinkles of forehead, *Prensa Med Arg* 51:1368, 1964.
Marino H: The forehead lift: some hints to secure better results, *Aesth Plast Surg* 1:251, 1977.
McKinney P, Mossie RD, Zukowski ML: Criteria for the forehead lift, *Aesth Plast Surg* 15:141, 1991.
Ortiz-Monasterio F, Barrera G, Olmedo A: The coronal incision in rhytidectomy: the brow lift, *Clin Plast Surg* 5:167, 1978.
Pitanguy I: Indications for and treatment of frontal and glabellar wrinkles in an analysis of 3,404 consecutive cases of rhytidectomy, *Plast Reconstr Surg* 76:157, 1981.
Pitanguy I, Silveria R: The frontal branch of the facial nerve: the importance of its variations in face lifting, *Plast Reconstr Surg* 38:352, 1966.
Powell N: *Proportions of the aesthetic face*, New York, 1984, Thieme-Stratton.
Reifkohl R: The forehead brow lift, *Ann Plast Surg* 9:55, 1992.
Rees TD, Wood-Smith D: *Cosmetic facial surgery*, Philadelphia, 1973, WB Saunders.
Rudolph R, Miller SH: Do forehead lifts lift or unfurl?, *Aesth Plast Surg* 16:1, 1992.
Santana MPS: Metodoligia craneomaxillofacial en ritidoplasty, *Cirugia Plast Ibero-Latinoam* 10(4), 1984.
Su CT, Morgan RF, Manson PN, Hoopes JE: Technique for division and suspension of the orbicularis oculi muscle, *Clin Plast Surg* 8:673, 1981.
Tessier P: Ridectomie frontale: lifting frontale, *Gaz Méd Fr* 75:5565, 1968.
Vasconez LO, Core GB, Askrew C, et al: Coronal facelift with endoscopic techniques, *Plast Surg Forum* XV:227, 1992.
Vecchione TR: Glabellar frown lines: direct excision, an evaluation of the scars, *Plast Reconstr Surg* 86(1):46, 1990.
Vinas CA, Caviglia C, Cortinas JL: Forehead rhytidoplasty and brow lifting, *Plast Reconstr Surg* 57:445, 1976.
Zide BM, Jelks GW: *Surgical anatomy of the orbit*, New York, 1985, Raven Press.

CHAPTER 4

Facial Rejuvenation: Technique and Rationale

Antonio Fuente del Campo

The subperiosteal facelift, based on the principle of relocation of the deep soft tissues of the face and restoration of their position and consistency, allows reestablishment of the relationship between the facial skeleton and the soft tissues that is altered over time by the gradual volumetric reduction of bone.[1,2]

This procedure has changed substantially since Tessier revolutionized the concept of face rejuvenation with his "mask lift,"[3] which was based on the subperiosteal detachment and traction of the deep tissues, thus achieving indirect skinlift. Psillakis[4] and Krastinova[5] contributed to popularize this procedure. Santana[6] was the first to broadly apply the principles of craniofacial surgery to rhytidectomy by doing more extensive subperiosteal detachments. Ramirez and co-workers[7] and Stuzin and co-workers[8] independently described the dissection between both sheets of the temporal fascia to avoid injuring the frontal branch of the facial nerve.

Maillard, Cornette de Saint Cyr, and Scheflan[9] described the use of the deep musculoaponeurotic system (DMAS) as a flap to pull and suspend the deep tissues of the lower half of the face. We[10-14] described the subperiosteal dissection of the mandible to correct the laxity of the deep soft tissues of the lower half of the face, and the "stepwise suspension" as a way to use the vertical traction applied in subperiosteal rhytidectomy to avoid preauricular incisions in many cases.

At the 1992 Annual Congress of the American Society of Plastic and Reconstructive Surgeons, held in Washington, D.C., Core and co-workers[15] and Liang and Narayanan[16] presented for the first time their concept of foreheadplasty by resecting the corrugator and procerus muscles with endoscopic techniques. Later, during the UCLA course held in Ixtapa, Mexico, in February of 1993, Isse[17] presented his own version of this procedure, which he called *endoforehead*. It was then, based on Isse's experience with the endoscopic approach, and on our own experience with subperiosteal facelift, that we designed our concept to perform the endoscopically assisted facelift.[18-22]

During the Second International Workshop on Aesthetic Surgery of the Face, held in Baltimore in April of 1993, we had the opportunity to study in cadavers the possibilities of this approach and to perform this procedure experimentally for the first time. Ramirez, who had also been trying to use the endoscope in forehead rejuvenation, joined the group. Since then, we have been working on the development of this approach and the instrumentation required to perform it.

The shift from an "open" to an endoscopic approach seemed a logical and natural step for me. The initial procedure I have described herein was based on vertical traction applied at the level of the coronal incision, and "stepwise suspension."[11] This allows use of the specific correction of the different areas and structures of the face, without depending on skin resection. This same concept and approach were easily replaced by the endoscopic procedure with the additional benefit of minimal incisions. It is interesting to see how a procedure that emerged at a certain moment with the input of several colleagues has rapidly made important headway, at the same time incorporating different and interesting variants, as illustrated in the chapters of this book.

The patients who request facial rejuvenation present different stages of aging. We have developed a classification system of grading rhytidosis as follows:

Grade I:	Initial midfacial laxity
Grade II:	Evident midfacial laxity and initial cervical laxity
Grade III:	Initial midfacial redundancy and evident cervical laxity
Grade IV:	Evident midfacial and cervical redundancies

Depending on the grade of rhytidosis, we perform only a subperiosteal facelift (basic procedure), or we combine it with a subcutaneous neck rhytidectomy, blepharoplasty, liposuction, or other complementary procedures. Our basic procedure consists of subperiosteal dissection, lifting of the deep soft tissues, stepwise suspension, indirect skin traction, and backward ear rotation.

SURGICAL PROCEDURE

With the patient under general anesthesia, or with local anesthesia and intravenous (IV) sedation, the procedure is begun by making two 1-cm parasagittal incisions in the frontal region, inside the hairline (Figure 4-1). Using a custom-designed, long, curved, malleable elevator (Figure 4-2), extensive subperiosteal dissection of the frontal region is performed around the supraorbital foramen through the access incisions, while the surgeon protects the supraorbital nerve from injury (Figure 4-3). The dissection is continued extensively toward the parietal and occipital regions and is extended toward the temporal regions in the subgaleal plane. At this point, the insertions of the frontooccipital muscle complex are released from

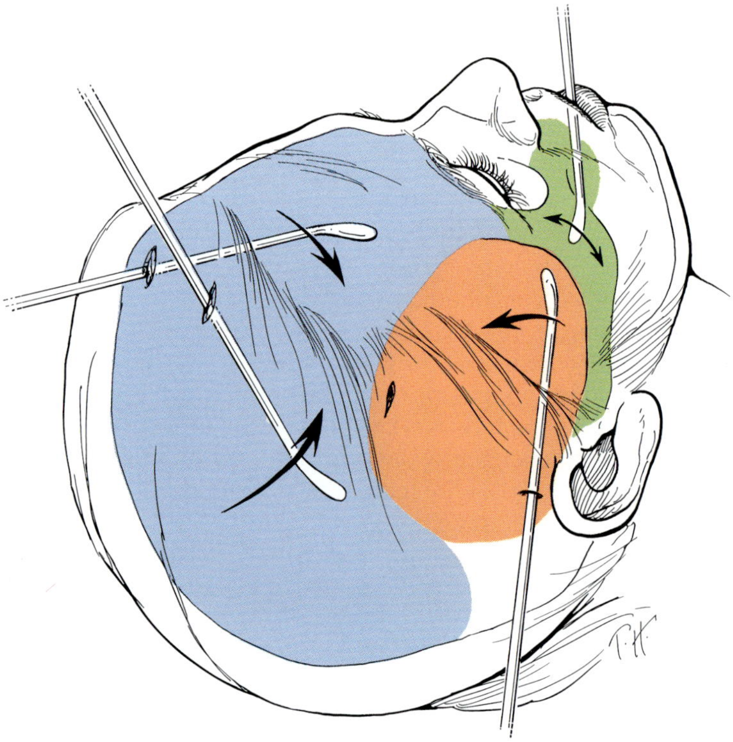

FIGURE 4-1
Incisions for endoscopic approach of a subperiosteal facelift, and the areas of dissection are shown.

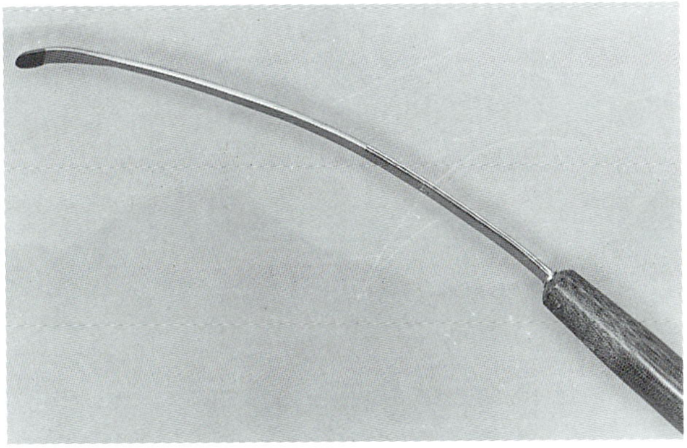

FIGURE 4-2
Long, malleable, subperiosteal elevator is shown.

the bone. As a result of this maneuver, the traction of this muscle caused by edema retracts the frontal skin and elevates the brows (the so-called "rubber-band effect").

The endoscope is introduced through one of the access incisions, and a long, isolated electrodissector (Colorado tip) (Figure 4-4) is inserted through the other access incision to score the periosteum and to effect electrocoagulation. While visualizing the inner surface of the flap, it is possible to score the periosteum horizontally above the level of the eyebrows and, if necessary, at other additional levels, from one temporal region to the other. This maneuver is particularly useful in patients with deep horizontal wrinkles of the forehead. It is important not to transect the frontalis muscle because it is the only muscle that elevates the brow. Partial resection or ablation of the depressor muscles of the brow (orbital part of the orbicularis, procerus, and superciliary corrugator muscles) is performed, either through these same incisions[15,16,18,22,23] or transnasally.[24]

Next, two more incisions are made in the temporal region, always inside the scalp area: one is made in an anteroposterior direction (1.5 cm) at the middle of the temporal region; the other is made vertically above the auricle (temporal

A

B

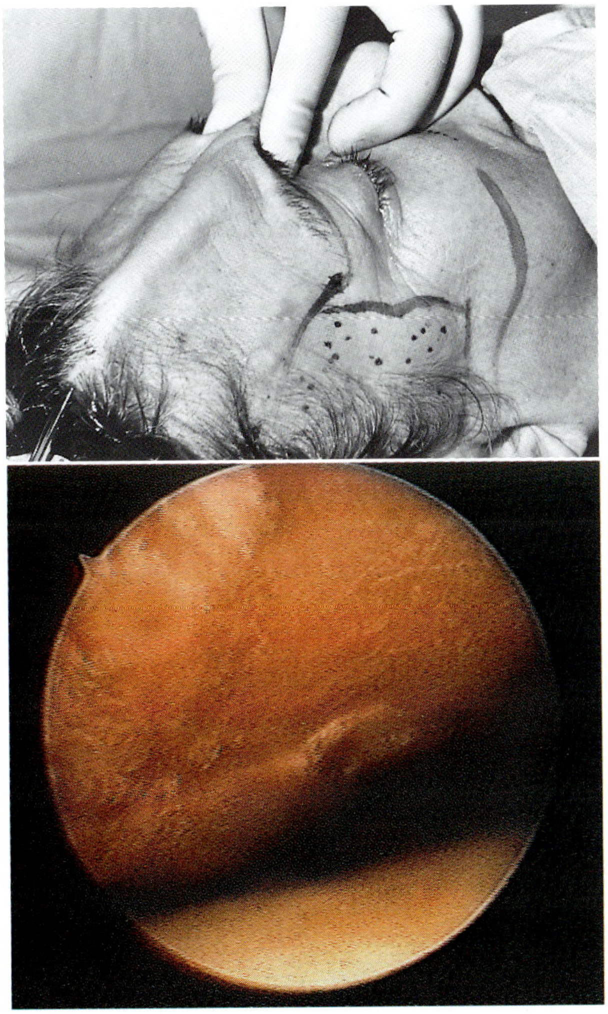

FIGURE 4-3
A, Subperiosteal dissection of the forehead and protecting nerves by placement of fingertips are shown. **B,** Endoscopic view of frontal bone and inner surface of flap.

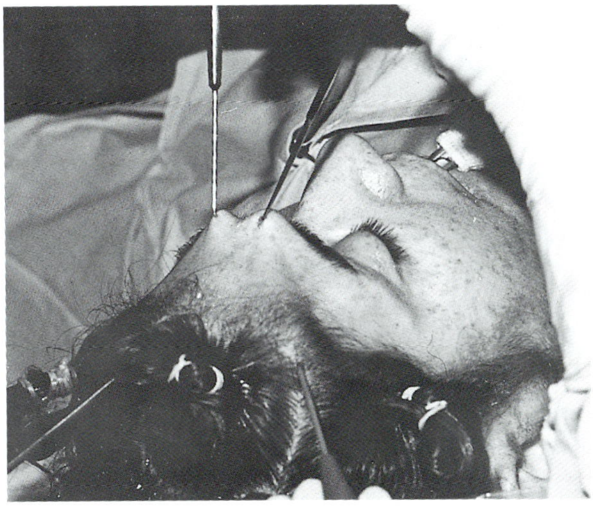

FIGURE 4-4
Shown are ablation of the depressor muscles and scoring of the periosteum with a long, isolated electrodissector, under endoscopic visualization.

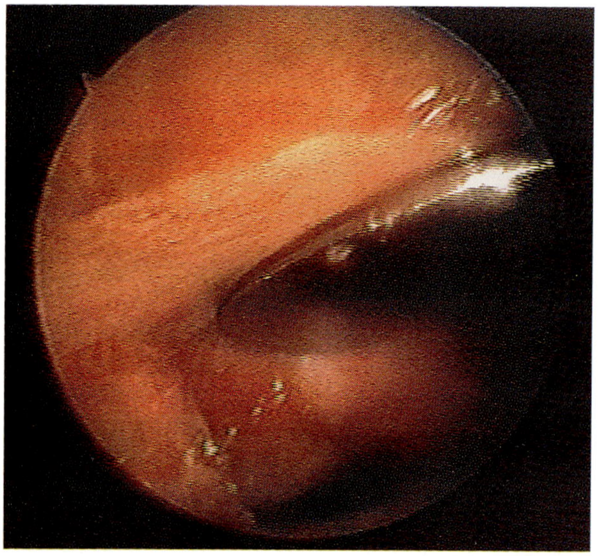

FIGURE 4-5
Endoscopic view of dissection between the parietotemporalis fascia and the superficial layer of the deep temporal fascia.

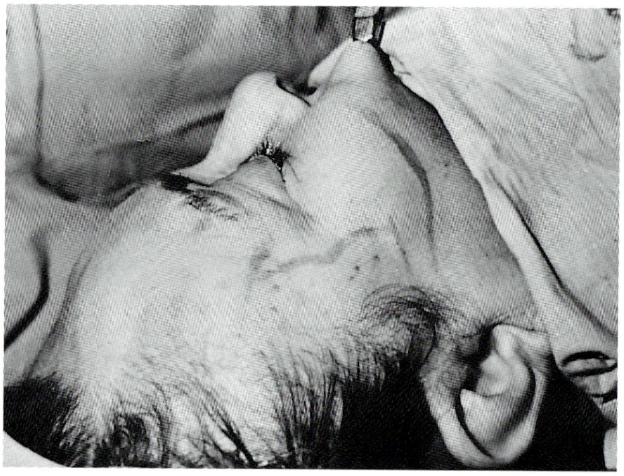

FIGURE 4-7
Subperiosteal dissection of the maxilla and the malar region through the Caldwell-Luc operation is shown.

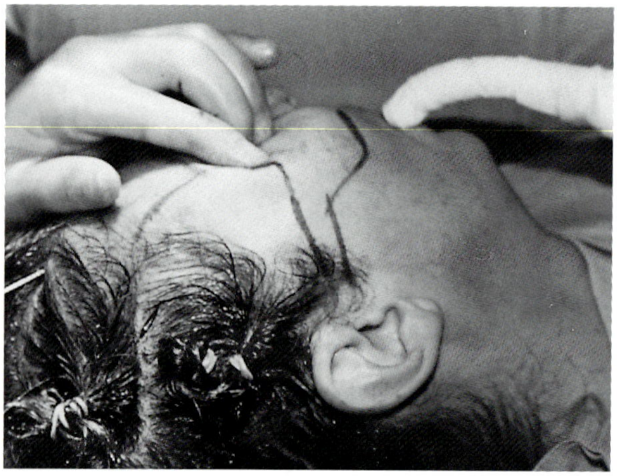

FIGURE 4-6
Subperiosteal dissection of the malar process of the frontal bone is shown.

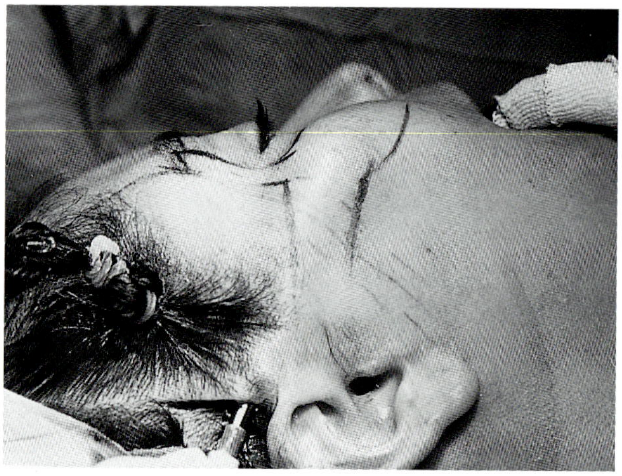

FIGURE 4-8
Subperiosteal dissection of the zygomatic arch through the supraauricular incision is shown.

inferior). Subgaleal dissection of this area is completed through these incisions, until reaching the superficial layer of the deep temporal fascia (Figure 4-5). This dissection is communicated with the subperiosteal dissection performed on the forehead. Through the parasagittal incisions, subperiosteal dissection is made to the malar process of the frontal bone and down to the malar bone (Figure 4-6).

The subperiosteal dissection of the maxilla and the malar region is performed through a 1-cm incision made in the superior vestibular sulcus at the level of the pyriform fossa (Figure 4-7). Through this route, a careful dissection of the pyriform area is carried out. Care is taken to avoid injury to the infraorbital nerve. Likewise, the inferior malar rim is dissected and the superficial insertions of the anterior belly of the masseter muscle are released. The vestibular route allows a faster, more effective, safer dissection in this area and provides a drainage route in case of bleeding or hematoma.

Through the inferior temporal incision the subperiosteal dissection of the zygomatic arch is completed from the back to the front (Figure 4-8). In

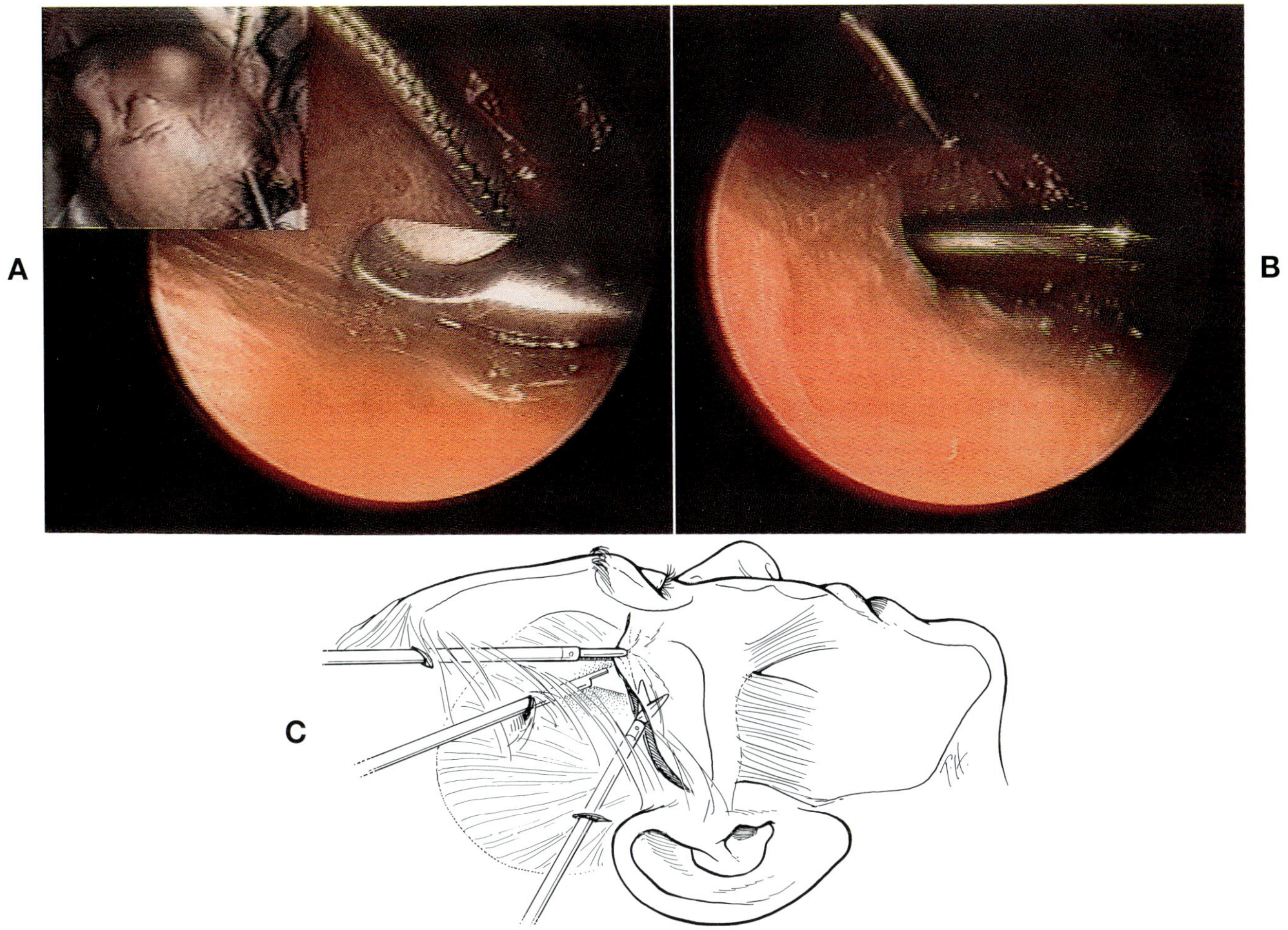

FIGURE 4-9
A, Endoscopic view of forceps grasping the superficial layer of the deep temporal fascia. **B,** Endoscopic view of scissors dissecting between the two layers of the deep temporal fascia. **C,** This maneuver is performed with the endoscope through the central temporal incision. Dissection forceps and scissors are introduced through the superior and inferior temporal incisions, respectively.

order to dissect between the two layers of the deep temporal fascia (Figure 4-9), the endoscope is introduced through the middle temporal incision to visualize the maneuvers, the dissection forceps are introduced through the parasagittal incision, and the scissors through the inferior temporal incision. The dissection is performed from above until reaching the superior border of the zygomatic arch. At this point the dissection is completed with an elevator from below, advancing upward subperiosteally from the zygomatic arch to the temporal region, between the two layers of the deep temporal fascia (Figure 4-10). Because of the location and direction of the frontal nerve, dissecting from below reduces the risk of nerve injury. At this point, the temporal and vestibular dissections are made to communicate, releasing the temporoparietalis and the temporal fascia from their bone attachments. Below the zygomatic arch a wide, blunt dissection with an oval, blunt dissector is performed over the cheek, between the posterior surface of the superficial musculo-aponeurotic system (SMAS) and the masseter muscle, reaching the lower third portion of the cheek (Figure 4-11).

With the dissection completed the stepwise suspension of the deep soft tissues is begun through a lower blepharoplasty incision. To achieve this, first a subciliary incision is made. Then subcutaneous dissection of the pretarsal region is performed, followed by blunt dissection between the fibers of the orbicularis oculi muscle to reach the levator labii muscles, medial to the infraorbital nerve, and the

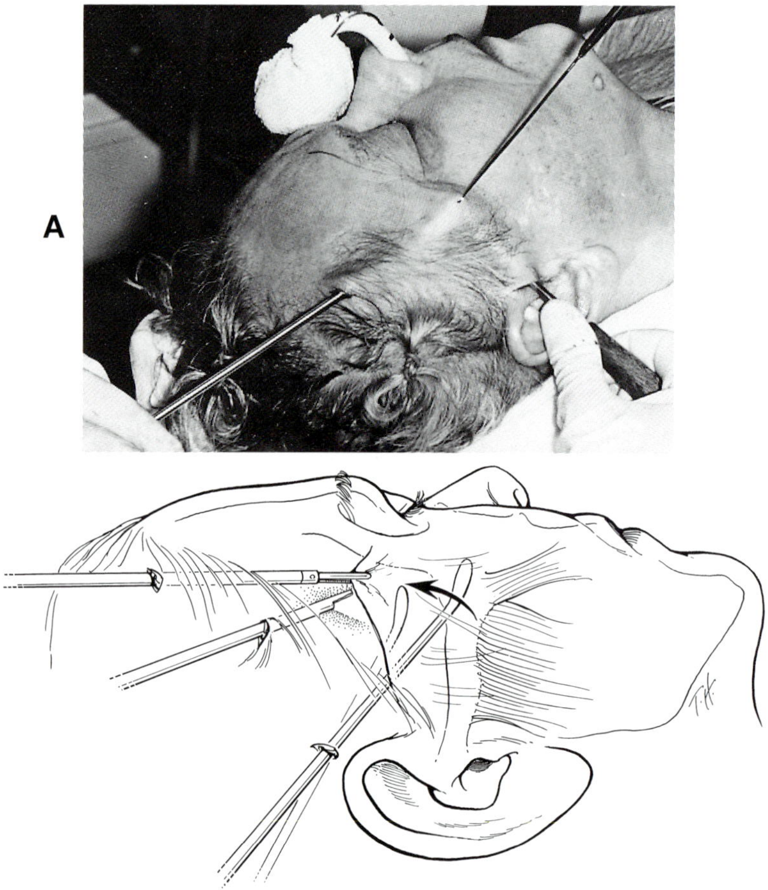

A

B

FIGURE 4-10
Subperiosteal dissection of the zygomatic arch is shown. **A,** Skin hooks forming a skin "tent" to facilitate the maneuver. **B,** The dissector comes upward from the zygomatic arch to the temporal region.

FIGURE 4-11
Oval, blunt dissector to dissect the cheek between the superficial musculo-aponeurotic system (SMAS) and the masseter muscle is shown.

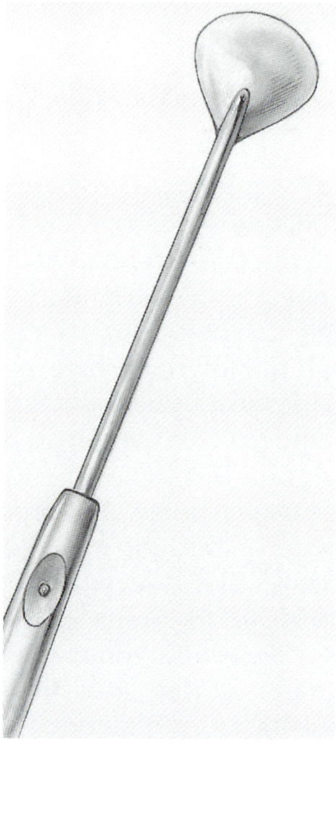

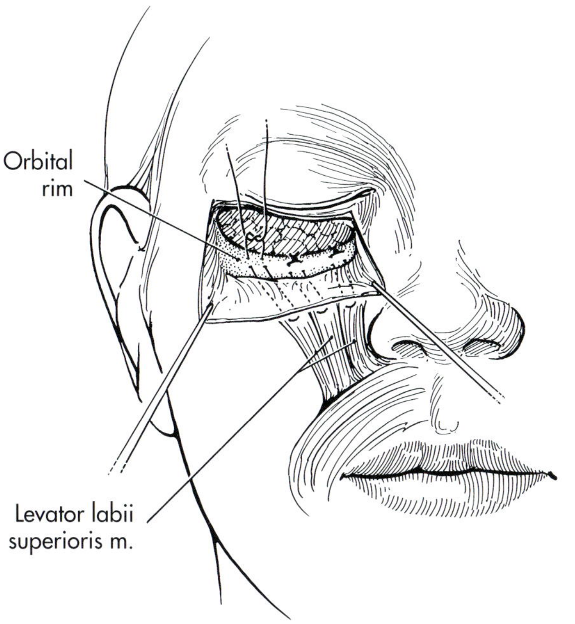

FIGURE 4-12
Shown are the levator labii muscles and the zygomaticus minor being lifted and sutured upward to the periosteum of the infraorbital rim.

A

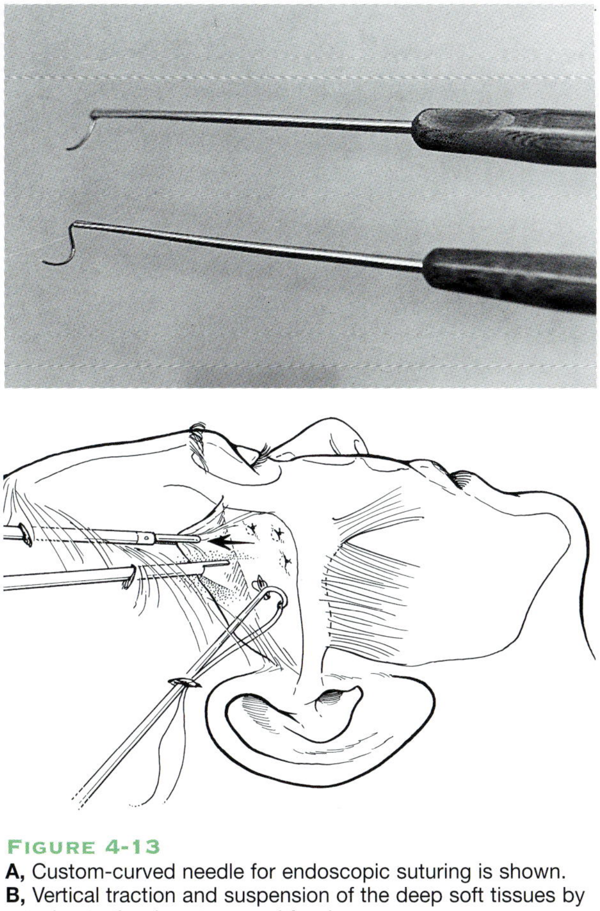

B

FIGURE 4-13
A, Custom-curved needle for endoscopic suturing is shown.
B, Vertical traction and suspension of the deep soft tissues by suturing to the deep temporal fascia.

zygomaticus minor laterally to it. These muscles are lifted and sutured upward to the periosteum of the infraorbital rim (Figure 4-12). Occasionally, it is necessary to drill holes in this structure for adequate fixation. This suspension corrects the nasolabial fold and lifts the medial part of the cheek and the malar bags. Because of the short distance between these muscles and the infraorbital rim, this maneuver is very effective, with a traction elevation ratio of 1.3:1.

The suspension of the cheeks is completed using a superior approach. The endoscope is introduced through the middle temporal incision, and the upper end of the superficial layer of the deep temporal fascia included in the flap is grasped with a forceps and pulled superiorly. Because of their continuity, the deep soft tissues and the skin of the face will also advance superiorly. Through the inferior temporal incision the superficial layer is sutured to the deep layer of the deep temporal fascia and to the temporal muscle itself, using 4-0 polyglactin 910 (Vicryl) on a custom-curved needle (Figure 4-13). Two to three stitches are placed at two or three different levels and are distributed along the upper border of the pulled fascia.

All the endoscopic maneuvers are facilitated by forming a skin "tent," using external traction with conventional skin hooks or specific skin retractors (Figure 4-14).[19-22]

Bleeding is usually minimal and easily controlled by compression, cold packs, and a long, insulated electrocautery.

If further elevation of the brows is desirable, percutaneous suspension of these structures to the frontalis muscle is performed.[25] Next, incisions on the scalp are sutured.

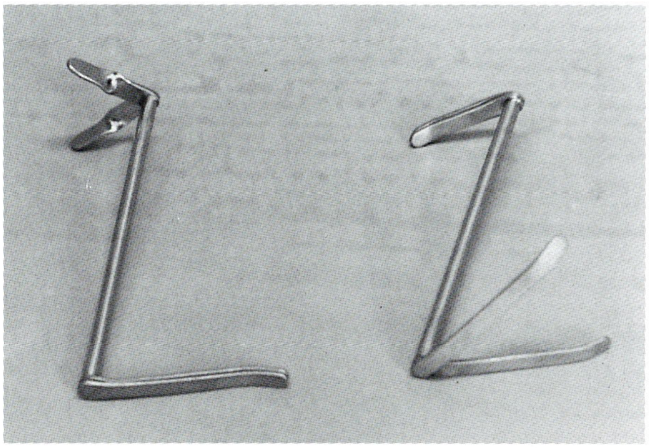

FIGURE 4-14
Double-action skin retractors for endoscopic procedures are shown.

To achieve fixation in the frontal area of the skin and of the new position of the eyebrows, we apply traction, combing the hair in a tight ponytail. In addition, the patient must wear an elastic band on the forehead for 10 days postoperatively.

CHEEKS AND NECK

In grade I rhytidosis the neck is almost unaffected; therefore, it is only necessary to perform liposuction of the subgenial region of the neck to correct its contour. The former is performed through a 5-mm incision behind the submental crease and the latter through a small incision placed inconspicuously behind the earlobe (Figure 4-15, *A*).

In the case of grade II rhytidosis, in which there is neck laxity, the correction is performed through a postauricular incision that runs upward and backward, approximately 0.5 cm above the retroauricular sulcus, and then descends diagonally through the mastoid region toward the neck (Figure 4-15). Through this a direct lipectomy and platysma dis-

A B C D

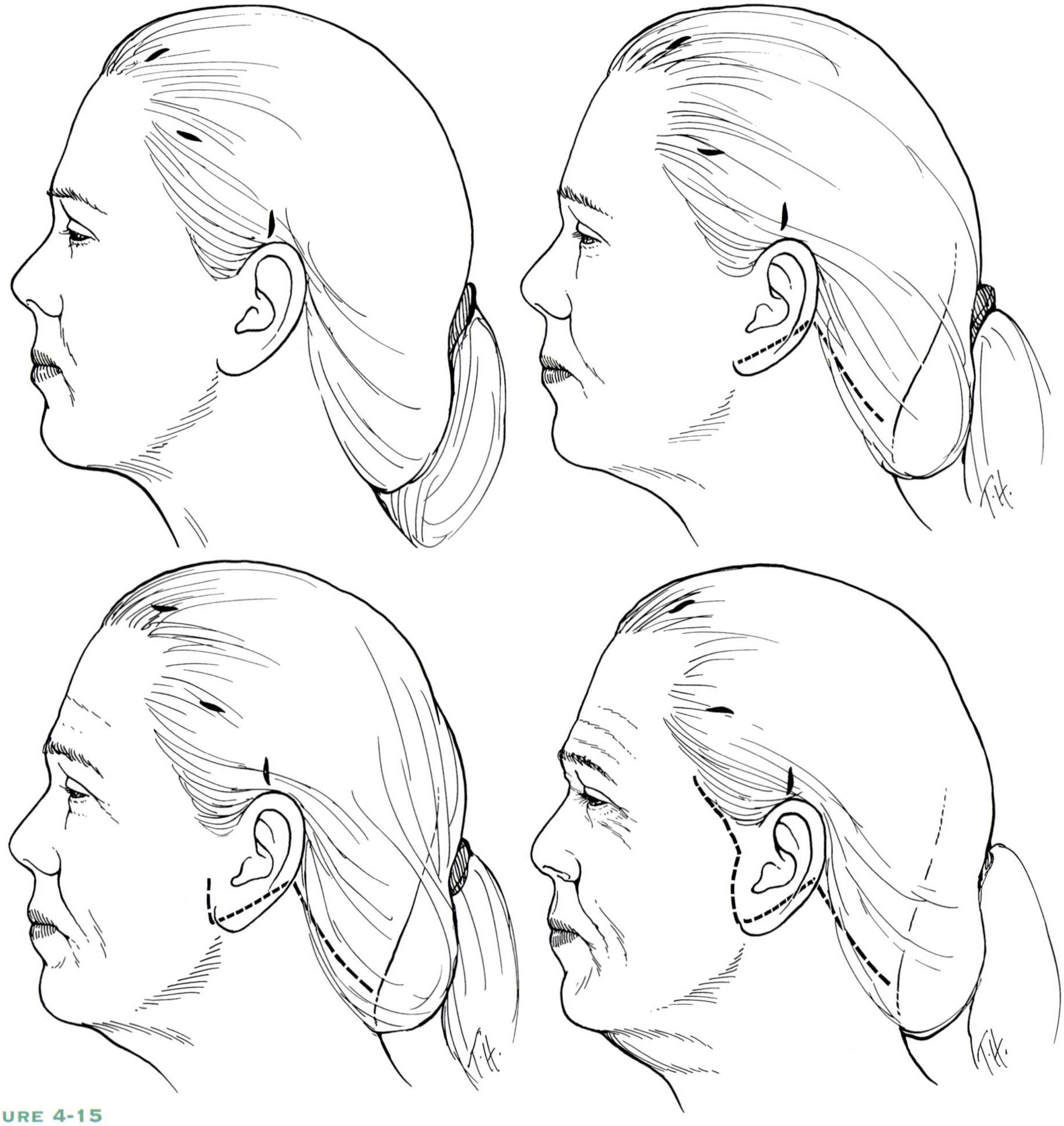

FIGURE 4-15
Incisions made for the basic endoscopic procedure and to treat the cheeks and neck of different grades of rhytidosis are shown. **A,** Grade I. **B,** Grade II. **C,** Grade III. **D,** Grade IV.

section can be performed. In the inferior vestibular sulcus a small, 1-cm incision is made through which subperiosteal dissection of the chin is performed, taking care not to injure the mentalis nerve. This maneuver releases the chin muscles and, indirectly, the superior and medial extensions of the platysma muscle, improving the jowls and the lines of expression by pulling this muscle backward through the neck incision. The laxity of the platysma can be corrected with any method that is considered appropriate to provide support and definition to this area.

The cutaneous redundancy in patients with grade III rhytidosis makes it necessary to resect the skin in the perilobular region of the ear to avoid formation of a rotational fold.

In addition to plicating the platysma, we plicate the superficial musculo-aponeurotic system (SMAS) in the preparotid and mandibular regions, with 4-0 Vicryl. The plication begins at the parotid level and advances on the mandibular region to the chin area. This simple maneuver reshapes the mandibular contour to correct the paragenial redundancy (jowls), and it also provides better contour of and

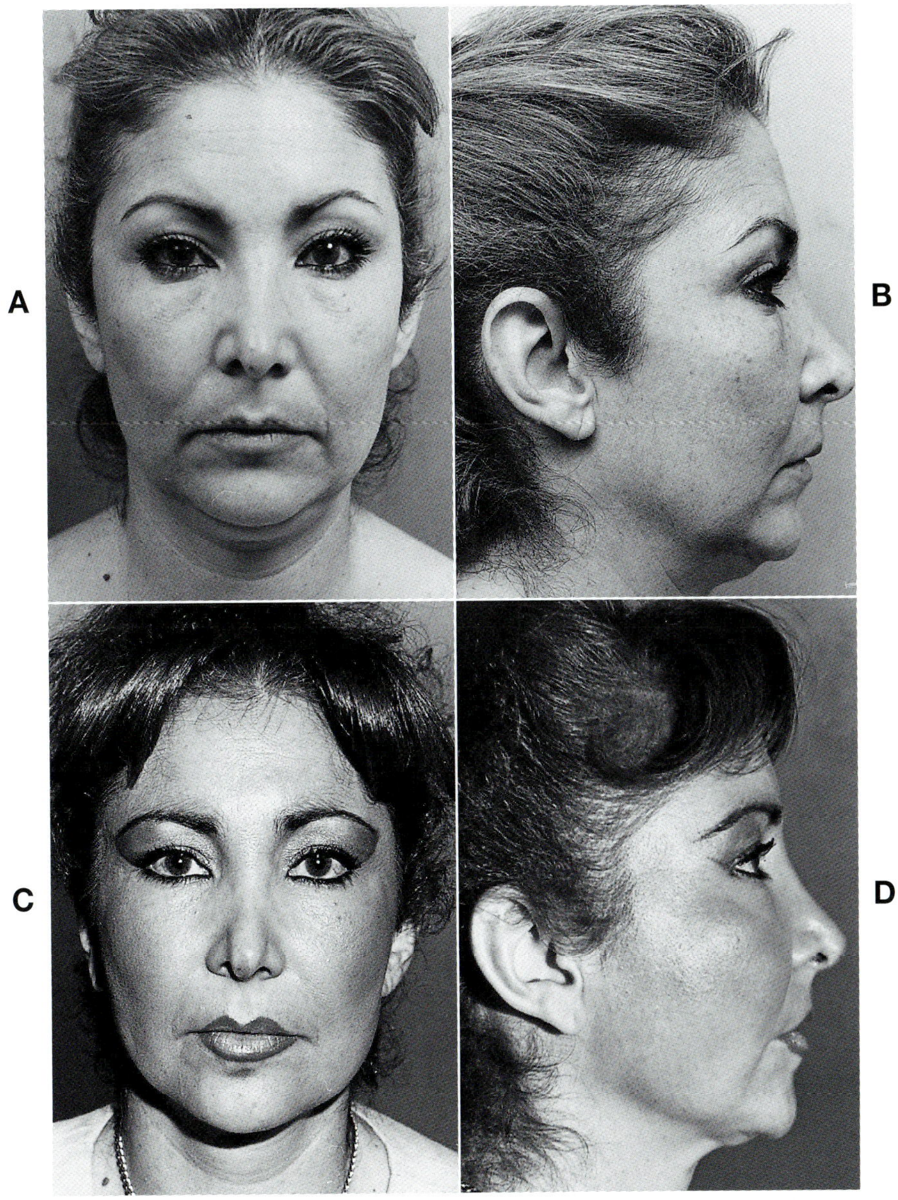

FIGURE 4-16
A,B, A 46-year-old woman with grade III rhytidosis is shown. **C,D,** Appearance 7 months after endoscopic facelift, subcutaneous necklift described for this grade of rhytidosis, inferior eyelid blepharoplasty, and submandibular suction-assisted lipectomy.

suspension to the parotid and submaxillary glands, which are frequently prominent or ptotic.

In patients with grade IV rhytidosis the marked skin redundancy in the cheeks and neck requires a preauricular incision. The preauricular incision surrounds the lobe and ascends vertically, following the pretragal sulcus. This is a natural fold that conceals the scar, without the need of more complex procedures, such as going into the tragus or another maneuver that might distort this structure. At the level of the helical root, the incision must be directed diagonally, forward and upward, entering 2 to 3 cm into the sideburn area, taking care to stay within the hair-bearing skin.

The subcutaneous dissection in the preauricular region is only 3 to 4 cm wide, which is sufficient for correcting the redundant skin in front of the ear. Approximation of the preauricular incision is with a continuous intradermal suture.

EYELIDS

In rhytidosis I and II the upper eyelids are frequently corrected by lifting the eyebrows to their correct position. If significant fat pockets are present, it is possible to remove them through small incisions in the palpebral skin, thus obviating the need for long cutaneous incisions along the upper eyelid. The traditional upper eyelid incision is indicated only when there is redundancy of skin and/or the orbicularis muscle. This is also a good approach to weaken the orbital part of the orbicularis oculi muscle and its depressor action to the brow.

The dramatic lifting that is achieved in the cheeks invariably produces skin redundancy in the lower eyelid, which requires resection. Such redundancy increases from 60 to 80% compared with what might be estimated preoperatively for a conventional blepharoplasty. The midfacial lifting counteracts the pull of gravity to the orbital septum and allows the periorbital fat to return to the original position in the orbit, which obviates the need to resect fat in most cases.

A strip of orbicularis oculi muscle, approximately 3 mm wide, is dissected and sutured laterally to the lateral canthus, providing excellent support and shape to the lower eyelid. In patients who require lifting of the lateral canthus, it is necessary to detach the canthal ligament from Whitnall's tubercle and then to affix it to the desired level by means of canthoplasty, with a nonabsorbable suture.

POSTOPERATIVE MANAGEMENT

When the open approach is used, patients develop more edema during the first 72 hours postoperatively than those who undergo conventional subcutaneous rhytidectomy. With the endoscopic approach the edema is significantly reduced and it dissipates rapidly. After 3 weeks, the results are evident.

Patients who have endoscopic facelift experience less pain, discomfort, and alteration of facial features. Instead, they have a sense of deep tension that is easily bearable. In the last 12 years we have treated 382 patients with different variations of the subperiosteal facelift, but all through the coronal approach. During the last 13 months we have performed the endoscopic procedure described in this paper on 28 patients. The results have been very similar to those obtained through the coronal approach and are considered very satisfactory by both the patients and the surgeons (Figure 4-16).

COMPLICATIONS

Among the complications observed with the endoscopic procedure, there has been temporal unilateral paralysis of the frontal branch of the facial nerve in 1 case, infraorbital hypoesthesia in 1 case, temporal paresthesia or hypoesthesia of the frontal region in 2 cases, and temporary lower eyelid ectropion in 1 case.

DISCUSSION

With the endoscopically assisted approach, the coronal incision has been avoided in all the cases, and the preauricular incisions were also avoided in almost 80% of patients (Figure 4-17). The subperiosteal procedure, based on the direct traction of the deep soft tissues without exerting direct tension on the skin, enables us to achieve natural results. With it, it is possible to avoid the "windswept look," which is so frequently seen with the "subcutaneous" or "cutaneous traction" rhytidectomy.

The dissection is made in an avascular plane so that the risk of bleeding, and therefore of hematoma, is almost nonexistent. The musculocutaneous flap is thick, with a rich vascular network, which makes the risk of cutaneous vascular compromise and necrosis very unlikely. For these reasons, it is an excellent option for those patients with vascular compromise from causes such as radiation, vascular disease, and smoking.

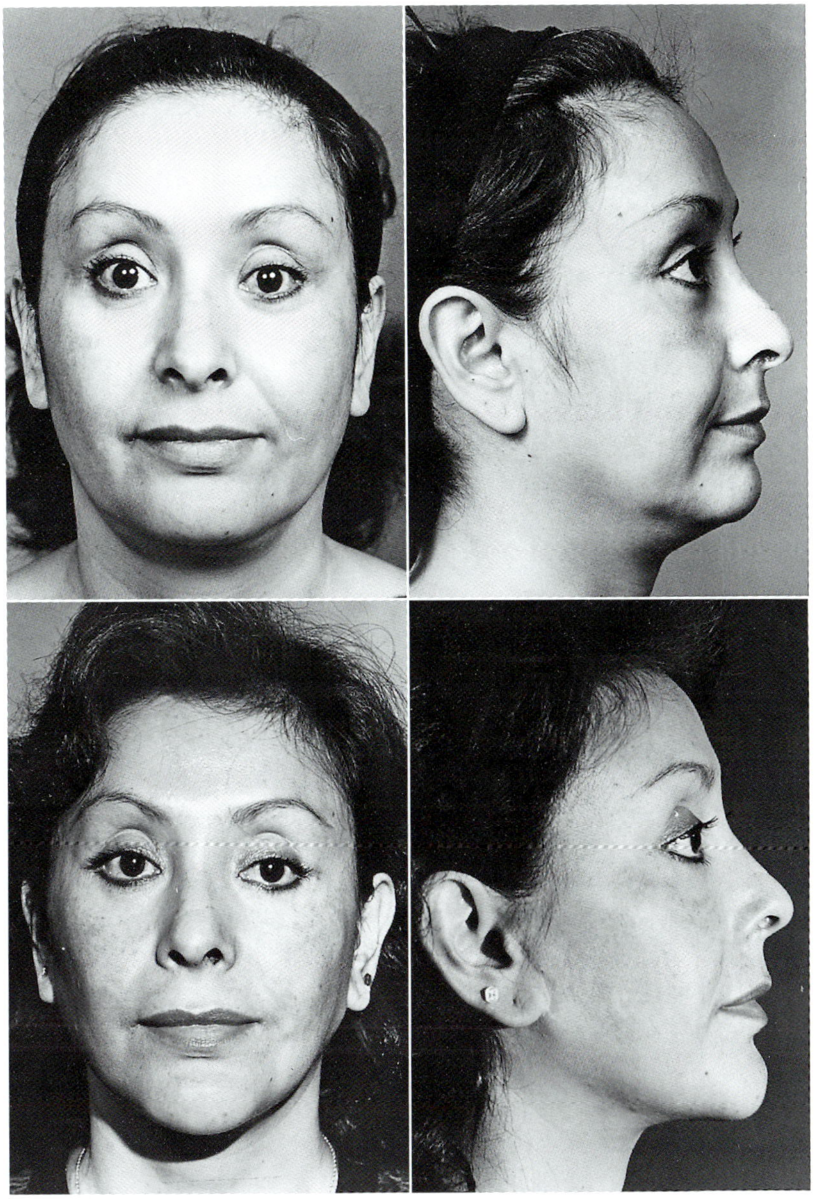

FIGURE 4-17
A,B, A 46-year-old woman with grade III rhytidosis is shown. **C,D,** Appearance 6 months after endoscopic facelift, combined with a limited subcutaneous rhytidectomy of the cheeks, subcutaneous necklift described for this grade of rhytidosis, inferior eyelid blepharoplasty, submandibular suction-assisted lipectomy, chin implant, and rhinoplasty.

This procedure frees up all the insertions of the muscles of facial expression, allowing for their redraping to the current skeletal volume and contour. At the same time, the stronger muscles self-adapt to a more natural relationship with their antagonist muscles, reestablishing a better facial muscle balance. This improves grooves, crests, depressions, and wrinkles.

The traction of the deep elements shifts the skin indirectly through the "retaining ligaments"[26,27] without altering their original relationship, a process that is not achievable when a subcutaneous rhytidectomy is performed.

The subperiosteal facelift specifically corrects the redundancy and ptosis of the deep soft tissues, which remain flabby and redundant beneath the skin of patients who have undergone only a subcutaneous rhytidectomy.

Subperiosteal suspension eliminates the redundancy of tissues in the inferior cheek quadrants and improves the volume and projection of the cheekbones, thus rendering a more youthful appearance.

The redundancy of the lower eyelids and the amount of skin to be resected increase significantly with this procedure. However, we have never experienced long-term postoperative lagophthalmos or ectropion. This fact confirms that, once suspended, the tissues stay in their relocated position.

Obviously, this procedure produces excellent results in young patients with discrete rhytidosis, but it is clear that its indications increase with age, as facial bone loss and ptosis of the deep soft tissues increase.

Patients being considered for secondary rhytidectomy are also excellent candidates for a subperiosteal facelift because of the substantial redundancy of deep soft tissues (which was not addressed by the previous facelift) and of their flabby, thin, poor-quality skin (Figures 4-18 and 4-19).

With the tension and position of the deep structures restored, the facial skin achieves a youthful

A,B

C

D,E

F

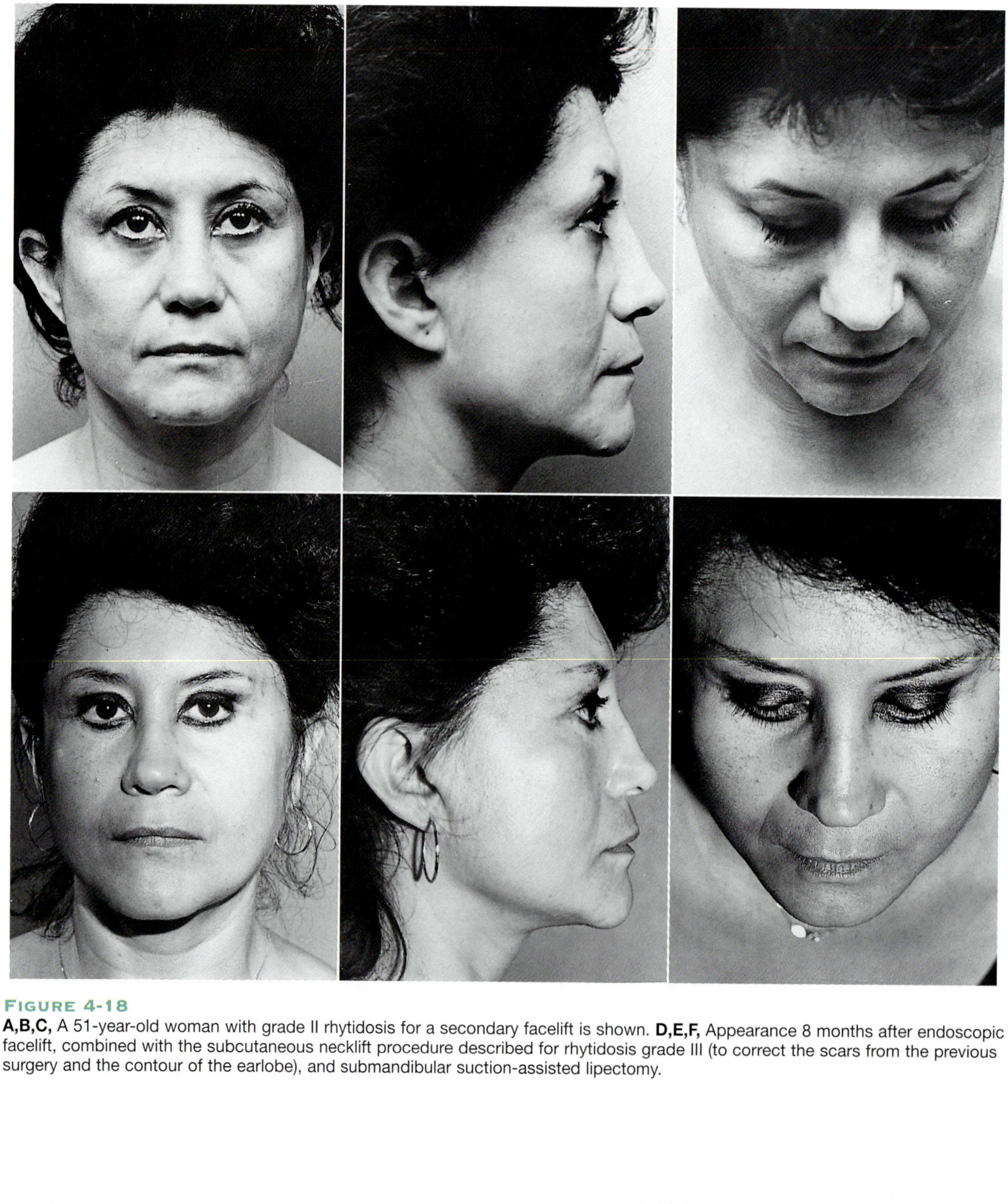

FIGURE 4-18

A,B,C, A 51-year-old woman with grade II rhytidosis for a secondary facelift is shown. **D,E,F,** Appearance 8 months after endoscopic facelift, combined with the subcutaneous necklift procedure described for rhytidosis grade III (to correct the scars from the previous surgery and the contour of the earlobe), and submandibular suction-assisted lipectomy.

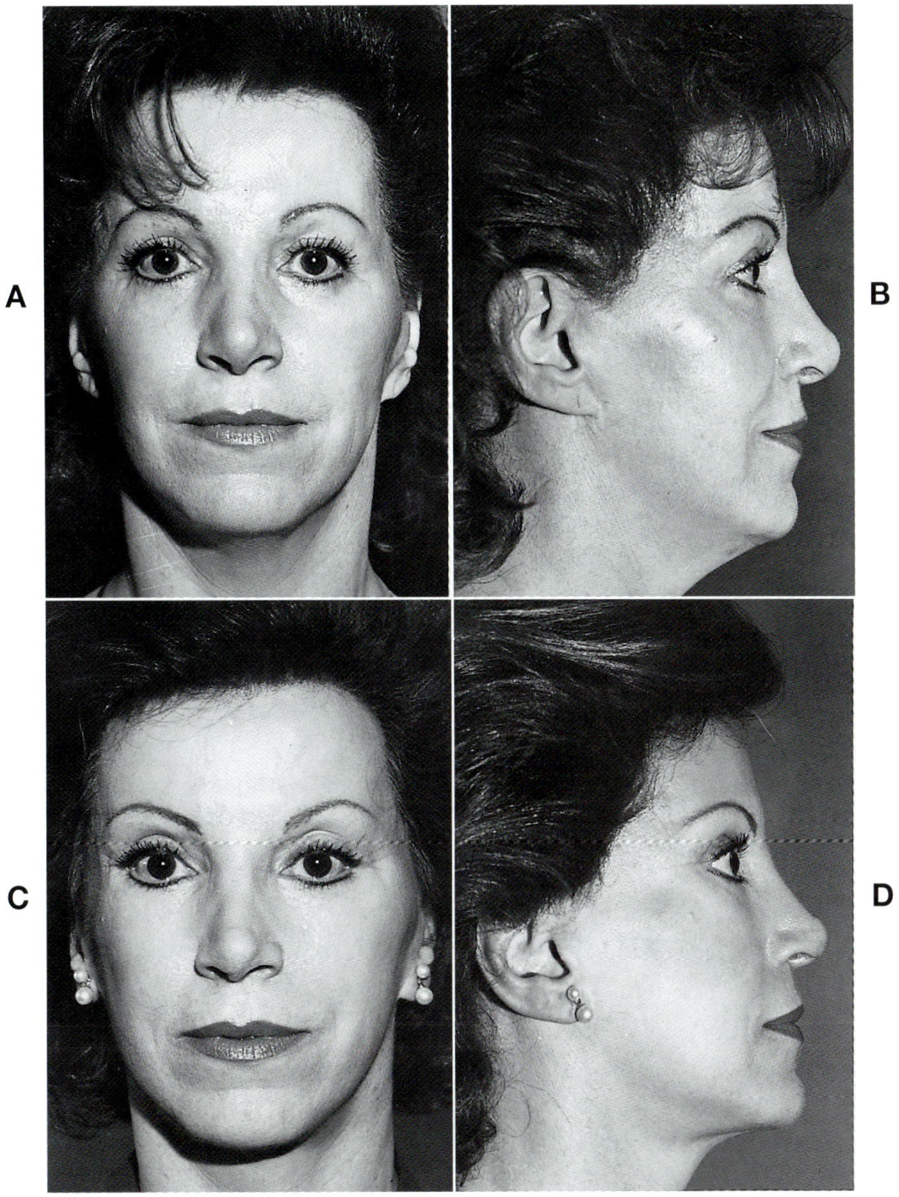

FIGURE 4-19
A,B, A 55-year-old with grade III rhytidosis for a secondary facelift is shown. **C,D**, Appearance 11 months after endoscopic facelift, subcutaneous necklift described for this grade of rhytidosis, and submandibular suction-assisted lipectomy.

and natural freshness. This cannot be accomplished by the subcutaneous rhytidectomy, where the traction load is borne entirely by the skin. Instead, with time, this tension may lead to additional skin atrophy.

On average, the open subperiosteal facelift requires 30 additional minutes of operative time compared with a subcutaneous coronal lift. Nevertheless, when compared to a procedure which also includes midfacial and neck rhytidectomy, the surgical time is reduced by approximately 45 minutes because there are no preauricular incisions to close, extensive subcutaneous dissections are not made, and the time necessary for hemostasis is minimal. For the same reasons, the endoscopic approach requires (after learning time) less operating time.

When support is restored to the deep soft tissues, the load on the skin is reduced. The integument, therefore, will need only serve as a cover and will not need to function as a supporting element, something for which it is not designed.

This increases the longevity of the results, as we have noted during 11 years of follow-up with some of our patients treated with open subperiosteal facelifts.

When these patients require a secondary procedure, it is possible to achieve excellent results with less aggressive operations and, even more importantly, without dramatically altering the features of the patient, an undesirable result frequently observed in patients who have undergone repeated subcutaneous rhytidectomies.

The endoscopically assisted subperiosteal facelift performed as an isolated procedure is indicated in patients with grade I rhytidosis. It is also indicated in grades II and III rhytidosis, where it is combined with subcutaneous rhytidectomy of the neck,[10-14] and in cases of secondary facelift. It is the procedure of choice in men in whom the traditional coronal incision is contraindicated due to alopecia.

The small incisions used through the endoscopic approach allow sufficient and effective access to perform the dissection and the suspension of the tissues released, obviating the use of the coronal incision, with its attendant discomfort and scarring. These patients do not experience hypoesthesia, or paresthesia in the frontal region, as can occur with bicoronal incisions.

The endoscopic approach reduces surgical trauma as well as postoperative edema. Since neither the veins nor the lymphatic vessels of this area are sectioned, swelling subsides faster and recovery time is shorter.

Although the endoscope has only recently been applied to this area of plastic surgery, we have obtained excellent results, with a high degree of patient satisfaction.

We feel that endoscopically assisted plastic surgery offers great advantages and broad perspectives. With appropriate training, the techniques are within the reach of all plastic surgeons.

We are convinced that this is only the beginning. The development of endoscopic surgery will open new horizons for our specialty, offering even greater possibilities.

REFERENCES

1. Isreal H: Age factor and the pattern of change in craniofacial structures, *An J Phys Anthrop* 39:111, 1973A.
2. Isreal H: Recent knowledge concerning craniofacial aging, *Angle Orthod* 43:176, 1973B.
3. Tessier P: Lifting facial sous-perioste, *Ann Chir Plast* 34:193, 1989.
4. Psillakis JM: Subperiosteal approach as an improved concept for correction of the aging face, *Plast Reconstr Surg* 82:383, 1988.
5. Krastinova-Lolov D: Le lifting facial sous perioste, *Ann Chir Plast* 34:199, 1989.
6. Santana PM: Metodologia craneomaxilofacial en ritidoplastias, *Cirugia Plast IberoLatinoamer* 10:322, 1994.
7. Ramirez OM, Maillard GF, Musolas A: The extended subperiosteal face lift: a definitive soft tissue remodeling for facial rejuvenation, *Plast Reconstr Surg* 88:227, 1991.
8. Stuzin JM, Wagstrom L, Kawamoto HK, Wolfe SA: Anatomy of the frontal branch of the facial nerve: the significance of the temporal fat pad, *Plast Reconstr Surg* 83:265, 1989.
9. Maillard GF, Cornette de Saint Cyr, Scheflan M: The subperiosteal bicoronal approach to total facelifting: the DMAS deep musculoaponeurotic system, *Aesth Plast Surg* 15:285, 1991.
10. Fuente del Campo A: *Face lift with no preauricular scars*. In Hinderer UT, editor: *Plastic surgery II*, Roterdam, 1992, Elsevier.
11. Fuente del Campo A: Face lift without preauricular scars, *Plast Reconstr Surg* 92:642, 1993.
12. Fuente del Campo A: Ritidectomia subperiostica. Un metodo de rejuvenecimiento facial sin cicatricez preauriculares, *Anales Medicos* 38:15, 1993.
13. Fuente del Campo A: Cirugia reparadora del envejecimiento facial sin cicatricez visibles, *Cirugia Cirujanos* 60:123, 1993.
14. Fuente del Campo A: *Subperiosteal face lift with stage suspension. A facial restoration method without preauricular scars.* In Psillakis J, editor: *Deep face-lifting techniques*, New York, 1994, Thieme.
15. Core GB, Vasconez LO, Askren C, Yamamoto Y, Gamboa M: Coronal face lift with endoscopic techniques, *Plast Surg Forum* XV:227, 1992.
16. Liang M, Narayanan K: Endoscopic ablation of the frontalis and corrugator muscles. A clinical study, *Plast Surg Forum* XV:54, 1992.
17. Isse N: Endoforehaed. The functional lift. Presented at the Symposium on Aesthetic Surgery of the Orbit, Eyelid and Ear, Ixtapa, Zihuatanejo, Mexico, February 17-19, 1993.
18. Fuente del Campo A: Endoscopic dissection and suspension in face lift. Presented at the III Workshop on Aesthetic Surgery of the Facial Skeleton, Tampere, Finland, September 6-10, 1993.
19. Fuente del Campo A: Ritidectomia subperiostica endoscopica, *Rev Colombiana Cir Plast* 4:19, 1994.
20. Fuente del Campo A: *Subperiosteal face lift, open and endoscopic approach.* In Owsley J, editor: *Syllabus of the Symposium on Aesthetic Surgery of the Face*, San Francisco, 1994.
21. Ramirez OM, Fuente del Campo A: *Facial rejuvenation: subperiosteal brow and face lift.* In Riley SR, editor: *Instructional courses*, St Louis, 1993, Mosby–Year Book.
22. Ramirez OM, Fuente del Campo A: Subperiosteal brow and face lift (endoscopic approach). Instructional course, 62nd Annual Meeting of the American Society of Plastic and Reconstructive Surgeons, New Orleans, September 19, 1993.

23. Isse N: Endoscopic facial rejuvenation: endoforehead, the functional lift. Case reports, *Aesth Plast Surg* 18:21, 1994.
24. Ramirez OM: Endoscopic techniques in facial rejuvenation. An overview, *Aesth Plast Surg* 18:141, 1994.
25. Fuente del Campo A: Centrofacial lifting, *Perspect Plast Surg* 7:87, 1993.
26. Bosse JP, Papillon J: Surgical anatomy of the SMAS at the malar region. In Transactions of the 9th International Congress on Plastic and Reconstructive Surgery, New York, 1987, McGraw-Hill.
27. Furnas DW: The retaining ligaments of the cheek, *Plast Reconstr Surg* 83:11, 1989.

CHAPTER 5

Facial Rejuvenation: Technique and Rationale

Ewaldo Bolivar de Souza Pinto
Patricia J. Erazo I.
Maria Fernanda Lopez

The ongoing pursuit to reduce the size of scars in conjunction with obtaining good results has led to continuing progress in the study and creation of new surgical techniques and strategies in the field of surgery, in general, and in plastic surgery, in particular, with the final common objective: a satisfied patient.

Since the beginning of 1993 we have been developing a new approach to facial rejuvenation surgery, characterized by the use of minimal incisions and the routine treatment of the deep structures of the face, with the help of videoendoscopy. We termed this technique *microfacelift with videoendoscopic aid.*[1]

We attribute the attainment of good results to the refinement of the indications for patient selection, improved surgical strategies and techniques, and the development of new surgical equipment, especially videoendoscopy.

In the beginning we had difficulties adapting to the videoendoscope and, because we were among the pioneers of this technique in Brazil, we proceeded cautiously. As time went by, however, the experience we acquired led us to use the instrument with more facility, obtaining better image definition on the video.

At present, facial rejuvenation surgery associated with the use of videoendoscopy provides new approaches, which emphasize the importance of treating the deeper structures of the face,[2] despite using smaller incisions and, at the same time, reducing the risk of nerve damage. Videoendoscopy has come to fit into this context perfectly, establishing its place in current and future plastic surgery.[1-3]

This chapter discusses our experience of more than 2 years with endoscopic facial rejuvenation techniques.

ANATOMY

It is obvious that the surgeon who is planning to perform plastic surgery, especially facial rejuvenation, should have ample knowledge of anatomy. Several areas in the face are generally considered to be "danger zones."[4] Their topography should be well known by the surgeon, who must exercise utmost care because carelessness in these regions could inflict serious damage to the patient. The sensitive nature of these danger zones derives from the fact that they contain one or more nerve branches directly adjacent to muscles, glands, and bones.

Facial rejuvenation surgery requires knowledge of the trajectory of the facial and trigeminal nerves, which are responsible for innervation of the face. With the advent of videoendoscopy, the risks of damaging nerve branches substantially decreased due to the direct visualization of the planes and the nerve structures of the face afforded by this technique.[4-8]

The trigeminal nerve is responsible for motor innervation of the masticatory muscles and the sensate innervation of the entire face. Through its first branch the facial nerve innervates the occipital and intrinsic ear muscle, and along its trajectory it penetrates the parotid gland. On leaving this gland, it branches out into the temporal, zygomatic, buccal, mandibular, and cervical divisions, which correspond to the motor branches of the facial mimic muscles.[6,7]

Various authors have described a triangular danger zone at the level of the temporal region.[4,5,7] Generally speaking, this is delineated by three lines that originate, respectively, 0.5 cm below the tragus, 2 cm above the tail of the eyebrow, and at the lateral orbital edge of the orbital region[4] (Figure 5-1). Subcutaneous undermining should be carried out only to the superior limit of this triangular area because invading it could damage the temporal branch of the facial nerve.

In the frontal region the galea inserts into the superior orbital rim, into the zygomatic process of the frontal bone and, at the same time, into the deep temporal fascia. Lower, it inserts into the zygomatic arch and medially into the glabella. The corrugator supercilii and the depressor muscles are strongly attached to the bone and the galea, which makes necessary their surgical separation at the periosteal plane in this region to accomplish free movement of the soft tissues.

While visualizing this zone directly with the help of the videoendoscope, the surgeon can perform a subperiosteal dissection with the supraorbital and supratrochlear nerves in clear view.

The superficial musculo-aponeurotic system (SMAS), described by Mitz and Peyronie in 1976,[9] covers the facial musculature and has four points of fixation: at the tragus; at the anterior edge of the external auditory canal; at the mastoid region, extending up to the nasogenial sulcus; and at the temporal region on the zygomatic arch, where the SMAS is attached to the periosteum. The latter area is ideal for plication because it is fixed to bone.[6,10,11]

In the region of the parotid gland the SMAS is thick and adherent, forming a safe and easily dissectable area. This corresponds to the intraparotid segment of the facial nerve. In this area the SMAS can be defined as a fibrous patch that extends from the tragus to the zygomatic muscles, where it is fixed, and to the risorius, the levator labii superioris, and the ala nasi muscles. These muscles are strongly inserted into the bony skeleton, from which they must be detached subperiosteally to be mobilized. This approach is possible at the level of the malar eminence by making a separation between the major and minor zygomatic muscles, detaching them from the malar eminence. Next, using a nonabsorbable suture (nylon), three stitches are made, sewing the minor suprazygomatic SMAS[12] onto the major suprazygomatic SMAS, always stitching below the zygomatic arch to avoid damaging the zygomatic nerve (Figure 5-2).

CLINICAL EVALUATION

In all plastic surgical procedures a fundamental understanding of the basic characteristics of the skin covering is necessary. Not the least of these is the ensemble of changes caused by the facial aging phenomenon. These changes are a result of many factors that lead to alterations in the deep anatomic structures of support, which make up the architecture of the tegument and whose deterioration is automatically reflected in the facial form and expression.

The progressive atrophy of the skin and subcutaneous tissue is produced by gravitational forces, internal changes (histologic and cellular), and external causes (environmental factors). These manifest themselves as aging changes in different segments of the face (Figure 5-3) such as frontal and glabellar wrinkles, accentuation of the grooves in the lateral eye region, ptosis in the caudal part of the eyebrows, ptosis of the eyelids, a decrease in the projection of the malar regions, accentuation of the nasogenial sulcus, changes in the nasolabial angle, a double chin, accumulation of fat and skinfolds in the cervical area, alteration of the mandibular angle, and others.[13,14]

In the preoperative selection of the patient, a complete physical and psychologic evaluation is necessary. Physical evaluation should include a detailed examination of the condition of the skin, the facial fat, musculature, and skeleton. Photographs and computer imaging are important auxiliary means of obtaining a better analysis of the entire face. The goal of the psychologic examina-

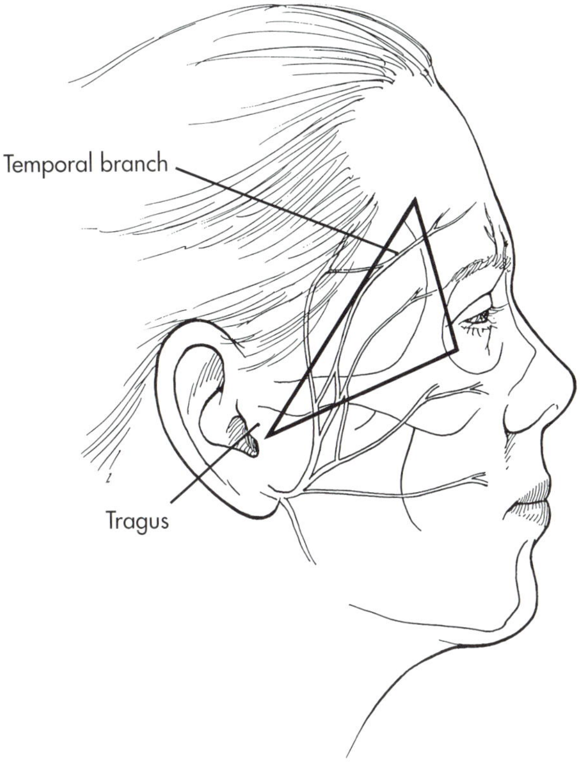

FIGURE 5-1
The triangular danger zone is shown.

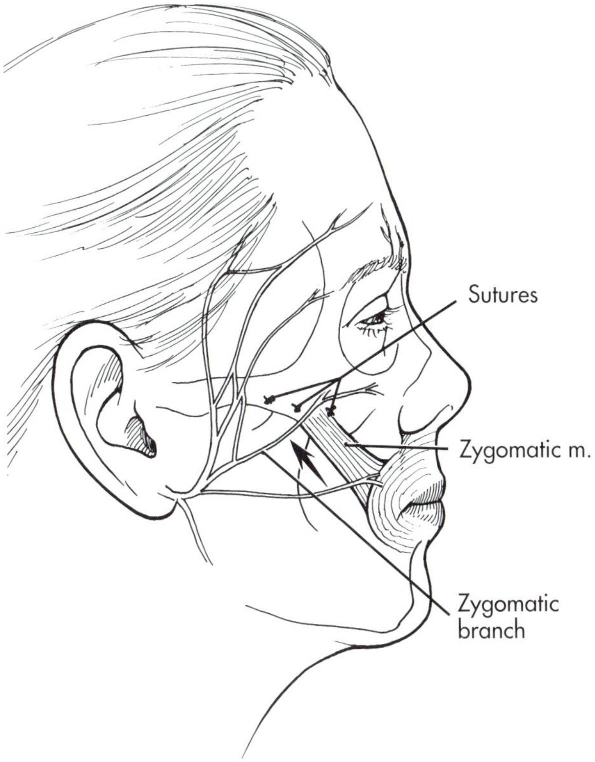

FIGURE 5-2
Superficial musculo-aponeurotic system (SMAS) suprazygomatic treatment is shown.

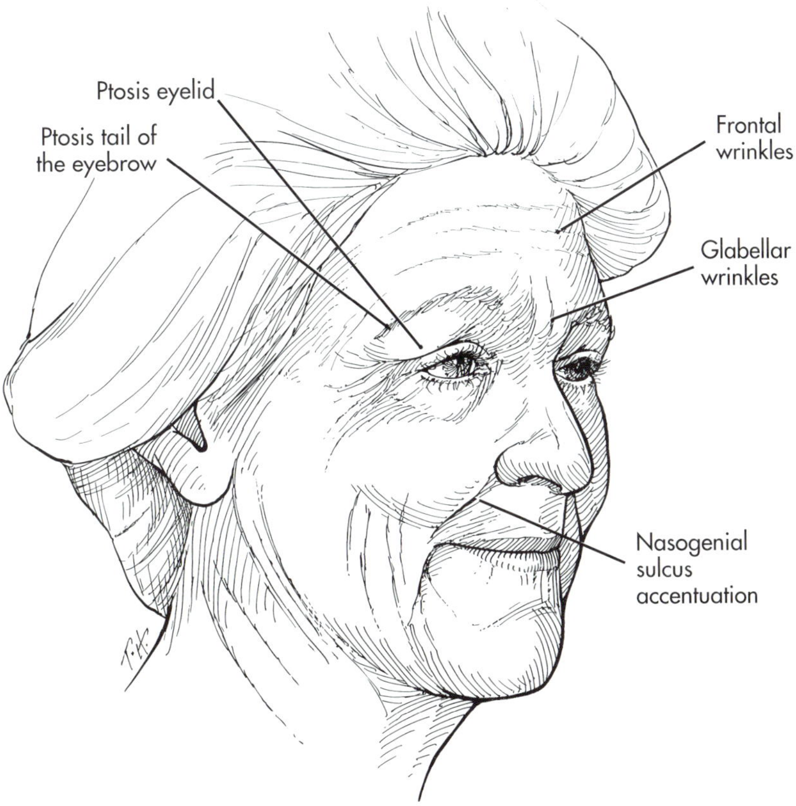

FIGURE 5-3
Different manifestations of the aging face are shown.

tion is to gain an understanding of patient's expectations vis-à-vis the improvement that the contemplated surgery can accomplish.

Based on our experience and on the evaluation of our results, we have arrived at a classification system that is divided into four categories, depending on the severity of the aging process and of the surgical treatment required accordingly:

Class 1 Treatment of the upper third of the face without skin resection, by means of endoscopic forehead lift only

Class 2 Treatment of the upper third of the face with endoscopy, in conjunction with treatment of the middle third of the face with skin resection and rotation of the flap (microfacelift).

Class 3 Treatment of the upper third of the face with endoscopy and facelift, with preauricular incision only (minifacelift).

Class 4 Treatment of the upper third of the face with endoscopy, associated with traditional facelift.

SURGICAL INSTRUMENTS

The surgical equipment is divided into two distinct groups according to the surgical phases performed: classic instruments, used to perform traditional rhytidoplasty; and endoscopic equipment, including the specially developed surgical instruments that are appropriate for this phase of the operation. Since the introduction of videoendoscopy into plastic surgery there has been constant progress in the development of new electronic and surgical equipment, with better image definition and facility of performance. This, in turn, has allowed for further refinement of the technique.

The electronic equipment used in our service consists of a color, high-definition videoendoscopy camera with automatic focus adjustment, connected to a no. 16 endoscope (4 mm) provided with mandril and protective cover at its distal extremity. The camera is connected to an automatically adjustable light source of 250 W, and the image is transmitted by a 14-inch, color, NTSC monitor that is connected to a VCR of the latest model, allowing for a clear image.

The success of videoendoscopic surgery depends on the use of the appropriate surgical equipment and on the physician's thorough knowledge of surgical anatomy and experience with the technique.

The auxiliary surgical equipment and instruments, which are constantly undergoing improvements to increase the surgeon's ease and quality of performance, can be divided into groups according to their function:

1. **Undermining instruments.** These vary in length (15 to 20 cm), width (3 to 5 mm), shape at their distal ends, and curvature. We prefer slightly concave undermining elevators for the periorbital region. They are used for undermining in the subperiosteal plane of the frontal region (Figure 5-4).
2. **Scalpels.** We prefer long-handled scalpels with no. 15 blades to perform periostomy in the treatment of the frontal region.
3. **Scissors.** We use scissors with "duck-bill" tips and long handles (20 cm), which permit precise cuts in the soft tissues and treatment of the periorbital musculature (Figure 5-5).

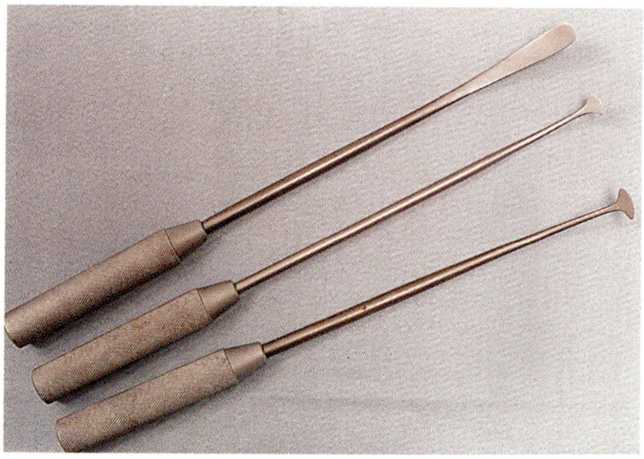

FIGURE 5-4
Undermining instruments are shown.

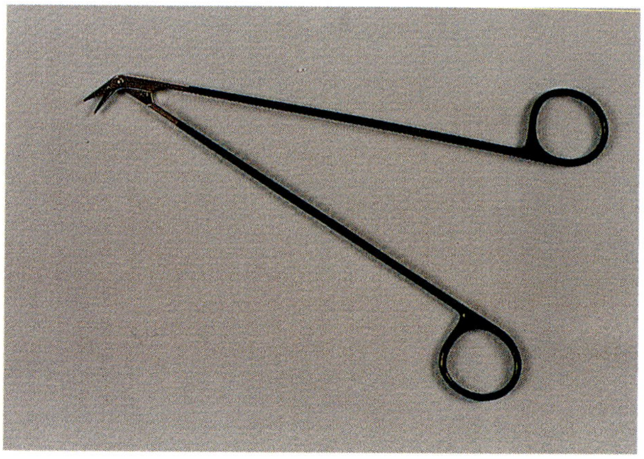

FIGURE 5-5
A pair of endoscopic scissors is shown.

4. **Resecting clamps.** These also vary in length (15 to 20 cm). Their function is in the surgical avulsion of the muscles in the region of the nasal root.
5. **Hemostatic clamps.** These are covered with insulating material to prevent burns.

PREOPERATIVE PREPARATION

The patient is routinely admitted the night before surgery, when the preanesthetic medication is begun under the supervision of the anesthesiologist. On the day of the surgery, the patient is taken to the operating room, where general anesthesia is administered. (We consider it unnecessary to shave the patient's hair preoperatively.) The head, face, neck, and upper portion of the thorax are cleansed with a povidone-iodine preparation (Betadine), while the ocular region is protected by the application of ophthalmic ointment. The external ear canals are cleaned and closed off with plugs. The operating drapes are affixed to the surgical fields with 3-0 monofilament nylon stitches in the hair-bearing skin.

Areas of incision and undermining (frontal, temporal regions and middle third of the face) are marked with methylene blue dye. These areas are infiltrated with a solution of 0.5% lidocaine and adrenaline (1:400,000). We consider the infiltration very important because, in addition to providing hemostasis, it helps with the dissection of the surgical planes.[14,15]

There are two distinct surgical phases, namely, performance of the microfacelift and the actual use of videoendoscopy.

MICROFACELIFT

During this surgical phase, which is aimed at the treatment of the middle third of the face, we use classic surgical instruments for rhytidoplasty. The microfacelift incision extends from the hairy skin of the temporal region (about 5 cm posterior to the hairline) to the upper tragus region (Figure 5-6). The incision has a maximum length of 7 cm and a slightly anterior concavity. Thus the supratragal incision of the microfacelift is different from both the traditional facelift (pretragal and retroauricular incision) and the minifacelift (pretragal incision).

The undermining begins in the temporal region, in the subgaleal plane (Figure 5-7), by positioning the scissors vertically to the plane of dissection, which allows for quick, safe, undermining movements. Hemostasis is always rigorous and is done with the electric scalpel for bleeding of the galeal edge. Metal clips are used to stop bleeding at the skin edge of the incision.

In the frontotemporal region the undermining is subcutaneous, avoiding deep dissection in the danger zone described previously, in order to avoid damage to the temporal branch of the facial nerve.

The undermining in the subcutaneous layer continues over the middle third of the face and extends to the periorbital region, malar area, nasogenial sulcus, and lateral corner of the buccal edge (Figure 5-8). This undermining is superficial to the zygomatic, buccal, and mandibular branches of the facial nerve. To obtain greater exposure in accessing these regions, a skin incision can be made in a horizontal

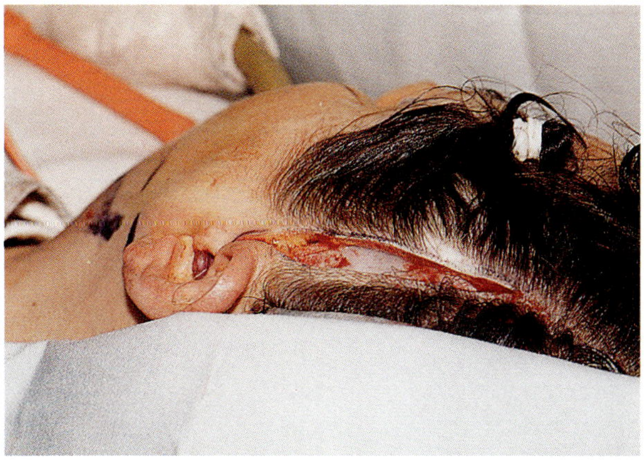

FIGURE 5-6
Microfacelift incision is shown.

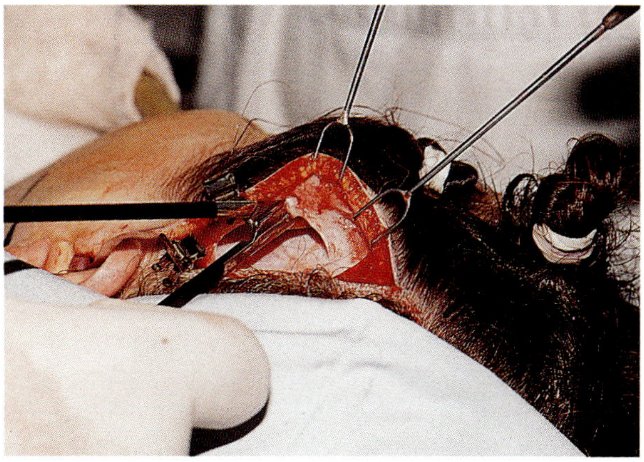

FIGURE 5-7
In the temporal region the subgaleal plane of dissection is shown.

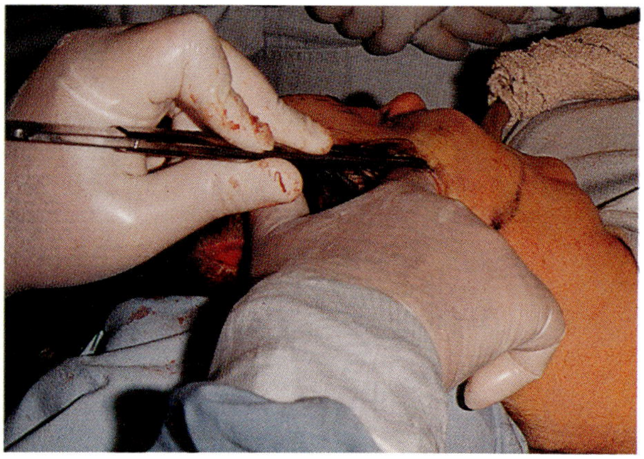

FIGURE 5-8
Undermining middle third section of the face is shown.

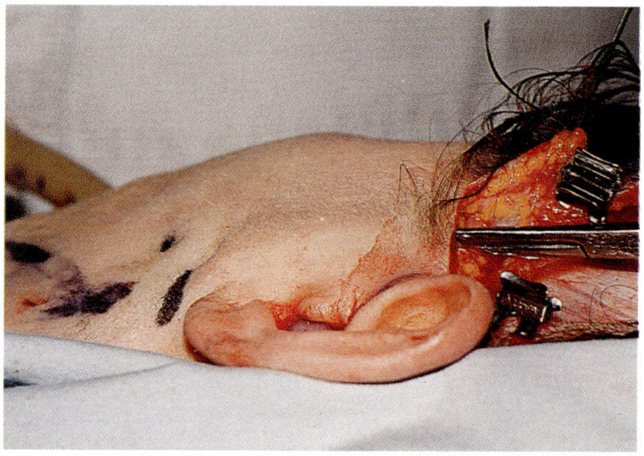

FIGURE 5-9
Incision of the sideburn is shown.

direction and superior to the tragus at the level of the sideburn, of about 2 cm in length. This incision also helps in repositioning of the hairline (Figure 5-9).

After completing the undermining and checking for hemostasis, treatment of the various structures begins as follows.

ORBICULARIS OCULI MUSCLE

This muscle is undermined in its lateral portion, spread, and sutured with 5-0 monofilament nylon. This surgical step improves the lateral periorbital wrinkles.

SUPERFICIAL MUSCULO-APONEUROTIC SYSTEM

Using the same temporal incision, the treatment of the SMAS is carried out via an incision previously traced with methylene blue dye, namely, two lines originating from a preauricular point. The first line runs parallel to the zygomatic arch, about 0.5 cm below it. The second, originating from the same point and located inferiorly in relation to the first, extends to 2 cm above the mandibular edge (Figure 5-10) The dissection of the SMAS must be carried out carefully as it proceeds anterior to the parotid border because of risk of injury to the zygomatic branches of the facial nerve. However, the supraparotid region is an area of greater safety because the SMAS is thicker there.

After dissection and hemostasis, tightening of the SMAS is carried out in a caudocranial direction, fixing it at the level of the tragus and of the zygomatic arch with nonabsorbable sutures. Then the excess SMAS is resected (Figure 5-11).

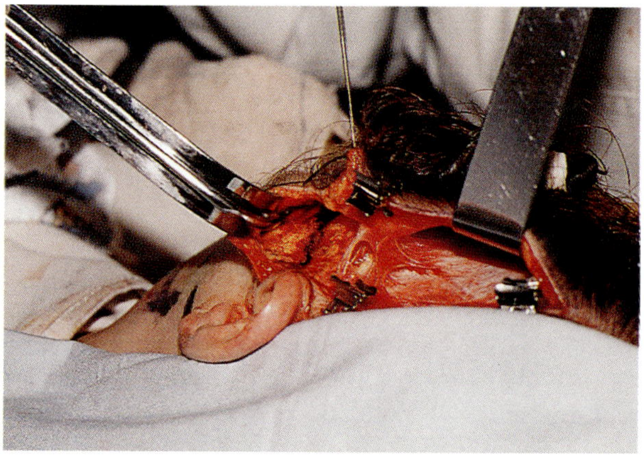

FIGURE 5-10
Marking the superficial musculo-aponeurotic system (SMAS) is shown.

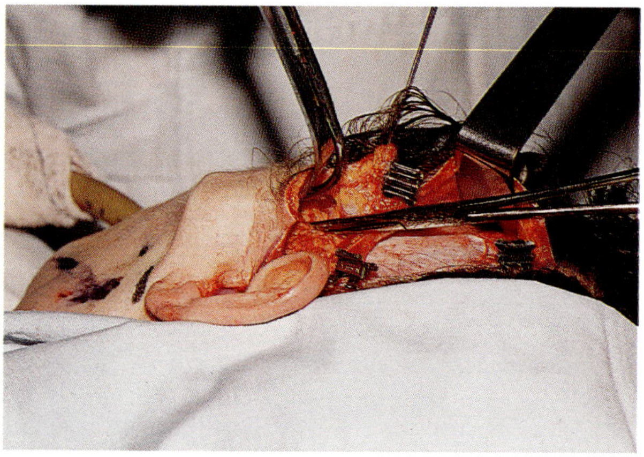

FIGURE 5-11
Tightening of the superficial musculo-aponeurotic system (SMAS) is carried out in the caudocranial direction.

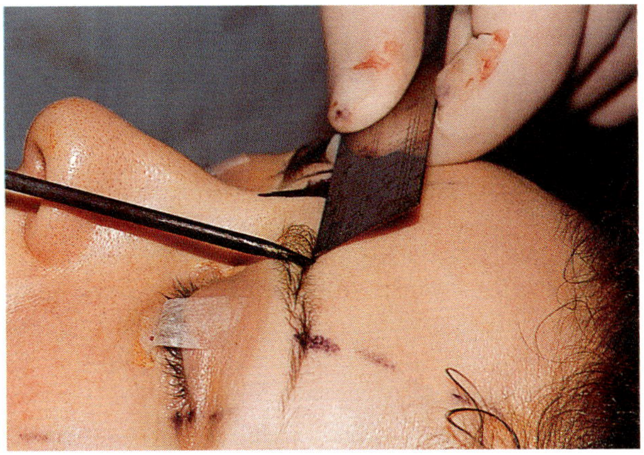

FIGURE 5-12
Marking the frontal area is shown.

VIDEOENDOSCOPY

The surgery proceeds with the treatment of the frontal region, directly visualized with the help of the videoendoscope. During this surgical phase all of the previously described electronic equipment and auxiliary surgical instruments is used.

Three incisions are made: the first is horizontal, open U-shaped, 2 cm long, and located in the midline of the forehead, posterior to the hairline. Two auxiliary incisions are placed laterally, each 1 cm long, and located above the frontal prominences. They are symmetrical. The videoendoscope will be used via these incisions for the treatment of the frontal regions and the tail of the eyebrow.

In addition to the incisions, the areas corresponding to the supratrochlear, supraorbital, and temporal branches of the facial nerve are marked in the frontal area (Figure 5-12). At first, the subperiosteal undermining of the superior portion of the forehead can be carried out blindly, respecting the preoperative markings which delineate the course of the nerves to be preserved (Figure 5-13). Caution must be used at the inferior portion of the forehead to avoid damaging the nerve branches previously outlined. At this point the endoscopic equipment is brought into the operative field, and the procedure is continued under endoscopic visualization.

During this surgical phase the surgeon himself manipulates the videoendoscope and undermines the periosteum, alternately using the central and lateral access incisions. The assistant intermittently irrigates with isotonic solution to maintain a clear and sharp operative view.

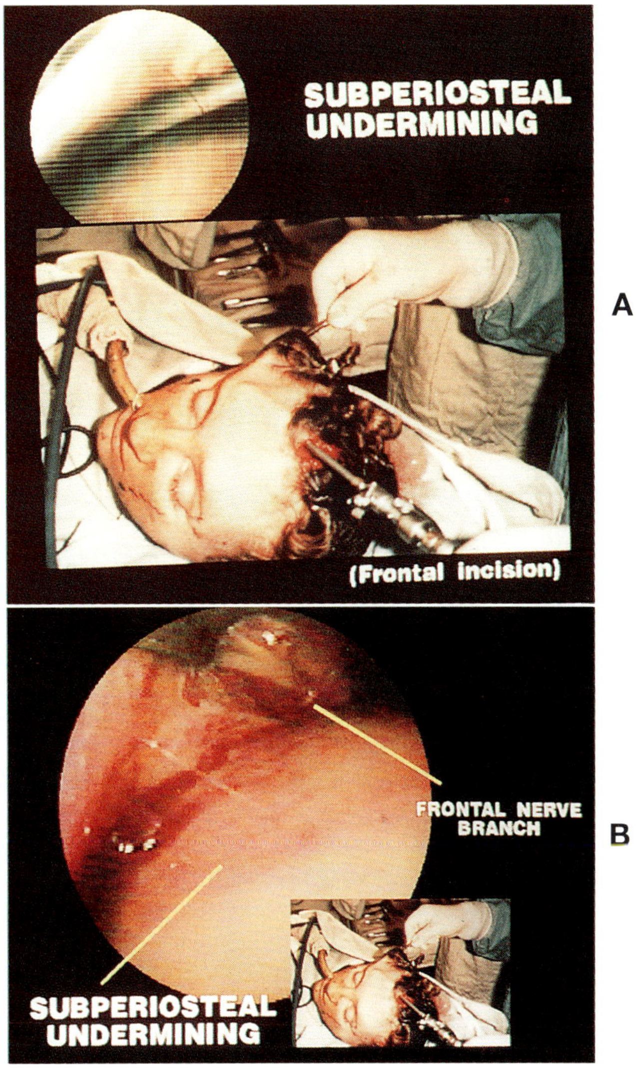

FIGURE 5-13
Videoendoscopic view of subperiosteal undermining. **A,** Frontal incision. **B,** Frontal nerve branch.

After the undermining, which is almost bloodless because of the subperiosteal level of dissection, the actual treatment of the frontal structures begins.

PERIORBITAL AREA

The undermining of the lateral third of the orbit obtained with this technique is ample, readily allowing elevation of the tail of the eyebrow. This results in a natural postoperative appearance, in contrast to the exaggerated cutaneous tightening characteristic of the results obtained with the traditional forehead lift techniques.

During this surgical stage tightening and fixation of the temporal SMAS are performed, imbricating it upon itself (Figure 5-14). The temporal incision made at the beginning of the microfacelift surgical phase is used as a means of access. With this stitch, the fixation in its new position of the tail of the eyebrow is achieved. After the appropriate repositioning of the skin (at the end of the surgery) better facial harmony is obtained.

MUSCLE MODIFICATION

We undermine blindly in a subperiosteal plane to the nasal root in the center, from there laterally—now with the aid of the endoscope—over the superior orbital rim, visualizing the supratrochlear nerves for their safe-guarding (Figure 5-15). Through this approach, next, the periosteum at the superior orbital rim is released with a knife, then the corrugator supercilii and the procerus muscles are surgically modified, respectively. To perform partial myectomy of these two muscles, which must be done as far inferior and as far lateral as possible, we use the delicate "duck-bill" scissors and resecting clamps (Figure 5-16).

Treatment of the frontal wrinkles consists of incisions made vertically and parallel to the frontalis muscle fibers, using a scalpel. The objective is to break the lines of force.

The use of videoendoscopy in the treatment of the frontal region through minimal incisions allows smoothing of the frontal and glabellar wrinkles and a natural and harmonious elevation of the eyebrows, especially in their lateral portion.

TAILORING OF SKIN FLAPS

The resection of skin begins after inserting the first fixation stitch, located at a level superior to the tragus (Pitanguy's "blocking" stitch of the traditional rhytidoplasty) (Figure 5-17). In the microfacelift, this is done after removal of the subcutaneous fat from the supratragal flap. Trimming of the skin follows, by resection of its excess, as the flap is pulled posteriorly and sutured. It is appropriate to point out here that in our experience the amount of skin resection in the microfacelift is minimal (Figure 5-18).

Adjustment of the skin is continued in a caudocranial direction, with anterior rotation of the

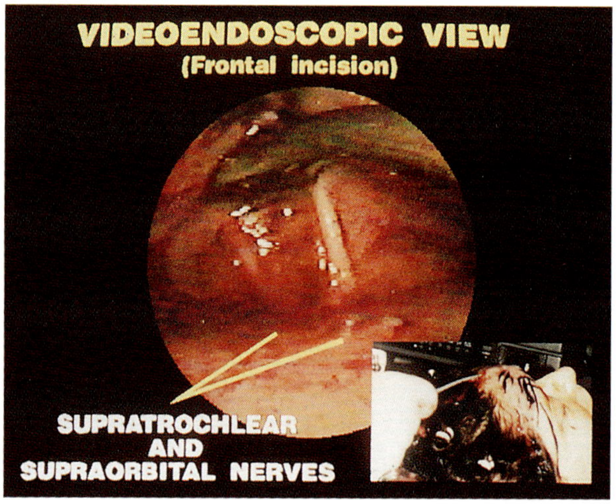

FIGURE 5-15
Visualization of the supratrochlear and supraorbital nerves is shown.

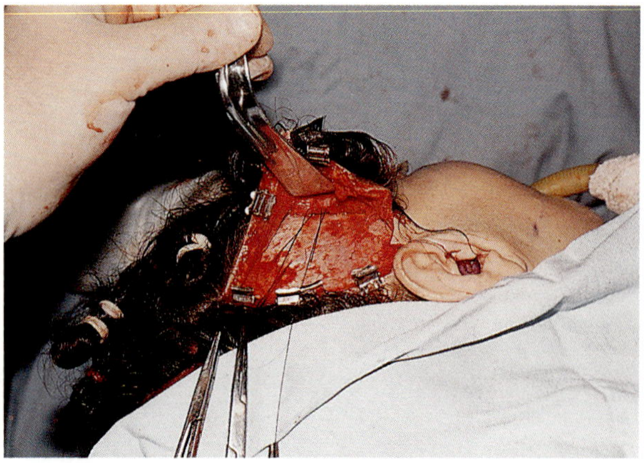

FIGURE 5-14
Fixation of the temporal superficial musculo-aponeurotic system (SMAS) is shown.

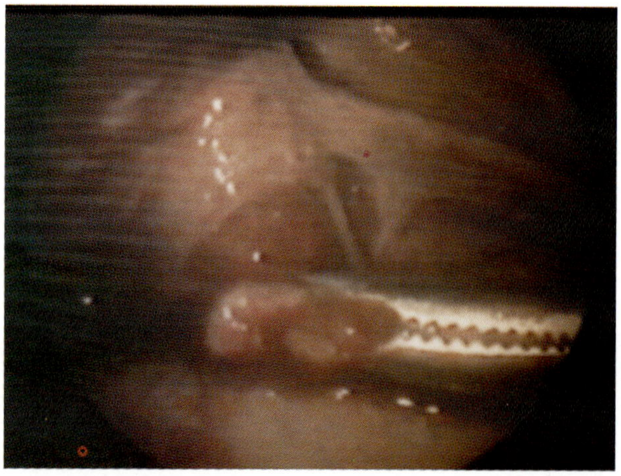

FIGURE 5-16
Endoscopic view of myectomy is shown.

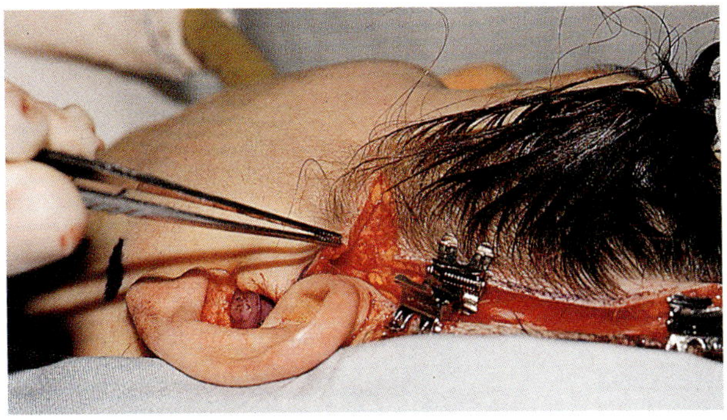

FIGURE 5-17
Pitanguy's blocking is shown.

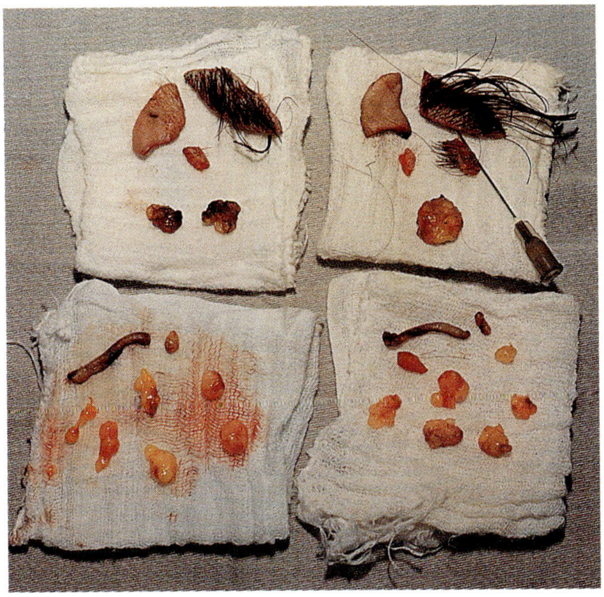

FIGURE 5-18
Skin resection is minimal.

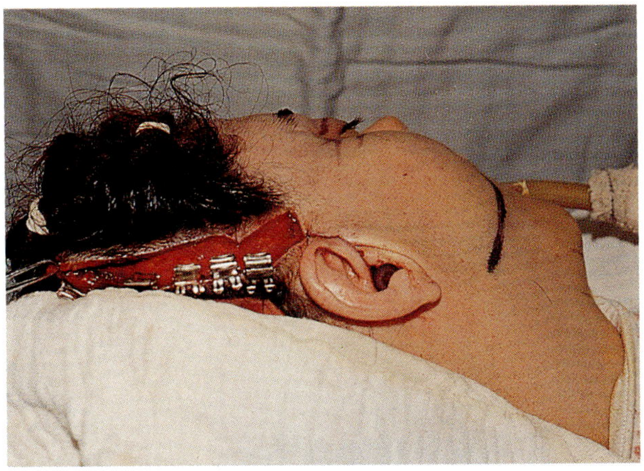

FIGURE 5-19
Caudocranial direction of the skin flap (temporal region) is shown.

superior part of the skin flap, in a direction parallel with the superior concavity of the temporal incision (Figure 5-19). A small triangular resection may be necessary, removing an area of about 1.5 to 2 cm from each side (Figure 5-20). At this point, the suture that raises the tail of the eyebrow is placed, which, because of the temporal SMAS modification as described earlier in the chapter, results in no skin tension.

Taking advantage of the supratragal horizontal incision made initially, now the inferior portion of the hairy skin flap is rotated in an anterior and inferior direction to achieve preservation of the sideburn (Figure 5-21). The suturing of this region is done with monofilament 5-0 half-buried stitches.

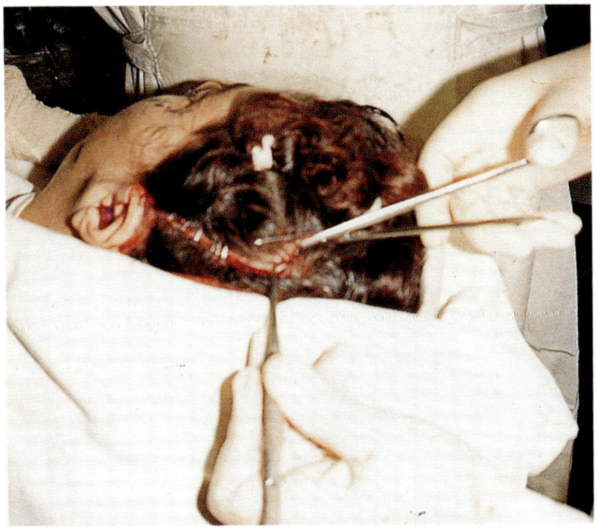

FIGURE 5-20
Small triangular resection is shown.

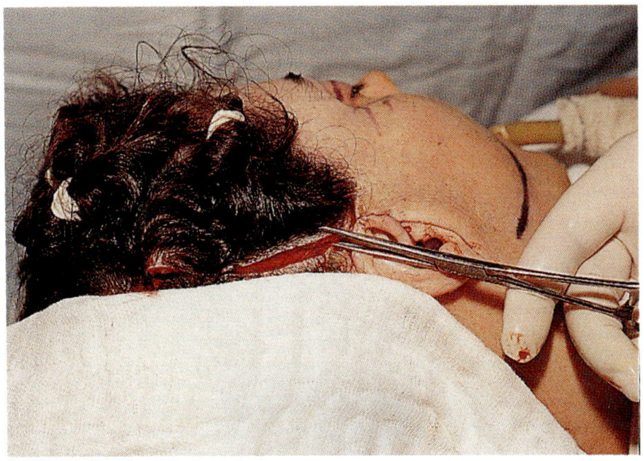

FIGURE 5-21
Rotation of the skin flap in the anterior and inferior directions is shown.

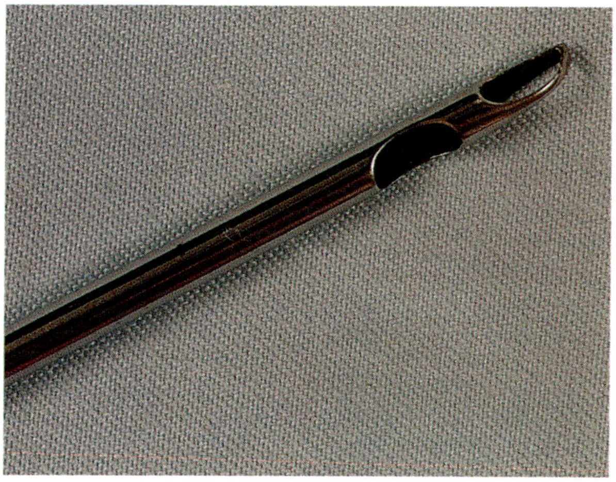

FIGURE 5-22
A Pinto cannula is shown.

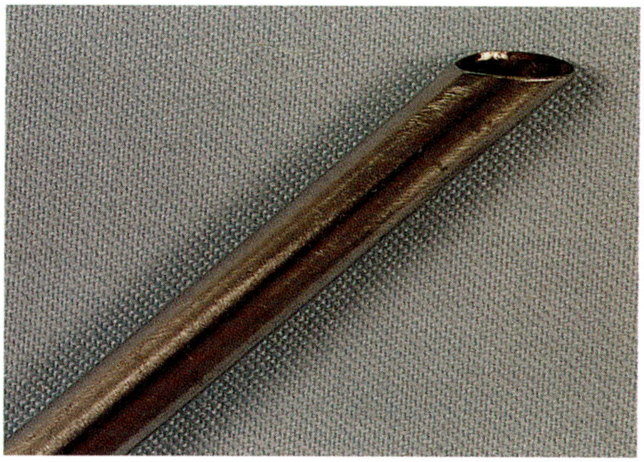

FIGURE 5-23
A Robles cannula is shown.

The hairy skin of the temporal region is then closed with staples or sutured with a simple running stitch using nonabsorbable material. The incisions used in the videoendoscopic phase are closed with a few interrupted sutures.

During the immediate postoperative period the preauricular skin demonstrates slight pleating, which usually disappears completely in the late postoperative period because of the relative elasticity and retractive capacity of the skin of young patients usually selected for this type of surgical approach (class 2). Rarely, we have noted an excess of cutaneous flaccidity present intraoperatively. In these patients, a minimal skin resection from the pretragal region is advisable, which leaves a final scar similar in length to that of the classic minifacelift.

We routinely use suction drains and gentle compressive dressings. Special attention is paid to bandaging the frontal region. The dressings here are maintained for 1 week to protect the undermined area.

The postoperative medication consists only of analgesics and antibiotics. The postoperative follow-up is the same as that used in traditional facial rejuvenation surgical procedures. Patients experience marked postoperative edema, which usually disappears in the middle of the second postoperative week. This technique allows the patient to resume general activities at the beginning of the second postoperative week.

COMPLEMENTARY SURGERIES

SUPERFICIAL LIPOASPIRATION

We often perform superficial lipoaspiration of the submental region and in the area of the mandibular angle using fine, 3-mm cannulas (Pinto-type and Robles-type perforating cannulas) (Figures 5-22 and 5-23). The liposuction is performed 1 cm below the mandibular angle, thereby avoiding injury to the marginal mandibular nerve. Most of our patients who undergo microfacelift do not present with indications to justify surgical manipulations of the platysma muscle.

BLEPHAROPLASTY

Another associated procedure is blepharoplasty, which we always perform after the microfacelift and the frontal endoscopic lift. In our experience the amount of resection of the upper eyelid skin is always smaller as a result of the lateral cutaneous pull achieved by the microfacelift.

RHINOSCULPTURE

There may be appropriate indication for rhinosculpture, which is determined preoperatively, independently of the performance of the microfacelift. Nevertheless, just with the videoendoscopic treatment of the nasal root we obtain an improvement in this region. In the case of a low radix, we fill this out with muscle flaps.

To fashion a nose more compatible in appearance with a youthful face we can also appropriately treat the nasolabial angle and/or the tip of the nose by means of a cartilage graft (auricular or septal). In our experience, however, this procedure is more frequently required in older patients undergoing classic rhytidoplasty (class 4).

CONCLUSION

Facelift surgery has undergone significant conceptual changes throughout the years as it has gone through different stages of evolution. Initially only the skin was lifted, then treatment of deep planes was incorporated, and finally we have arrived at the subperiosteal approach. The present-day treatment of deep layers with facial videoendoscopy is done through smaller incisions, using auxiliary techniques in conjunction such as superficial lipoaspiration and blepharoplasty. The results obtained are more harmonious, resulting in greater patient satisfaction.

REFERENCES

1. de Souza Pinto EB: XXX Congresso Brasileiro de Cirurgia Plástica. Microfacelift com auxílio endoscópico, Curitiba, 1993.
2. Adamson JE, Horton CE, Crawford HH: The growth pattern of the external ear, *Plast Reconstr Surg* 36:466, 1965.
3. Isse NG: Endoscopic facial rejuvenation: endoforehead, the functional lift. Case reports, *Aesth Plast Surg* 18:21, 1994.
4. Seckel BR: *Facial danger zones: avoiding nerve injury in facial plastic surgery,* St Louis, 1994, Quality Medical Publishing.
5. Pitanguy I, Ramos AS: The frontal branch of the facial nerve: the importance of its variations in face lifting, *Plast Reconstr Surg* 38:352, 1966.
6. Larrabee WF Jr, Makielski KH: *Facial sensory innervation.* In *Surgical anatomy of the face,* New York, 1993, Raven Press.
7. Larrabee WF Jr, Makielski KH: *Facial nerve.* In *Surgical anatomy of the face,* New York, 1993, Raven Press.
8. Larrabee WH Jr, Makielski KH: *Forehead and brow.* In *Surgical anatomy of the face,* New York, 1993, Raven Press.
9. Mitz V, Peyronie M: The superficial musculoaponeurotic system (SMAS) in the parotid and cheek area, *Plast Reconstr Surg* 58:80, 1976.
10. Rees TD: *The SMAS and the platysma.* In *Aesthetic plastic surgery* Vol II, Philadelphia, 1980, WB Saunders.
11. Larrabee WF Jr, Makielski KH: *Superficial musculoaponeurotic system.* In *Surgical anatomy of the face,* New York, 1993, Raven Press.
12. Morales P, Castro R, ERREA E, Nociti J: Suprazygomatic SMAS in rhytidectomy, *Plast Reconstr Surg* 8:181, 1984.
13. de Souza Pinto EB: Transactions VIII International Congress Plastic Surgery. Refinements in Rhytidoplasty, Canada, 1983.
14. de Souza Pinto EB, Queiroz W, Muniz AC, Prado Filho FSA, Ruiz RO: *Ritidoplastia.* In Robe, editor: *Atualização em Cirurgia Plástica Estética,* São Paulo, 1993, Tournieux A.A.B.
15. de Souza Pinto EB, Trivellini LR, Abdalla SC, Assad Junior F, Yepez IM: *My preferences in rhytidoplasty.* In Toledo S, editor: *Annals of the International Symposium Recent Advances in Plastic Surgery,* São Paulo, 1989.

SUGGESTED READINGS

Aston S: Platysma-SMAS cervical rhytidoplasty, *Clin Plast Surg* 10:507, 1983.

Castañares S: Forehead wrinkles, glabellar frown and ptosis of the eyebrows, *Plast Reconstr Surg* 34:406, 1964.

Hamra ST: The three-plane face lift dissection, *Ann Plast Surg* 12:268, 1984.

Larrabee WF Jr, Makielski KH: *Facial musculature.* In *Surgical anatomy of the face,* New York, 1993, Raven Press.

Liang M, Narayanan K: Endoscopic ablation of the frontalis and corrugator muscle: a clinical study, *Plast Surg Forum* XV:54, 1992.

Owsley J: Platysma-facial rhytidectomy, *Plast Reconstr Surg* 60:843, 1977.

Psillakis JM, Rumley TO, Camargos A: Subperiosteal approach as an improved concept for correction of the aging face, *Plast Reconstr Surg* 82(3):383, 1988.

Vasconez LO, et al: Coronal facelift with endoscopic techniques, *Plast Surg Forum* XV:227, 1992.

CHAPTER **6**

Facial Rejuvenation: Technique and Rationale

Luiz S. Toledo

The advent of liposuction marked the beginning of the minimal incision approach in surgical procedures designed to alter facial and body contours. At first, obtaining good skin retraction after suctioning the fat was possible only in selected patients, that is, those who were young with localized fat deposits and good skin tone.

Superficial liposuction broadened this indication to include older patients, with a more flaccid skin tone. Working in the superficial layer of fat allowed for better skin retraction.[1] With superficial liposculpture—the combination of superficial liposuction and fat injection—a great improvement of the sagging facial structure is obtained, and it may be used to treat patients who would have otherwise undergone traditional rhytidoplasty. Light fruit-acid peels, introduced in the early 1990s, complement this procedure by ameliorating fine wrinkles, without resorting to skin resection.

It was in 1992 that the plastic surgeon finally incorporated the endoscope into his armamentarium,[2-6] among the last surgical specialists to do so. The endoscope complements the minimally invasive techniques that have been used to postpone or substitute rhytidoplasty. We can now treat facial muscles by simple dissection and suture while the camera allows us to check hemostasis, thereby increasing the safety of closed procedures.

The endoscope lends itself to use in other areas of the body, in such procedures as breast augmentation, mastopexy, and abdominal plication. The results of these procedures will have to stand the test of time. All these new techniques, however, have one goal in common: there must be no skin excess at the end of the procedure. This is where superficial liposculpture complements the endoscopic approach by enhancing skin retraction.

We treat the face in three separate sections, that is, the forehead, midface, and neck, whether simultaneously or separately, depending on the case. The forehead approach is subperiosteal, whereas the midface and neck approaches are subcutaneous. We classify endoscopy as a minimally invasive procedure; therefore, we prefer to use local anesthesia, which obviates the need for hospitalization, substantially lessens the risk of postoperative edema and bruising, leaves no visible scars, and allows a fast return to routine activities.

Dr. Toledo has donated his share of the proceeds from the sale of the endoscopic instruments that carry his name to UNICEF, São Paulo.

The purpose of this procedure is to achieve a substantial improvement in the patient's appearance, while avoiding morbidity and a long recuperation. Our combination of procedures together with local anesthesia and intravenous (IV) sedation have been most satisfactory in our experience from the viewpoint of surgical outcome. Patients undergoing this type of procedure in the morning can go home before noon. This is particularly important for our patients from out of town (almost 50%) who are concerned about the length of recovery time and thus the length of their stay in São Paulo.

We can also offer more extensive treatment, which may have longer-lasting results but also implies general anesthesia, hospitalization, and a longer recovery time—something our patients avoid.

TECHNIQUE

ANESTHESIA

After monitoring the patient, we use a combination of sedation, local anesthesia, and tumescent technique. We start IV sedation with fentanyl (Fentanyl*), 0.5 to 2.0 μg/kg, and maintain it with midazolam (Dormonid*), 0.02 to 0.08 mg/kg. Tenoxican (Tylatil*), 20 mg IV, is used to prevent postoperative pain and methoclopramida (Plasil*), 10 mg IV, to prevent nausea. We use naloxone (Narcan*), 0.04 to 0.4 mg, and flumazenyl (Lanexat*), 1 ml of a 0.5-mg solution diluted in 10 ml, injected slowly intravenously to reverse sedation at the end of the surgery.

Local anesthesia for the forehead and the skin incisions is a solution of 1% lidocaine, 20 ml; epinephrine (1:200,000 dilution); and 3% sodium bicarbonate, 2 ml. For the rest of the face we inject subcutaneously a tumescent solution of 2% lidocaine, 10 ml; epinephrine (1:1000), 0.5 ml; saline, 160 ml; and 3% sodium bicarbonate, 5 ml.

INSTRUMENTS

For facial liposculpture we use a 3-mm gauge, 15-cm long, pyramid-tipped cannula, a 1.5-mm gauge, 15-cm long, flat-tipped cannula with two holes, and 10-ml Luer-Lok syringes (Figure 6-1).

For endoscopy we use a Chakoff endoscopy system (Figures 6-2 to 6-7), periosteal elevators, dissectors, scissors, dissecting forceps with cautery, a 30-degree and a 0-degree telescope with irrigation sheath, a Toledo dissecting/retraction sheath, an endoscopic needle-holder, and a suture-passer. The telescope is connected to the Hyper-Had camera, the xenon light source, a Sony medical monitor, an Agfa slide-maker, a Super VHS VCR, and a Sony video printer.

*These are brand names in Brazil.

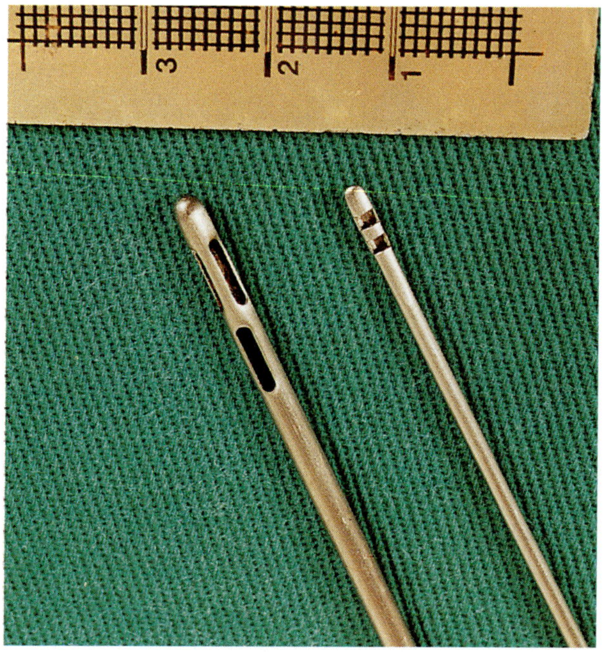

FIGURE 6-1
(Left) A 3-mm gauge, 15-cm long, pyramid-tipped cannula (the Tulip Company) that is used for deep facial suction is shown. *(Right)* A 1.5-mm gauge, 15-cm long, flat-tipped cannula with two holes (Grams Medical) that is used for superficial suction of the neck and jowls is shown.

A

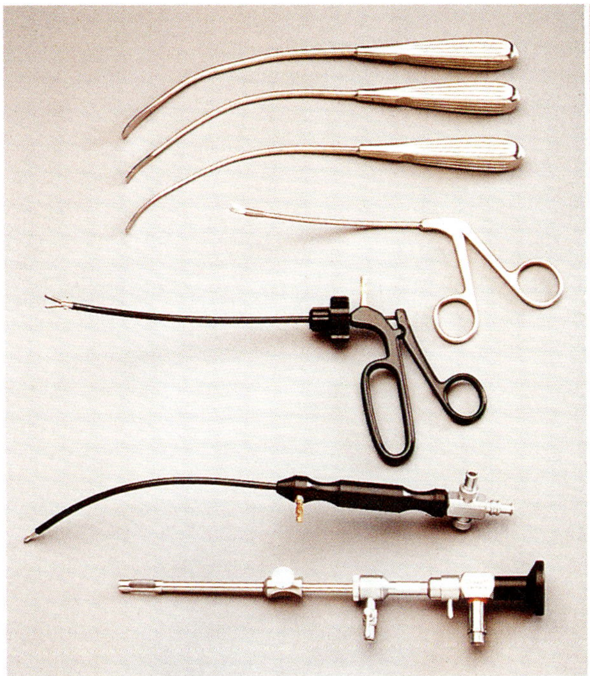

B

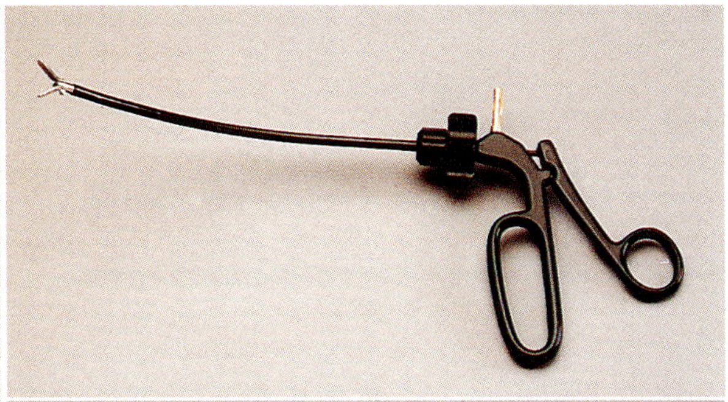

C

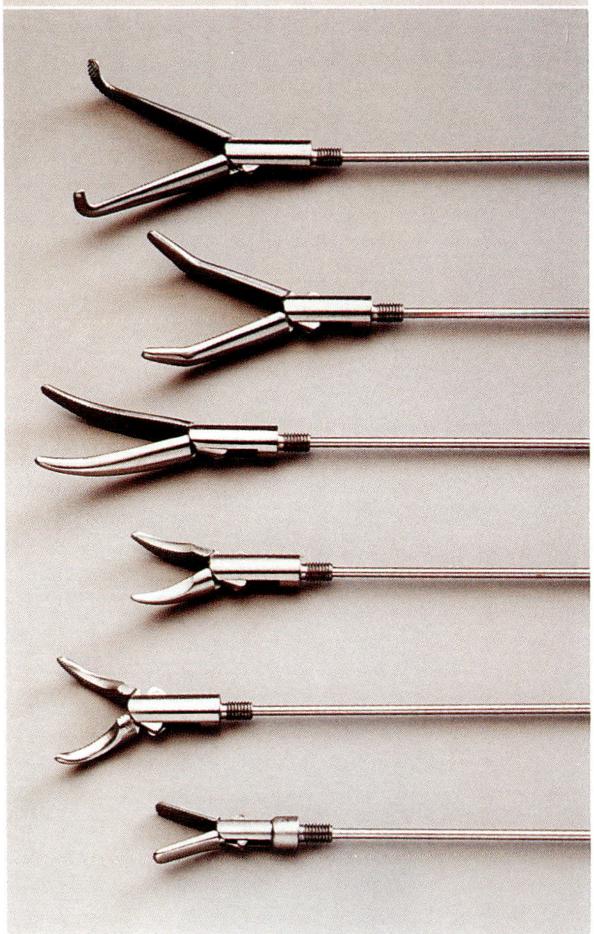

FIGURE 6-2
A, The Chakoff endoscopy system is shown. From the top: periosteal elevators, dissectors, scissors, dissecting forceps with cautery, a dissector/cautery with smoke suction, a telescope with irrigation sheath, and a Toledo dissecting/retraction sheath. **B,** Dissecting curved forceps needle-holder, with cautery. **C,** Interchangeable tips.

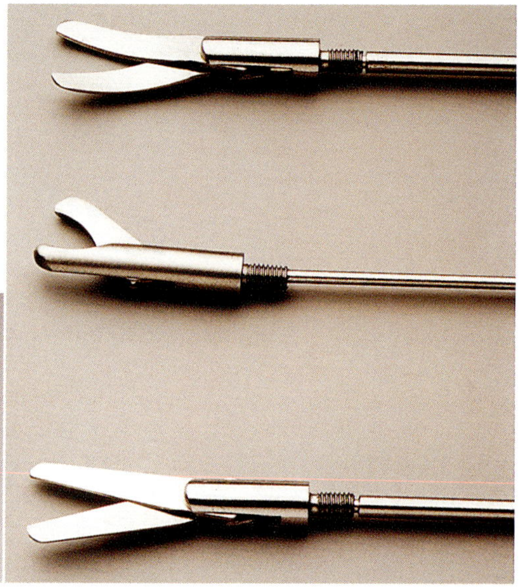

B

FIGURE 6-3
A, Dissecting straight forceps/scissors, with cautery are shown.
B, Interchangeable tips.

A

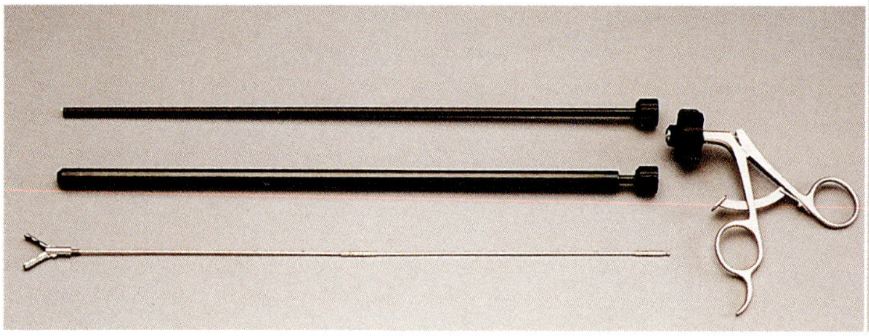

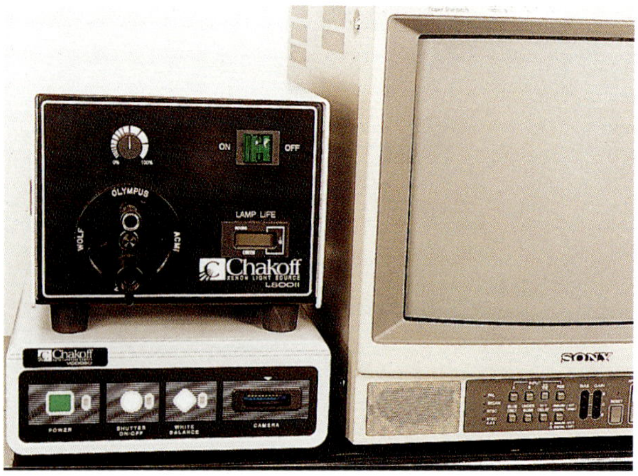

FIGURE 6-4
The documentation system is shown. Sony medical monitor, Chakoff xenon light source, and Chakoff Hyper-Had camera.

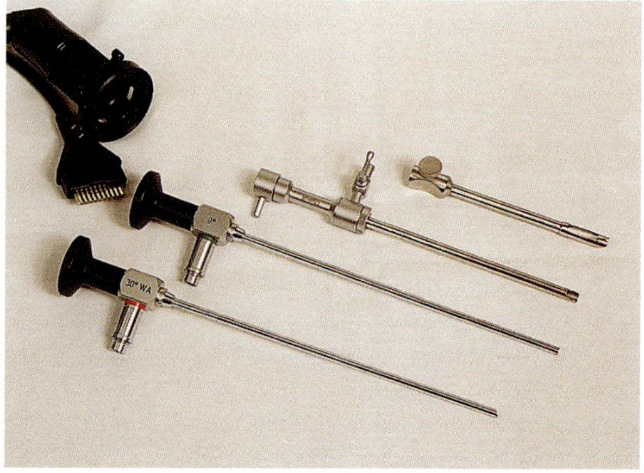

FIGURE 6-5
Shown are a 4-mm gauge, 30-degree tip telescope that is used in forehead lifts and a 0-degree telescope with irrigation and dissection/retraction sheath used in the face and cervical regions.

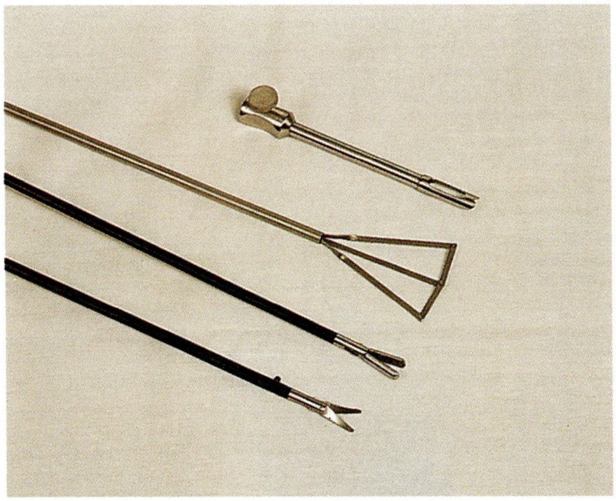

FIGURE 6-6
From the top: a dissection/retraction sheath that is used in the face and cervical regions, a kite retractor used to elevate the skin of the face and neck during hemostasis and plication, and a coated endoscopic hemostat and scissors are shown.

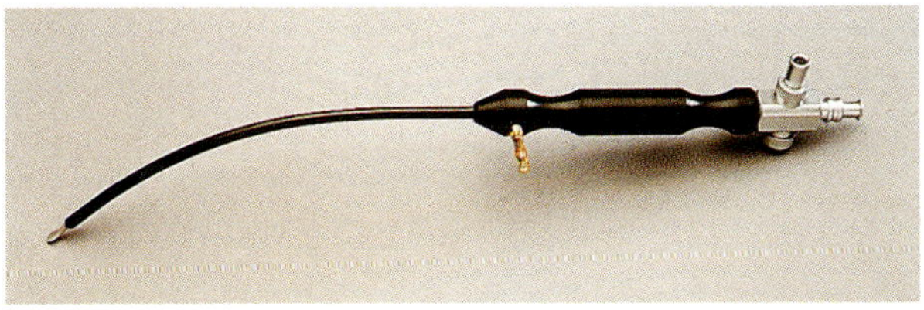

FIGURE 6-7
This coated endoscopic dissector/cautery with smoke suction is a very useful instrument in the dissection of the orbital rim.

THE FOREHEAD

If we are treating only the medial part of the forehead, we make only three 1.5-cm incisions, one medial and two lateral, placed in the scalp, 5 mm from the hairline and perpendicular to it. If we treat in conjunction the lateral part of the forehead and want to elevate the tails of the eyebrows, we add two temporal 2-cm incisions, parallel to the hairline, 1 cm in the scalp.

Before dissecting the forehead we free the scalp from the aponeurosis of the occipitofrontalis muscle. This allows for elevation of the forehead, which is pulled by the occipital part of the muscle once the periosteum is cut and the muscle attachments in the frontal part are freed.

Subperiosteal dissection of the forehead is performed using periosteal elevators. It is important to free the scalp between the incisions, allowing a clean operating field.

If we are treating only the medial part of the forehead, we stop the dissection upon reaching the temporal muscles. When we are using the temporal incisions as well, we dissect down to the level of the temporal muscle and proceed from a lateral to a medial direction just above the superficial layer of the deep temporal fascia, until we reach the medial subperiosteal dissection.

Dissection is blind down to 2 cm from the orbital rim. We then insert the endoscope to guide the dissection. Through one incision we insert a 4-mm, 30-degree tip telescope with irrigation and retraction sleeves. Through another incision we introduce an elevator and dissect under the periosteum. We use a no. 15 blade or the endoscopic scissors to incise the periosteum and reach the muscles.

We clean the field with saline irrigation, either continuously or with a syringe. Bleeding vessels are cauterized with coated forceps.

Next, we identify the corrugator muscles, usually of dark red color, dissecting to the edge of the orbital rim, first laterally then medially to the supraorbital bundle. We free the cephalic medial attachments of the orbicularis muscles and the depressor supercilii. We reach the whiter procerus muscles and free them from the nasal bone. We have the choice of either freeing these muscles or removing part of them if they are hypertrophic and wrinkle the forehead excessively. The frontalis muscles can be partially cut to weaken their action and avoid an undesired overelevation of the eyebrows.

Laterally, we incise the periosteum and free its attachments to the orbital rim, until we reach the desired elevation of the eyebrows. Our patients do not like the eyebrows too high (Figures 6-8 and 6-9). We can obtain an initial elevation of 1 cm by just freeing the muscles. This will reduce to a 7- or 8-mm elevation after only 1 year, which is usually sufficient. If more elevation is desired, it is possible to suture the structures to a screw or to the bone itself; we prefer not to do so. We keep the structures in place with a compressive dressing for 3 days and leave Penrose drains in for 24 hours. The procedure can be performed in 30 to 35 minutes.

THE MIDFACE

In 1989, we were taught the Jacques Faivre[7,8] triple facelift, which included a subpalpebral lift. This is a procedure in which, through a lower blepharoplasty skin incision, the premalar region is dissected subperiosteally and sutured to the periosteum of the orbital rim. This eliminates the excess skin from the lower eyelid and also elevates the nasolabial fold. This is a fabulous procedure that can give very good results. It is not, however, a "light" procedure; it involves general anesthesia and a long recovery time.

We prefer a subcutaneous endoscopic dissection, through two 1.5-cm incisions, one temporal in the scalp, and another behind the earlobes. Through these two incisions we can dissect the mid-third of the face to the nasolabial fold and perform hemostasis with the insulated forceps. We use a 0-degree endoscope with irrigation sheath, a Toledo dissecting/retraction sheath to separate the skin from the submuscular aponeurotic system (SMAS) (it is not possible to use the forehead 30-degree telescope, with the dissecting sheath). With an endoscopic needle-holder we plicate the SMAS to the temporal aponeurosis with the help of a suture-passer. We do not suction fat from the malar zygomatic area, but only from the jowls, when necessary, and from the neck, below the jaw line. Two or three stitches placed here will give a satisfactory elevation of the premalar fat pad, with improvement of the nasolabial fold and filling out of the malar depression (Figure 6-10).

THE CERVICAL REGION

We treat the neck through 3-mm incisions in the mastoid regions and another incision in the submental area. These incisions should be short so that we do not lose the vacuum when suctioning with the syringe. We start with superficial liposculpture to recontour the area using a 3-mm gauge, 15-cm long, pyramid-tipped cannula, adapted to a 10-ml Luer-Lok syringe. We remove the deeper fat layer and then, with a 1.5-mm gauge, 15-cm long, two-holed, flat-tipped cannula, we improve the result by working on the superficial plane of the jowls and neck, closer to the skin, to obtain uniform retraction. At this point it is important not to skeletonize the neck area, always leaving a uniform layer of fat attached to the platysma. After suctioning fat, the cannula is worked with the holes facing the dermis, scraping the skin, provoking the even, controlled retraction of the area. The three incisions are extended to 1.5 cm, sagging of the skin and platysma is treated through a complete video endoscopic dissection, using the 0-degree telescope with an irrigation sheath (Figure 6-4), a Toledo dissecting/retraction sheath to separate the skin from the platysma, performing hemostasis and plication. For plication we use a no. 0 Gore-Tex sling suture, which is placed in the periosteum of the mastoid, buried in the insertion of the externocleidomastoid muscle and passed through the cervical mental angle with the help of a suture-passer, between the platysma and the skin to the contralateral side. The suture placement in the mastoid area should not be too tight. The patient, being awake, can help with the adjusting of the tightness of the sling, by swallowing freely and yawning with ease. This avoids postoperative discomfort and the necessity of having to release the suture, as it has happened twice. The skin incisions are sutured with two or three 5-0 nylon stitches, which are removed within 5 days.

An elastic dressing is worn for 24 hours, after which we prescribe five sessions of manual lymphatic drainage, performed by our estheticians every other day. This lessens the edema and bruising (Figure 6-11). This rejuvenation treatment is usually combined with fat injections that are performed in three stages, every 2 months, with small quantities injected into the malar, nasolabial, and glabellar areas.

Use of corrective makeup is helpful in patients with busy schedules. During the last few years we have added light chemical peels to our facial rejuvenation program. These peels improve fine wrinkles and age spots and give a youthful, healthy appearance to tired skin. Alpha-hydroxy-acid peels are done in fortnight visits and can also be prescribed as daily creams.

CONCLUSION

Videoendoscopic facial rejuvenation is not a substitute for rhytidoplasty, but it can be very beneficial, especially for younger patients (30 to 45 years of age), who seek improvement with a fast recovery time. Excess skin will need to be removed sooner or later to achieve a superior result. Some patients, however, will never opt for an extensive facelift and are pleased with the results obtained with the videoendoscopic technique. This may represent a permanent change in our practice. There is

FIGURE 6-8
A,B,C, Preoperative view of a 42-year-old female patient. **D,E,F,** View 24 hours postoperatively, with the drain still in place after an endoscopic forehead lift. We performed a subperiosteal dissection and releases of corrugator, procerus, orbicularis, and depressor supercilii muscles. There was satisfactory elevation of the eyebrows, with little morbidity. Skin resection and blepharoplasty were not done. **G,H,I,** Six-month postoperative view of the same patient. There was a 2-mm drop in the ultimate position of the eyebrows.

A,B

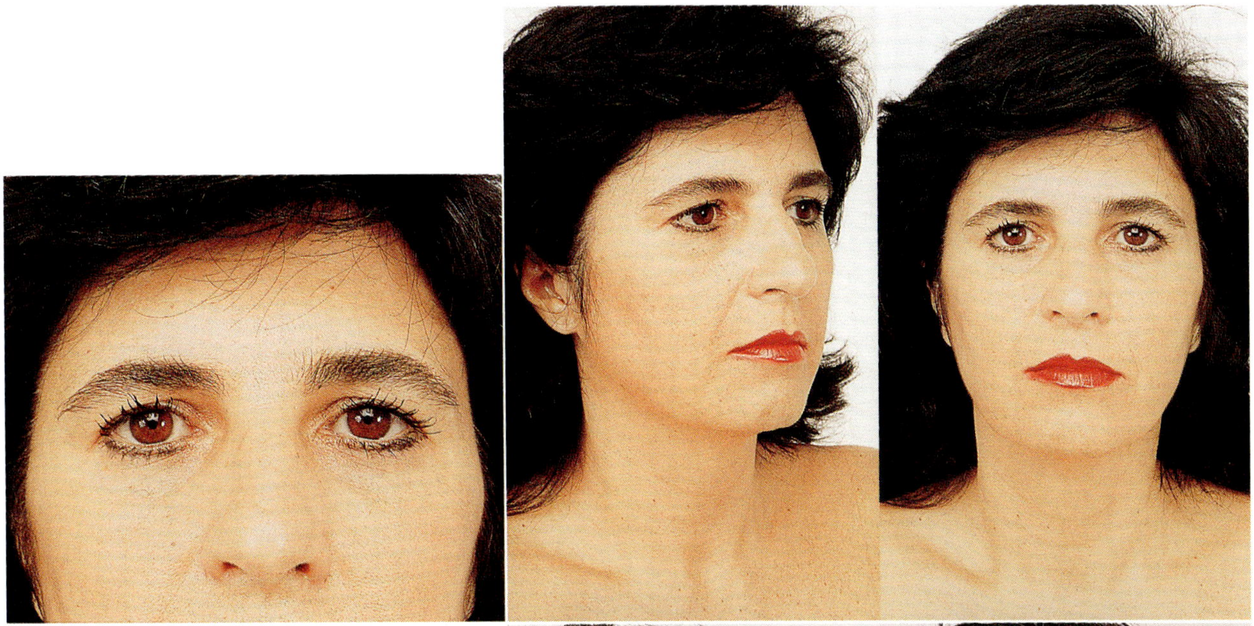

C

D,E

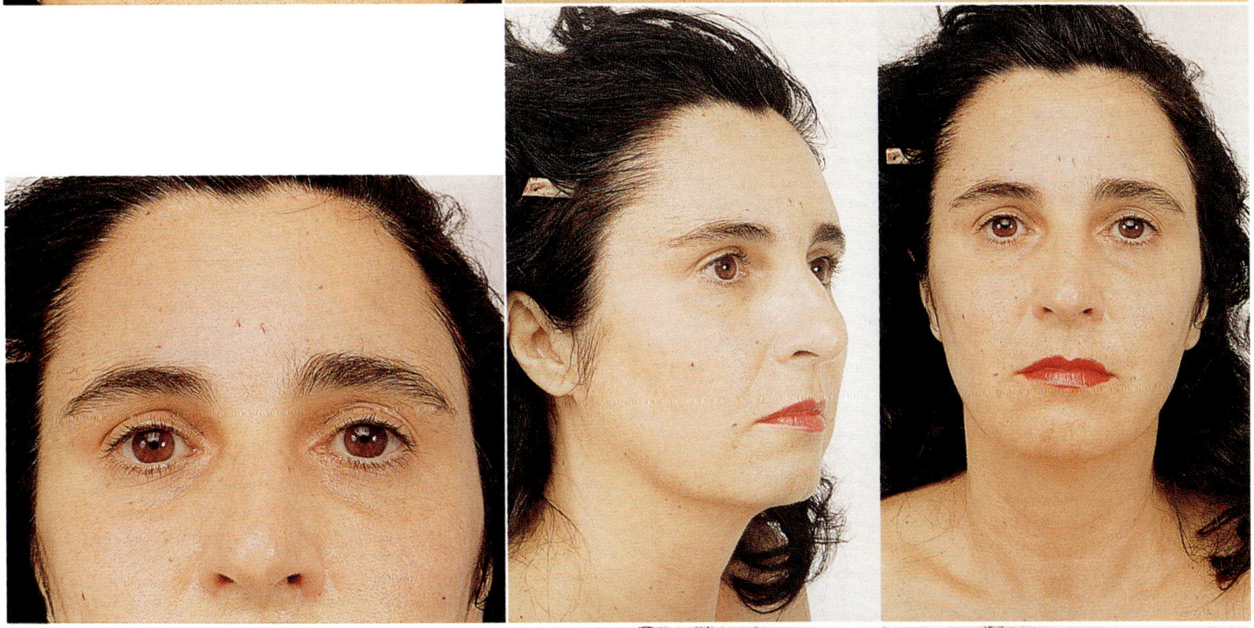

F

G,H

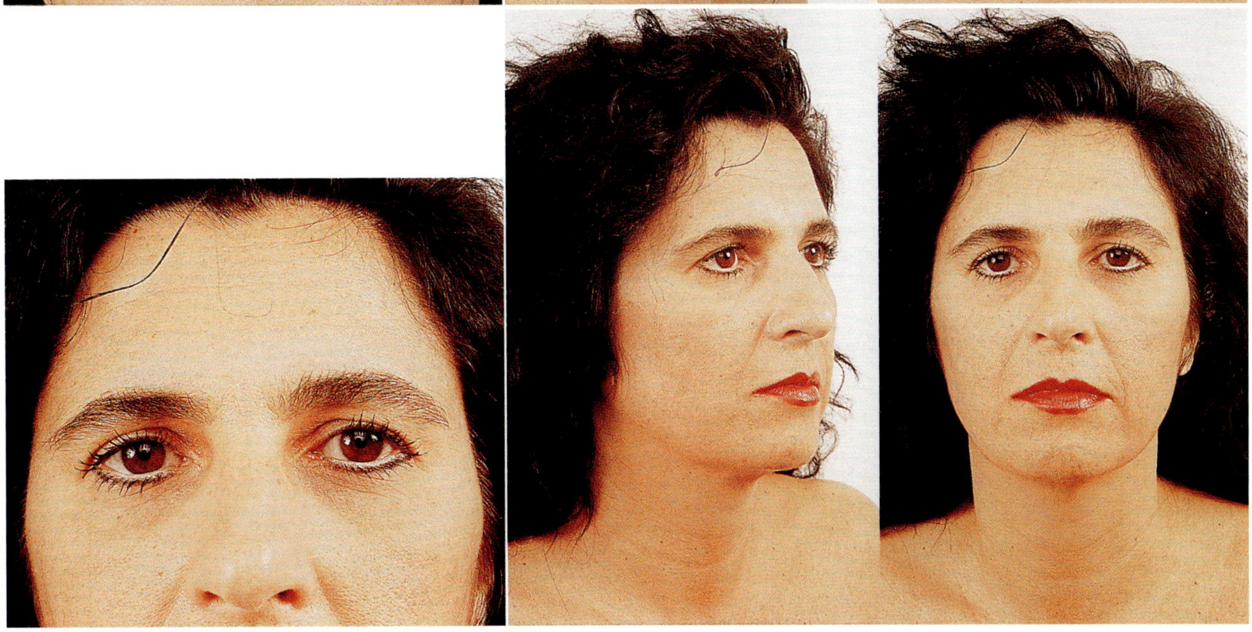

I

FIGURE 6-9
The interrupted line shows the level at which the subperiosteal dissection sections the periosteum and reaches the muscles. The solid line shows the level of dissection of the muscles from the orbital rim and nasal bone.

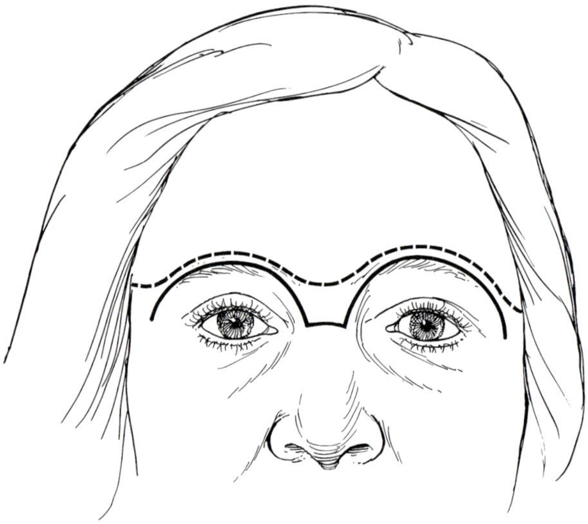

A

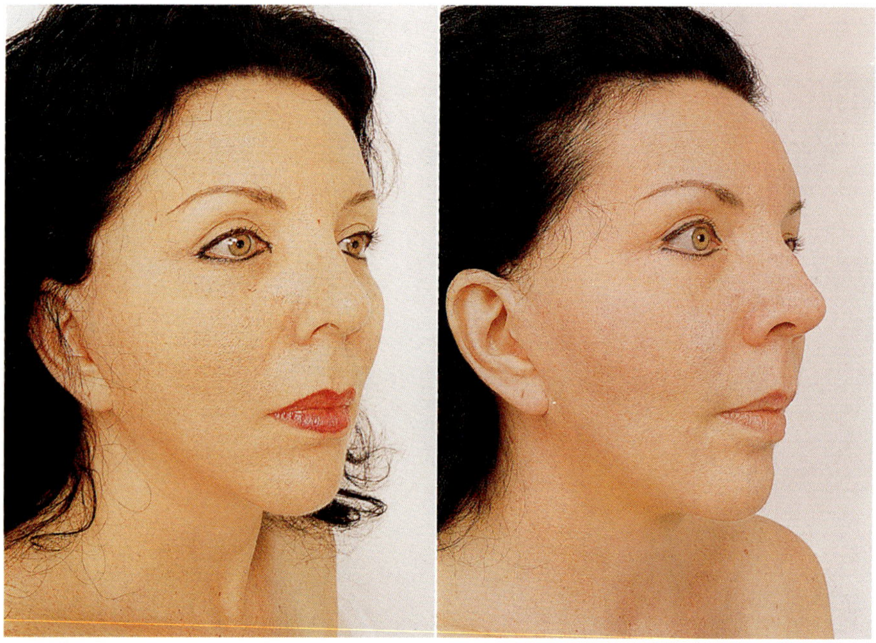

B

FIGURE 6-10
A, Preoperative view of a 49-year-old patient who had a rhytidoplasty at 35 years of age. Patient complained of malar ptosis, but did not wish to undergo another traditional rhytidoplasty. **B,** Postoperative view at 14 months, after a malar subcutaneous endoscopically assisted facelift. **C,** Shown are the positions of the two or three stitches that elevate the malar fat pads, improving the nasolabial folds.

C

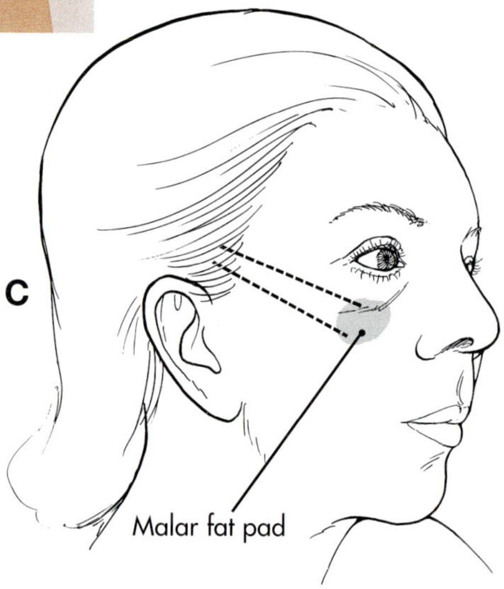

A

B

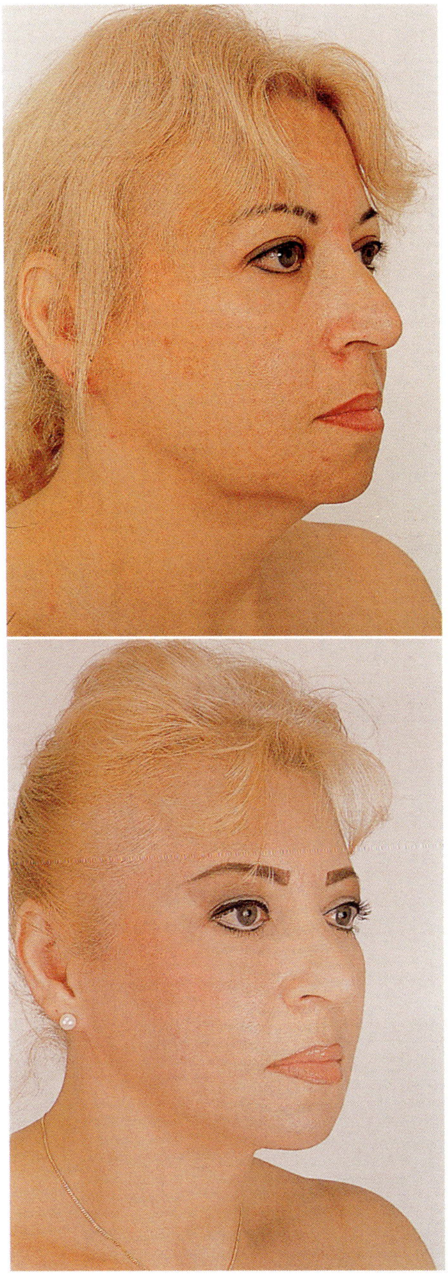

FIGURE 6-11

A, Preoperative view of a 48-year-old patient with malar and cervical ptosis who wanted rejuvenation but not facelift scars. **B,** One-year postoperative view, after malar and cervical subcutaneous endoscopically assisted facelift, plus facial liposculpture. No forehead lift and no blepharoplasty were done. The difference in skin quality is not simply a result of using makeup, but is also due to the home glycolic acid program used for over 6 months.

Continued.

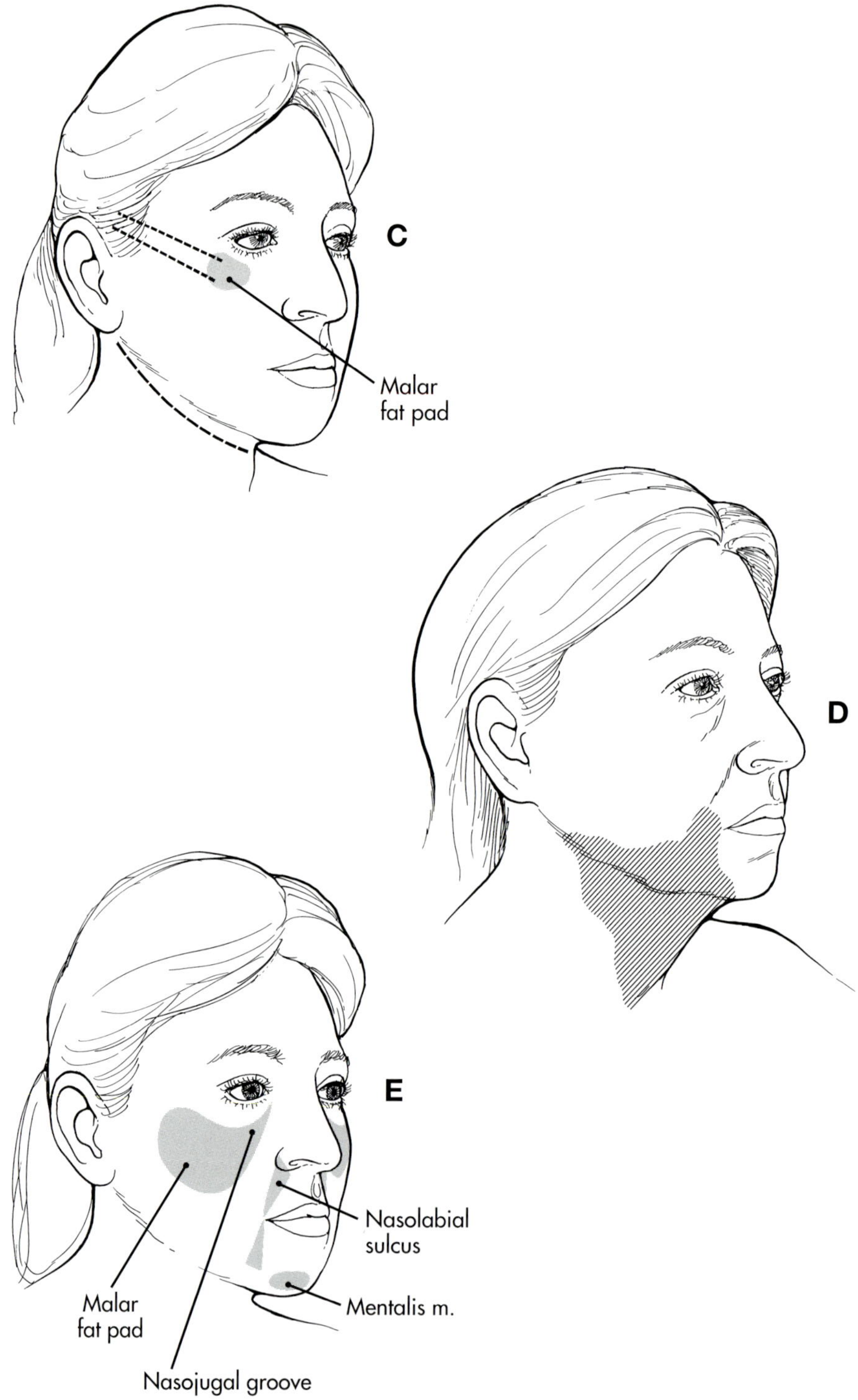

FIGURE 6-11, CONT'D

C, Shown are the positions of the two sutures that elevate the malar fat pads, improving the nasolabial folds. Also shown is the position of the no. 0 Gore-Tex cervical suture. **D,** Seventy-six ml of fat were suctioned from the cervical and jowl areas. **E,** The patient had three consecutive fat-injection procedures in the nasojugal (0.5 ml per side), malar (1.5 ml per side), nasolabial (2.5 ml per side), and mental (2 ml) areas. The last injection was given 9 months before the photograph was taken.

objection in a certain category of patients, especially those in the public eye, to the rhytidoplasty scars and the "loss of character" in the postoperative appearance. We should avoid creating facial appearances that do not match the voice, body habitus, and attitudes of the person. The procedures described in this chapter may not be appropriate for all patients but are definitely suitable for a select group of patients with their own set of requirements and expectations.

REFERENCES

1. Toledo LS: Syringe liposculpture. A two year experience, *Aesth Plast Surg* 15:321, 1991.
2. Toledo LS: Video-endoscopic facelift. Presented at the Brazilian Society of Plastic Surgery, Jornada Carioca Meeting, Rio de Janeiro, Brazil, August 5, 1993.
3. Toledo LS: Video-endoscopic facelift, *Aesth Plast Surg* 18:149, 1994.
4. Vasconez LO, Core G: Endoscopic techniques of coronal lifting. Video tape no. 436-A. UAB Division of Plastic Surgery, 1992.
5. Isse N: Endo-facial training seminar, Newport Beach, CA, EUA, June 11,12, 1993.
6. Ramirez O: Endo-facial training seminar, Newport Beach, CA, EUA, June 11,12, 1993.
7. Faivre J: *The triple facelift.* In Toledo LS, Pinto EBS, editors: *Annals of the International Symposium "Recent Advances in Plastic Surgery"—RAPS/90—São Paulo, Brazil,* Marques Saraiva Graf e Edit SA, March 28-30, 1990.
8. Faivre J: The triple facelift. Current approach, *Arch Otolaryngol Head Neck Surg* 117(1):47, 1991.

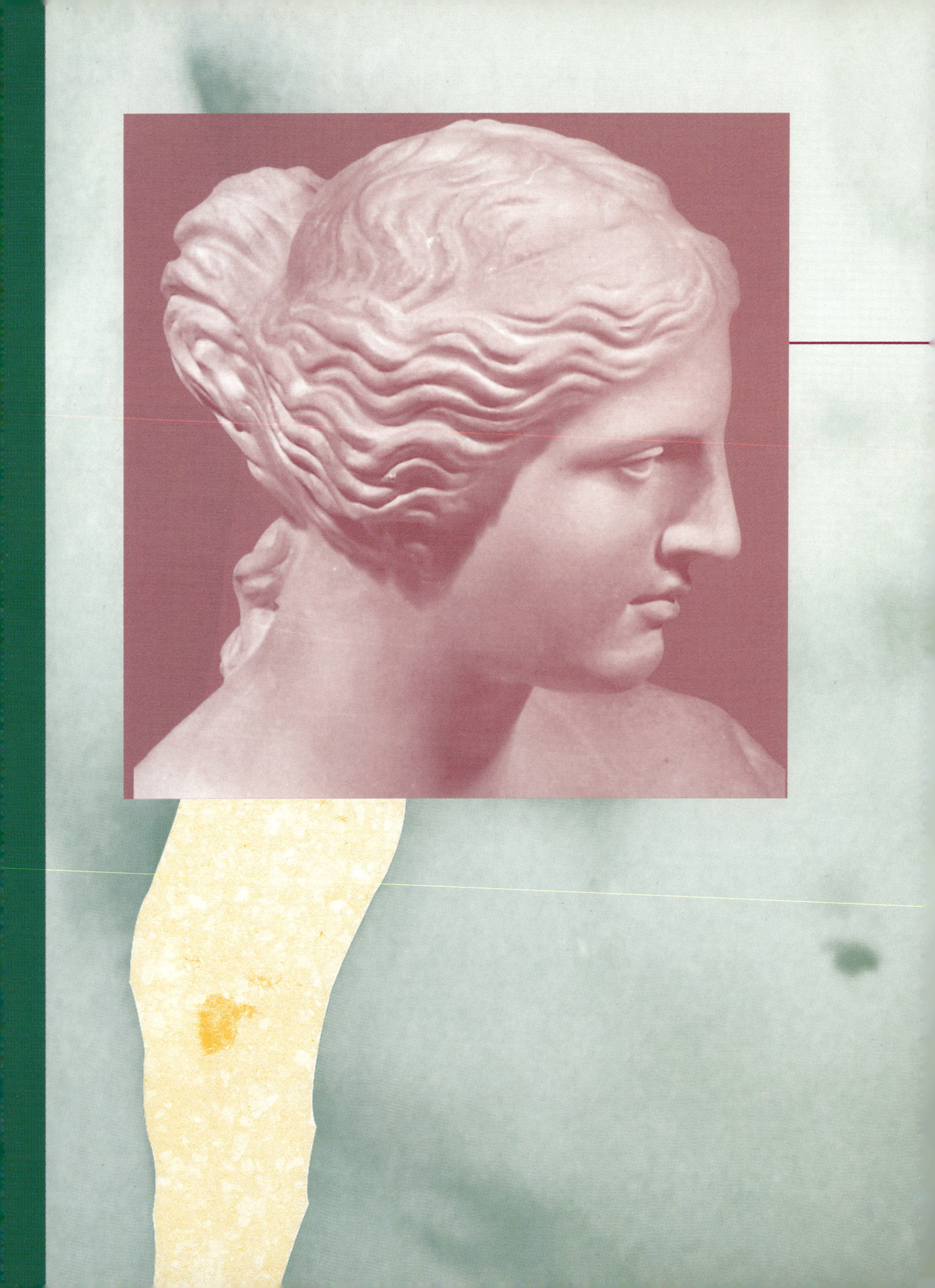

PART II

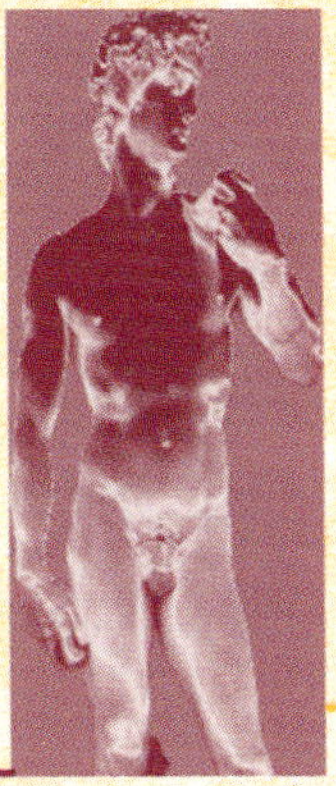

BODY SCULPTING

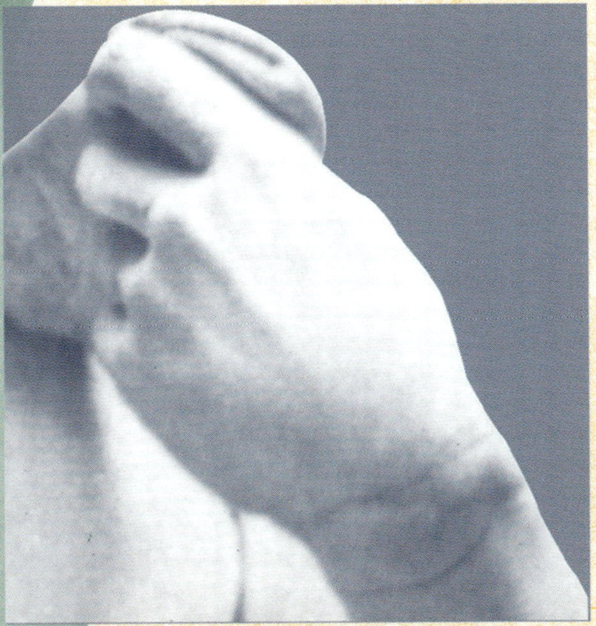

CHAPTER 7

Anatomic Considerations

Joseph P. Hunstad
Peter Bela Fodor

Anatomic considerations play an essential role in endoscopically assisted body contouring from the planning stage of each procedure and throughout its execution to achieve a predictable outcome.

The ability to visualize the anatomy of the operating field three-dimensionally is critical to the consistent and reliable performance of all surgical procedures. A keen understanding of anatomy is *important* in "open" procedures, in which the operating field is fully visualized; however, when the field of view is significantly restricted, as is the case in endoscopic procedures, this understanding becomes *crucial*.

With the magnification achieved during endoscopic surgery, each procedure becomes a sequence of small segments being visualized seriatim, whose sum represents the entire picture of a given operation. It is precisely the knowledge and understanding of anatomy that connects these disjointed segments in the surgeon's mind into a fluid continuum encompassing the integrity of the operating field, which is partly within and partly without the momentary field of vision. This chapter explores the range of anatomic considerations pertaining to body contouring in a generalized fashion and focuses on distinct, individual areas that are important during the actual performance of endoscopic procedures.

BREAST

Topography

The female breast's symmetrical, conically shaped, cutaneous appendages consisting of fat and glandular parenchyma occupy a significant portion of the anterior and lateral chest wall (Figure 7-1). The breast parenchyma itself extends from the clavicle superiorly to and below the inframammary crease inferiorly. In the costal plane this corresponds to the area extending from the second or third to below the sixth or seventh costal cartilages. Histologically, the presence of breast parenchyma extends medially across the midline; clinically, however, it is seen to begin just off the midline of the sternum, extending over the costochondral junction laterally to a line posterior to the anterior axillary line. The breast parenchyma itself can be present at and beyond the lateral border of the latissimus dorsi.[1-5]

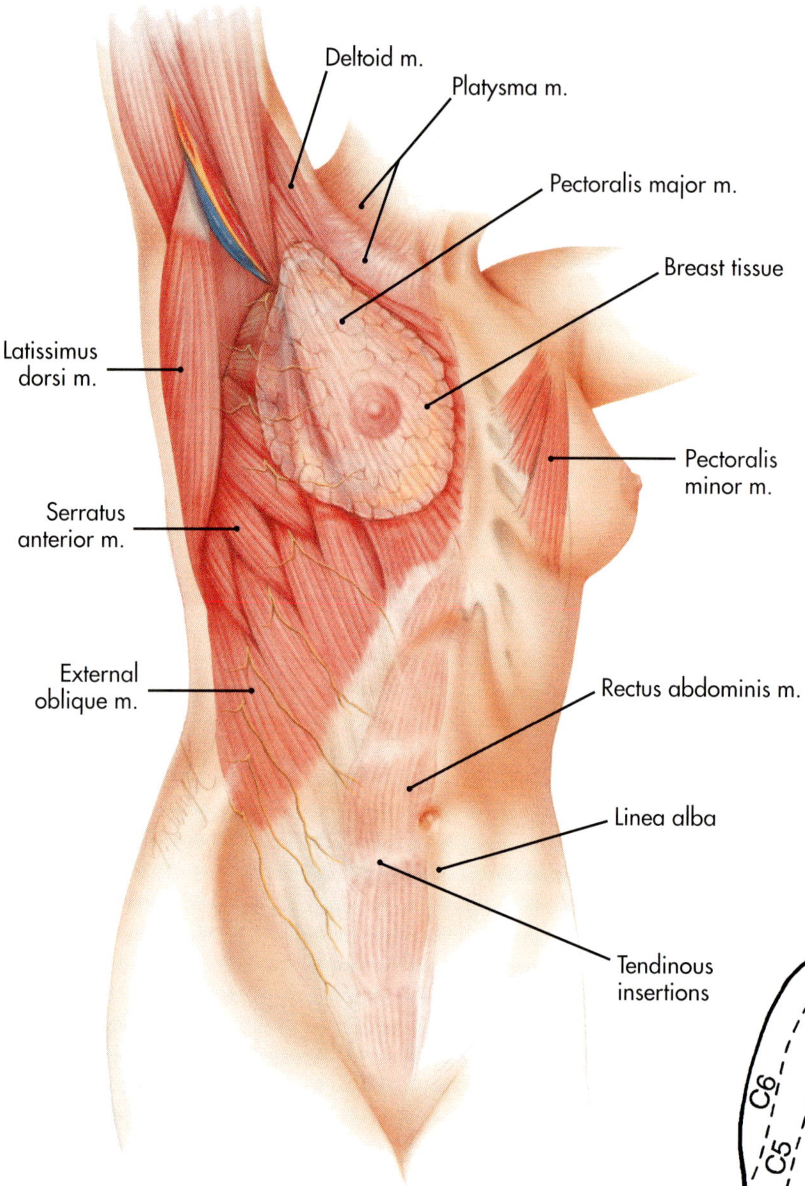

FIGURE 7-1
The topography of the breast is shown. The breast parenchyma overlies important muscle groups of the anterior chest wall. The axillary tail of the breast and the lateral aspect of the pectoralis major muscle form the anterior axillary fold. The platysma, the pectoralis major, serratus anterior, and external oblique muscles, and the rectus sheath lay immediately beneath the breast itself. Deep to the pectoralis major muscle, separated by a loose areolar "potential" space, are the subclavius and pectoralis minor muscles.

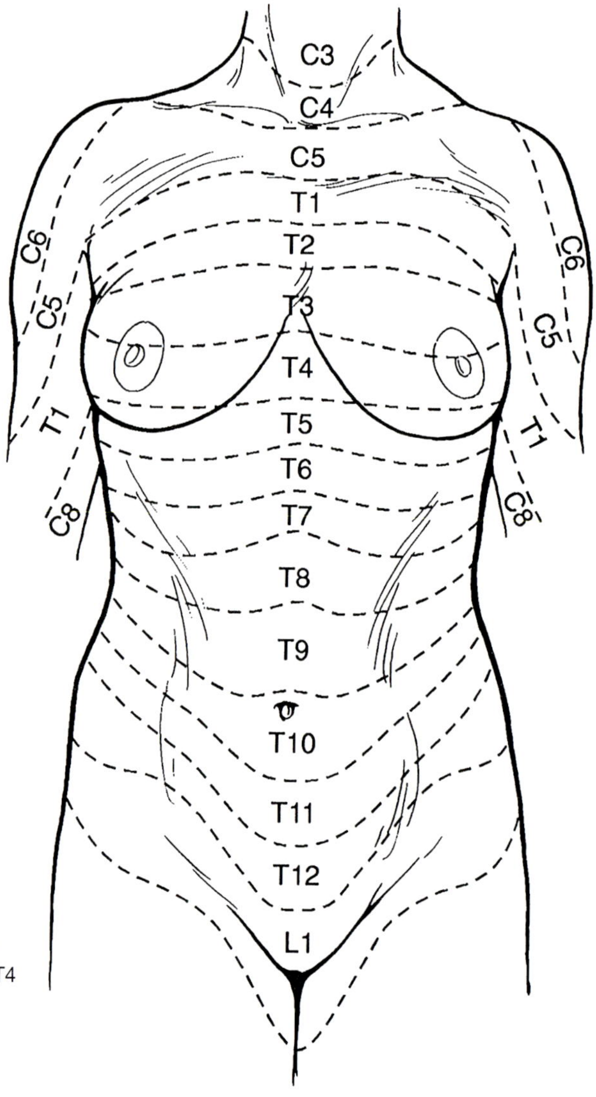

FIGURE 7-2
The dermatome pattern of sensory innervation of the breast and abdomen is shown. The nipple–areolar complex lies at T4 and the umbilicus at T10.

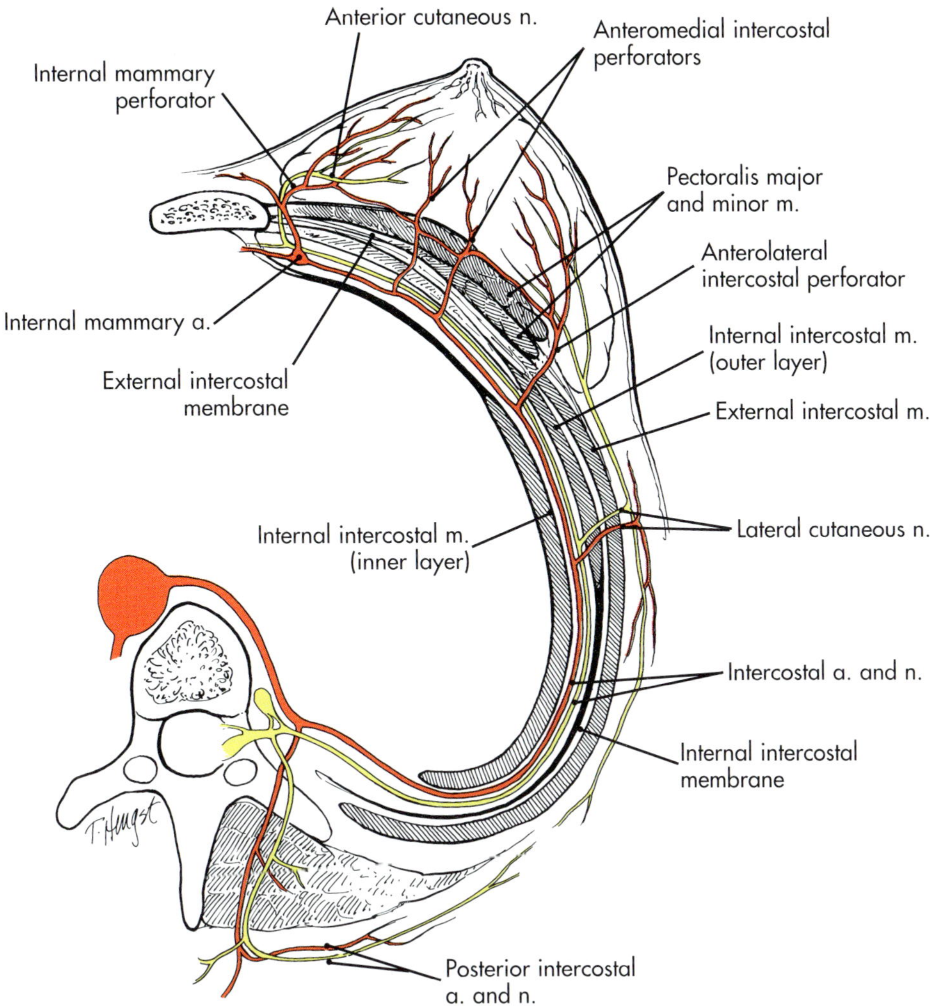

FIGURE 7-3
The anatomy of the intercostal space is shown. The intercostal nerves exit from the spinal canal and immediately sends forth the dorsal ramus. This continues anteriorly as two major branches, the anterolateral cutaneous and the anteromedial cutaneous nerves. The anterolateral cutaneous nerve divides into medial and lateral branches in the lateral thoracic region; the anterior medial cutaneous nerve divides into medial and lateral branches in a parasternal location. The sensory innervation of the breast skin is derived from the anterior branch of the anterolateral intercostal nerve and the lateral branch of the anteromedial intercostal nerve. They course within the breast parenchyma itself to supply sensory fibers that innervate the overlying skin.

SENSORY INNERVATION

Sensory innervation of the breast is extremely important; therefore its preservation is desirable in all breast surgery. The skin of the breast is innervated segmentally via a dermatome pattern (Figure 7-2). Intercostal nerves arising from the spinal cord at levels T2 through T6 send forth two major branches (Figure 7-3). One is the anterolateral cutaneous nerve, which emerges between segments of the serratus anterior at the anterior axillary line. The other is the anteromedial cutaneous nerve, which accompanies perforating branches of the internal mammary artery, which arise from beneath the rib margin at the lateral border of the sternum and course somewhat diagonally into and through the pectoralis major origin to innervate the skin of the medial portion of the breast.[1,5,6-9] Each of these cutaneous nerves, the anterolateral and the anteromedial, divides into two branches, coursing laterally and medially, respectively, as their names indicate. The central portion of the breast is innervated from levels T3 through T5 via the anterior branch of the lateral cutaneous and the lateral branch of the anteri-

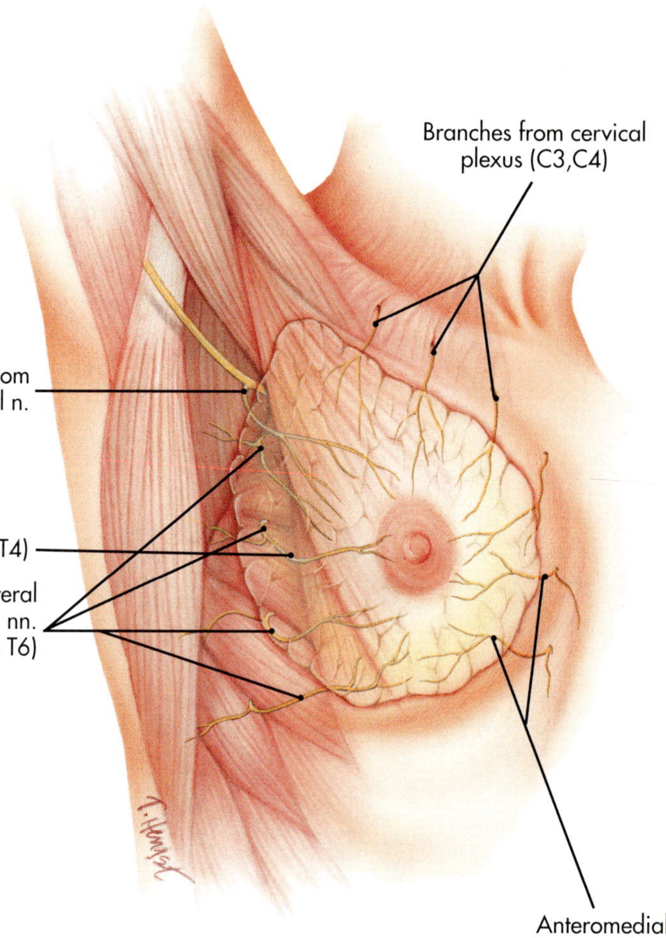

FIGURE 7-4
As shown here, the sensory innervation to the breast arises from the anteromedial nerves T3 to T5 and the anterolateral nerves T2 through T6. The superior aspect of the breast is innervated by branches coursing through the platysma and over the clavicle from the cervical plexus. The sensory innervation of the nipple–areolar complex is derived from the anterior branch of the fourth anterolateral intercostal nerve.

or cutaneous nerves (Figure 7-4). The anterior branch of the fourth lateral cutaneous nerve has been described as "the nerve to the nipple" because it often supplies sensation to the nipple–areola complex (Figure 7-3).[1-4] Care must be taken to avoid disruption or avulsion of these lateral cutaneous nerves during the blunt dissection performed to create the submuscular pocket for breast augmentation. A medial-to-lateral motion will gently stretch and push the nerves in a lateral direction without disrupting them, preserving the sensory innervation of the breast. Supraclavicular nerves C3 and C4 course over the clavicle to innervate the skin of the upper portion of the breast (Figure 7-4).[4,6,7,9,10]

SKIN, SUBCUTANEOUS TISSUE, AND LIGAMENTS

The glandular structure of the breast is contained within two distinct fascial layers. The superficial layer, which is immediately adjacent to and at times indistinguishable from the deep layer of the dermis, begins as an extension of the superficial fascia at the level of the inframammary crease. It extends over the entire surface of the breast to rejoin these layers of fascia at the level of the clavicle (Figure 7-5). The deep layer of the superficial fascia, the posterior "capsule" of the breast, forms the most posterior aspect of the gland, arising from the superficial fascia at the level of the inframammary crease and then rejoining the superficial layer of this fascia superiorly at the level of the clavicle.[1,11] This deep

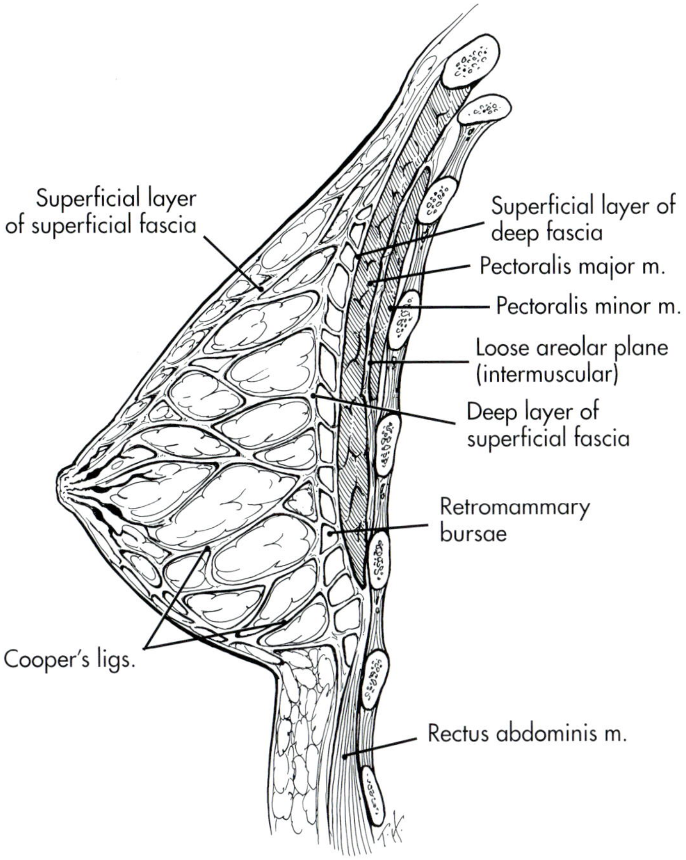

FIGURE 7-5
The fascial anatomy of the breast is shown. The superficial fascia divides at the level of the inframammary crease into superficial and deep layers. The deep layer overlies the loose areolar potential space known as the retromammary bursae; the superficial layer is intimate with the skin itself. Between these two layers arise Cooper's ligaments. Deep to the retromammary bursae is the overlying fascia of the pectoralis major muscle and superior aspect of the anterior rectus sheath.

fascial layer is strong and distinct. Immediately beneath this fascial layer there is a loose areolar plane, commonly known as the retromammary bursae. It is at this anatomic plane that the breast itself moves freely over the pectoralis major muscle, the medial aspect of the serratus anterior muscle, and the uppermost portion of the rectus abdominis and external oblique muscles during exercise and muscular contraction. This fascia is thickest in the most inferior portion, where it is quite inelastic. It thins and becomes more elastic over the pectoralis major and serratus regions. Without appropriate surgical release, the thicker, inelastic quality of the inferior aspect of the fascia in this region leads to high-riding implants in both reconstructive and aesthetic breast surgery.

Cooper's ligaments are fibrous connections extending perpendicularly between the dermis and the superficial layer of the superficial fascia of the breast to the deep layer of the superficial fascia, and even to underlying muscle fascia (Figure 7-5).[1,2,3,8]

UNDERLYING MUSCLE GROUPS

Beneath the deep layer of the superficial fascia comprising the posterior capsule of the breast there are many major muscle groups (Figure 7-1). These include superiorly the inferior aspect of the platysma (its origin), the pectoralis major muscle, the lateral portion of the serratus anterior muscle, the superior aspect of the rectus sheath (rectus abdominis muscle), and the superior aspect of the external oblique muscle. The platysma takes its origin from the fascia over the pectoralis major and deltoid muscles and ascends into the neck to be inserted into the skin of the lower face and mandible. The lateral border of the pectoralis major muscle (in addition to the tail of the breast as it courses upward on the lateral aspect of the pectoralis major) forms the anterior axillary fold. The origin of the pectoralis major muscle is superiorly from the anterior aspect of the medial clavicle, continuing on the lateral sternal border, and ending inferiorly at the seventh costal cartilage. Its fibers also originate directly from the anterior surface of the second through sixth costal cartilages medially, and inferiorly from a small slip that arises from fibers of the anterior layer of the rectus sheath. Adherent pectoral fascia covers the muscle. This begins at the clavicular origin and extends inferiorly to become continuous with the fascia of the abdominal wall. The pectoralis major muscle is inserted into the crest of the greater tubercle of the humerus.[2,5,9]

The pectoralis minor muscle, immediately beneath the pectoralis major muscle and overlying the ribs, originates from the upper outer anterior surface of the third, fourth, and fifth ribs. It attaches to the coracoid process of the scapula. A loose areolar potential space exists between the pectoralis major and minor muscles. This areolar plane separates freely during an axillary approach, allowing the space to be entered surgically for implant placement for augmentation and reconstructive purposes.[1-3,7,8,12]

Superior to the pectoralis minor and beneath the pectoralis major muscles is the small subclavius muscle, originating from the first rib and inserting into the subclavian groove of the clavicle. The serratus anterior muscle occupies the superior lateral aspect of the thorax, beneath the pectoralis major and minor muscles. It originates from the anterior and superior borders of ribs one through eight, and is inserted into the inframedial and inferior borders of the scapula. It forms the medial wall of the axilla. The inferior slips of this muscle origin interdigitate between slips of the external oblique muscle.[1-3,5-7,9]

MOTOR NERVE INNERVATION

The motor innervation to the muscle underlying the breast is quite varied (Figure 7-6). The cervical branch of the facial nerve (cranial nerve VII) innervates the platysma. The pectoralis major muscle is innervated by the lateral pectoral nerve (innervating the upper, medial half of the muscle) and the medial pectoral (innervating the lower, lateral half of the muscle). The lateral pectoral nerve is so named because it arises from the lateral cord of the brachial plexus, and the medial pectoral nerve is so named because it arises from the medial cord of the brachial plexus.[5] In point of fact, the lateral pectoral nerve innervates the more medial portion of the pectoralis muscle, and the medial pectoral nerve innervates the more lateral portion of the pectoralis major muscle. The medial pectoral nerve exits the pectoralis minor muscle to enter the pectoralis major superiorly and then innervates the lower portion of the muscle. The lateral pectoral nerve courses in conjunction with the thoracoacromial vessels to enter the pectoralis major muscle along its deep superior surface, immediately beneath the clavicle. This neurovascular structure, although adherent to the undersurface of the muscle, can be injured from aggressive dissection or retraction during endoscopic pro-

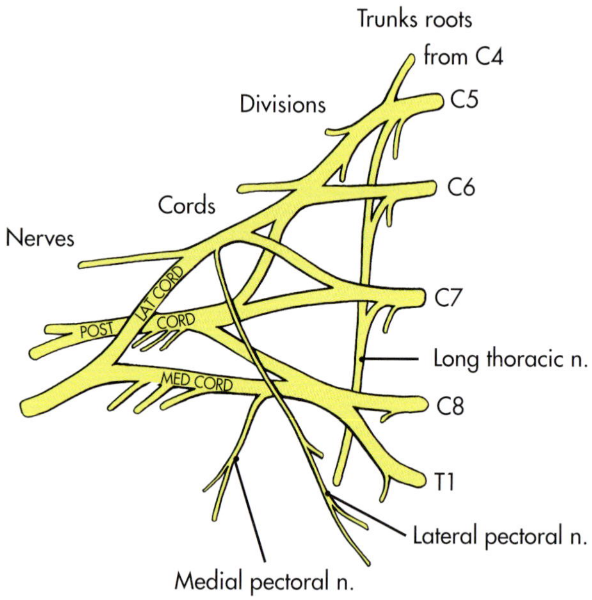

FIGURE 7-6
The motor nerve innervation for the anterior chest musculature is shown. The lateral pectoral nerve, which innervates the superior medial aspect of the pectoralis major muscle, arises from the lateral cord or the brachial plexus. The medial pectoral nerve (lateral to the lateral pectoral nerve) arises from the medial cord and is so named. It innervates the inferior and lateral aspects of the pectoralis major muscle. The long thoracic nerve innervates the serratus anterior muscle. The intercostobrachial nerve, supplying sensation to the upper inner-arm, courses through the axilla.

cedures. The serratus muscle is innervated by the long thoracic nerve and the subclavius is directly innervated by a small branch from the upper trunk of the brachial plexus.[2,3,5,8,9]

BLOOD SUPPLY

The blood supply to the breast is derived from four sources (Figure 7-7). The internal mammary vessels contribute large perforating branches that course beneath the rib margin at the costal border, supplying the medial aspect of the breast. These perforating branches course diagonally as they pierce the space between the costal cartilages, ascend anteriorly and laterally into the pectoralis major muscle, then arborize subsequently into the breast parenchyma and subdermal plexus of the skin. These are resilient vessels as can be attested to by their continued patency following blunt transaxillary breast augmentation. During the blunt dissection for creation of the submuscular pocket for breast augmentation, by sweeping medially and upward the parasternal internal mammary perforator branches can be stretched and still preserved. With endoscopic surgery, they can be individually identified and preserved. If, however, dissection to decrease the intramammary distance requires their division, the blood supply to the pectoralis and overlying breast tissue is not jeopardized because of the significant overlap and redundancy of the multiple vascular territories. The lateral thoracic artery, known as the external mammary artery, supplies vascular branches to the lateral aspect of the breast.

In addition, the third, fourth, and fifth inter-

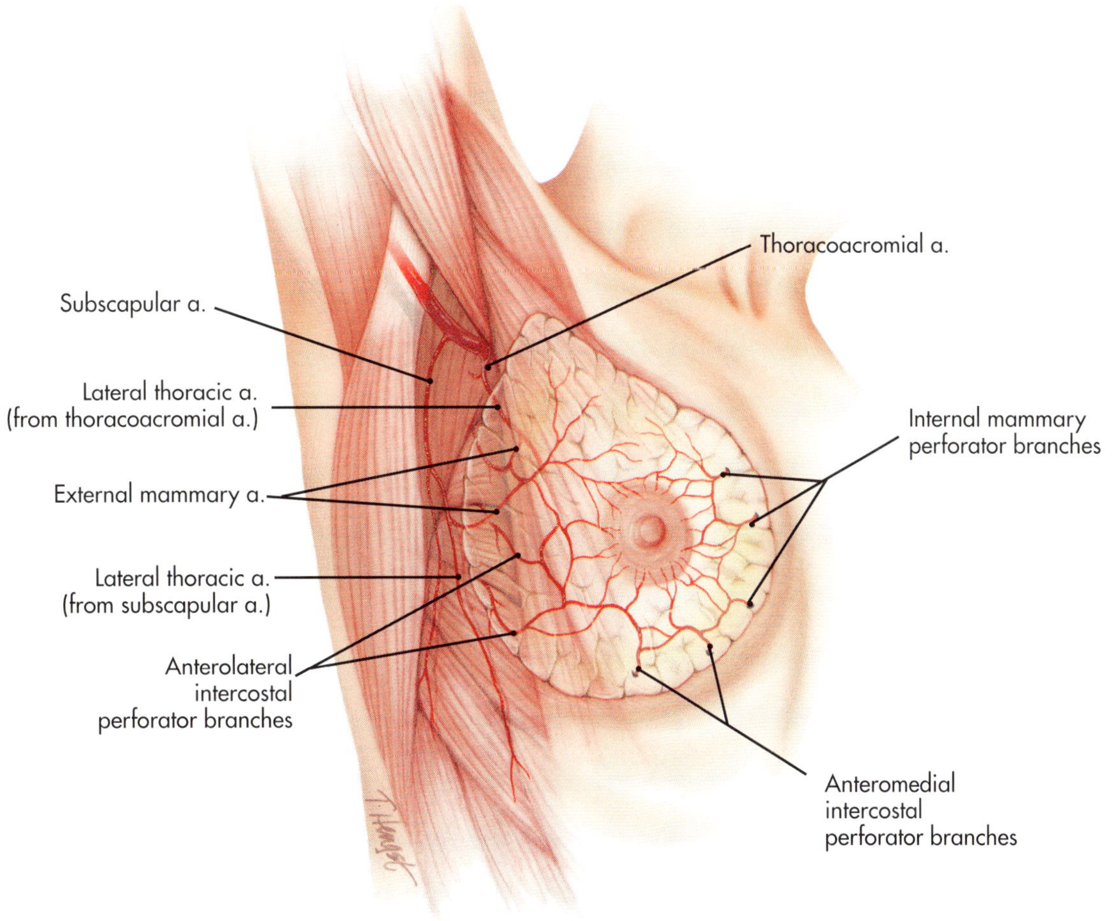

FIGURE 7-7
The blood supply of the breast is derived chiefly from large perforator branches coming from the internal mammary artery, which contribute more than 60% of the blood supply to the breast. The anterolateral intercostal perforator branches supply the lateral aspect of the breast, and the superior aspect of the breast is supplied by the external mammary artery, a continuation of the lateral thoracic artery. The supreme thoracic artery and the pectoral branch of the thoracoacromial artery supply the uppermost portion of the breast.

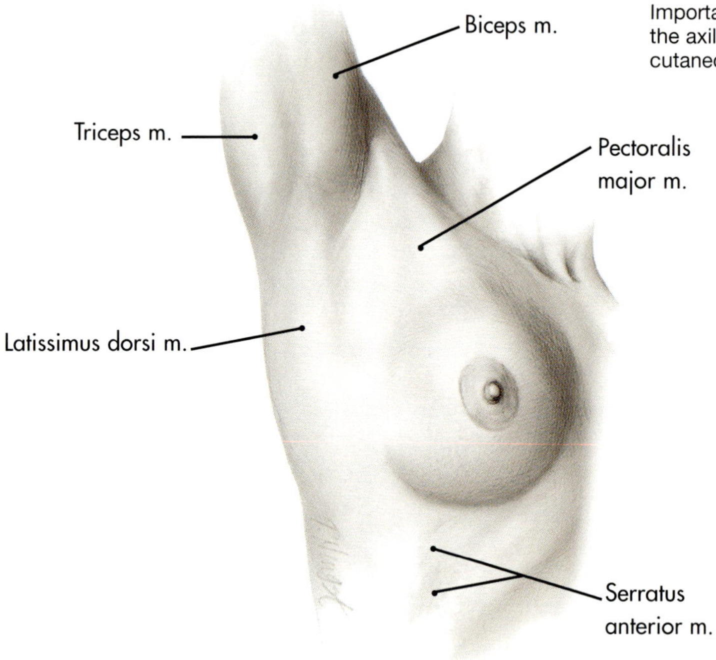

FIGURE 7-8
Important structures in the axilla include the brachial plexus, the axillary vein, the long thoracic nerve, the anteriolateral cutaneous nerves, and the intercostobrachial nerve.

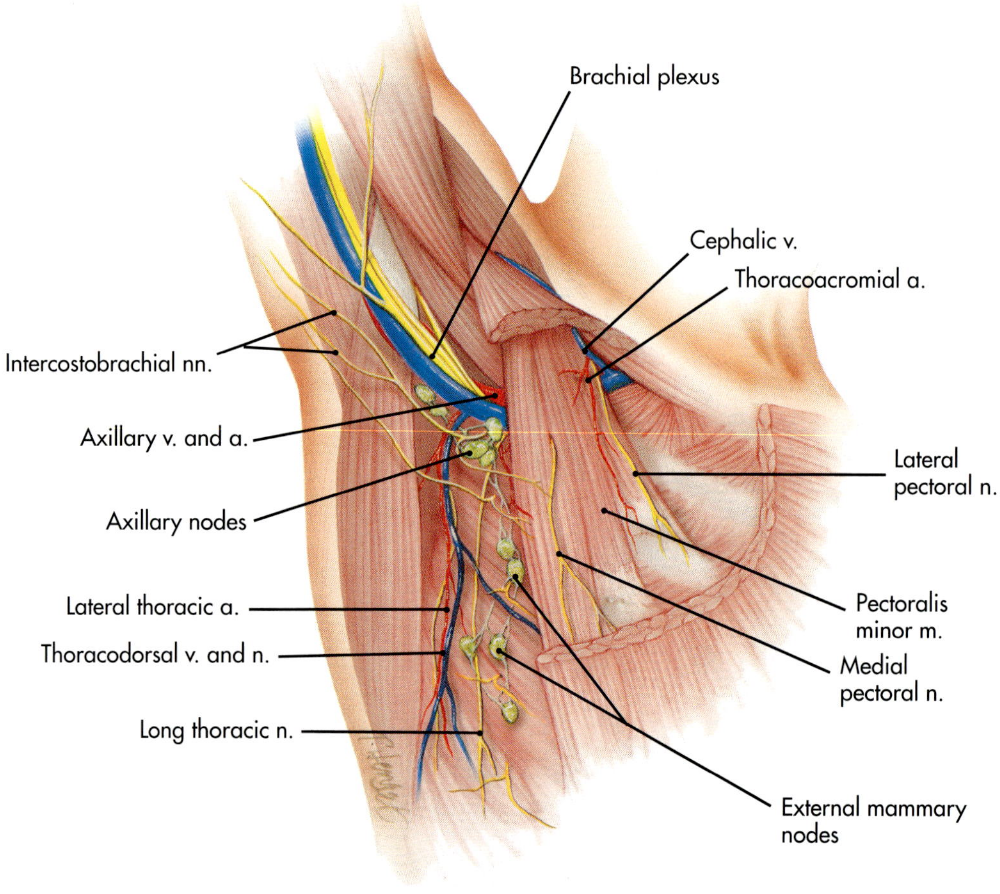

costal arteries send forth anterior lateral and anterior medial intercostal perforating vessels. Finally, branches from the supreme thoracic and pectoral branch of thoracoacromial artery supply the upper pole of the breast.*

LYMPHATICS OF THE BREAST

Lymphatic drainage of the breast is divided into two major basins. The majority of the lymphatic drainage is directed toward the tail of the gland into the axilla. Some of the lymphatic drainage from the central portion of the breast can go directly into the intramuscular nodes (of Rotter) and then into the axillary nodes, or directly into the subscapular nodes and then into the axillary nodes. This nodal basin subsequently drains into the clavicular nodal basin. The internal mammary nodes drain the medial and central aspects of the breast. They are based along the route of the internal mammary arteries.[1,5,7] The lymphatics of the breast parenchyma richly intercommunicate ("Grand Central Station" fashion) in the center of the gland at the nipple–areola complex.

AXILLA

The axilla is a pyramid-shaped recess, whose floor is delineated by the axillary fascia (Figure 7-8). The anterior wall is composed of the pectoralis major and minor muscles; the posterior wall is composed of the scapula and scapular musculature. The serratus anterior muscle forms the floor of the pyramid. The anterior axillary fold is composed of the lateral border of the pectoralis major muscle and Spence's tail of the breast.[1,4] The posterior axillary fold is composed of the teres major and the latissimus dorsi muscles. Many important structures lodge in the axilla: the axillary lymph nodes and the axillary artery and its accompanying vein. The brachial plexus is also found in the apex of the axilla. A number of important sensory nerves, including the intercostal brachial cutaneous nerve and the medial brachial cutaneous nerve, also course through this area. These nerves travel within the axillary fat pad to supply sensation to the upper arm.[5-7,9] They course superficially within the subcutaneous tissues just posterior to the superior aspect of the pectoralis major muscle. Care should be taken to avoid dissection high in the axilla or aggressive upward retraction, either of which could injure these important structures within the axilla. It is not necessary to divide these nerves during the axillary dissection associated with modified radical mastectomy. Knowledge of their location is helpful for the maintainance of sensation to the inner aspect of the upper arm and thorax after breast surgery. Similarly, during the axillary approach for endoscopic breast surgery, their preservation is essential.

*References 1,3,4,7,9,13.

ABDOMEN

TOPOGRAPHY

The boundaries of the abdomen are the costal margins superiorly, the pubic crest inferocentrally, the inguinal ligaments inferolaterally, and the iliac crests laterally (Figure 7-9). Surface anatomic features of note include the umbilicus, which is located at the midline between the anterior superior iliac spines and also at a level between the third and fourth intervertebral discs. The abdominal midline, between the xiphoid process and pubic crest, corresponds to the underlying linea alba, which is the central aponeurotic junction of the abdominal

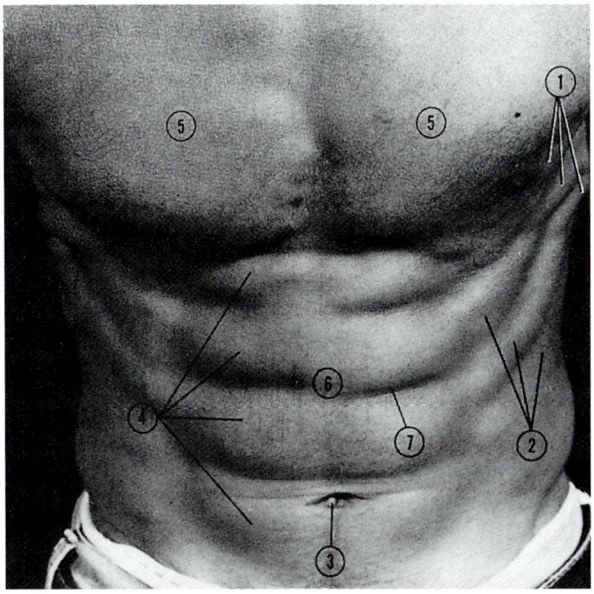

FIGURE 7-9
The abdominal surface anatomy is shown. Important surface anatomic characteristics directly relate to important underlying musculature. 1 Serratus anterior muscle. 2 External oblique muscle. 3 Umbilicus. 4 Rectus abdominis muscle. 5 Pectoralis major muscle. 6 Linea alba. 7 Tendinous insertions.

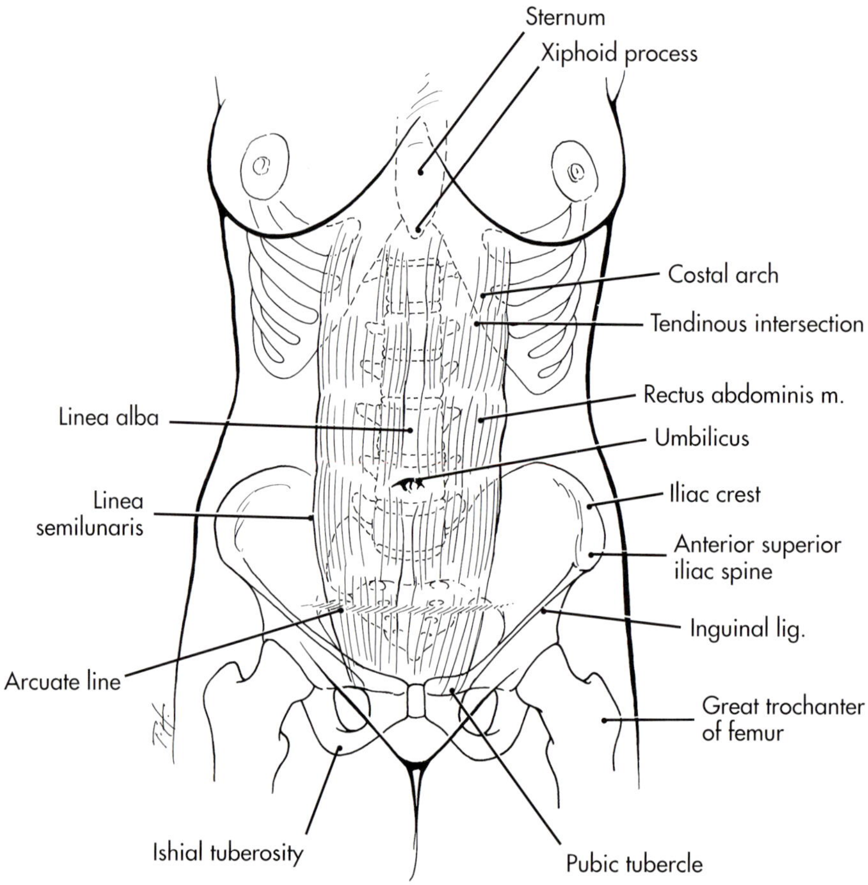

FIGURE 7-10
Deep anatomic structures of the abdomen are shown. Important anatomic landmarks beneath the skin's subcutaneous tissue can be readily visualized and palpated. These include the midline xiphoid process, the costal margins, the anterior superior iliac crest, the pubic tubercle, the inguinal ligament, and the linea semilunaris (the lateral border of the rectus abdominis muscle).

musculature. This midline separates the abdomen into two mirrored halves. The underlying abdominal musculature creates specific topographic characteristics (Figure 7-10). These include the rectus muscle bulges, which are formed by the transverse tendinous inscriptions (insertions) of the rectus muscle. The lateral border of the rectus muscle, corresponding to the lateral border of the rectus sheath, is known as the linea semilunaris. Lateral to this line exists the broad, flattened, lateral abdominal region, which corresponds to the underlying external oblique muscle. The xiphoid process, costal arches, iliac crest, anterior superior iliac spine, and pubic tubercle are the readily palpable bony anatomic landmarks.[5-8]

SENSORY INNERVATION

The cutaneous sensory innervation of the abdomen is segmental via a dermatome pattern in a manner similar to the sensory innervation of the breast (Figure 7-3). These nerves originate from the spinal cord and divide immediately into a dorsal root to supply sensation to the posterior aspect of the trunk (via medial and lateral branches) and into a ventral ramus, which continues anteriorly and gives off the so-called lateral cutaneous branch. This again divides into anterior and posterior branches. Finally, the continuation of the anterior branch divides into medial and lateral terminal branches. This "segmental" sensory pattern corresponding to dermatome distribution is consistent throughout the abdominal wall.[2,3,6-8]

Specific anatomic structures of reference include the innervation of the nipple–areolar complex (previously mentioned) at the level of T4, the umbilicus at the level of T10, and the inguinal and pubic areas corresponding to the lowest thoracic (T12), lumbar, (L1 to L2), and sacral dermatomes (S1, S2, S3) (Figures 7-1 and 7-4). In

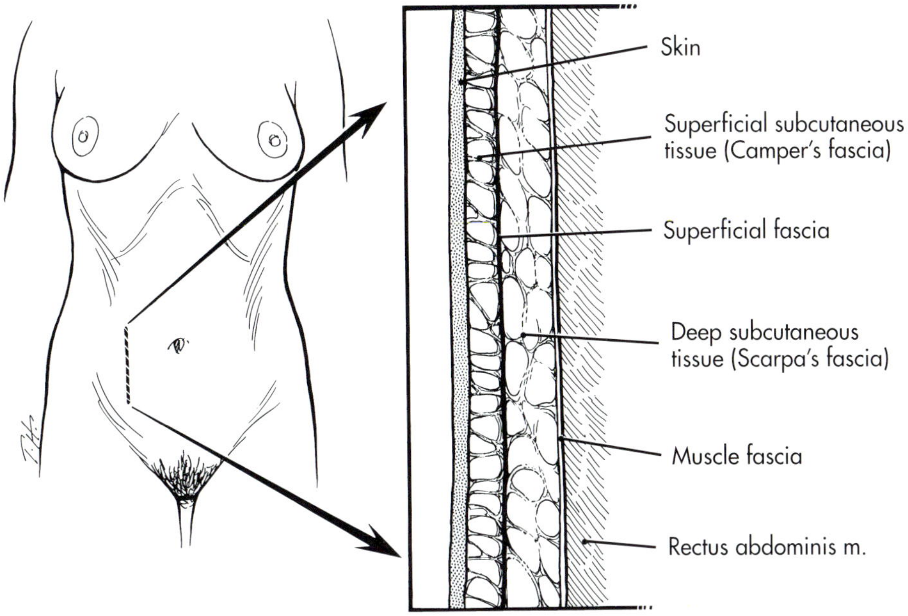

FIGURE 7-11
The superficial fascia is a strong, discrete layer that is continuous from the inguinal ligament inferiorly to the inframammary crease superiorly. It separates the superficial fat from the more loosely organized deeper fat layer.

addition, the iliohypogastric nerve (L1) provides sensation to the superpubic region.[2-5,7]

SKIN, SUBCUTANEOUS TISSUE, AND LIGAMENTS

Underlying the abdominal skin, within the subcutaneous fat, are two distinct fat layers separated by a thin yet strongly resilient fascia (Figure 7-11). This fascial layer (within the subcutaneous tissue itself) forms a continuous sheet and is known as Scarpa's fascia.[2,3,5,11] It extends from the level of the inframammary fold to the lowermost portion of the abdominal region to the level of the inguinal crease. Inferiorly, it becomes continuous with the inguinal ligaments. Superiorly, it ascends to a point above the costal arches and partially contributes to the formation of the inframammary crease. Scarpa's fascia is an integral part of the system of fascial condensations termed by some, and emphasized by Lockwood, as the *superficial fascial system*.[11,14] As pointed out by Fodor, the entire superficial fascial system is the human derivative of the panniculus carnosus that is widely present in primates.[15] The above-mentioned Scarpa's fascia is a well-defined layer of impressive strength. During abdominal operations, closing this fascia as a distinct layer can help prevent formation of a depressed scar, which otherwise can be created by the postoperative retraction of this anatomic structure. In addition, this surgical maneuver transfers tension away from the skin closure and results in a finer scar.

MUSCULATURE

The musculature of the abdominal wall is composed of a number of large paired muscles (Figure 7-12). This creates a symmetric configuration of the abdomen, with a central separation created by the midline linea alba. The rectus abdominis muscles are perhaps the most important and best studied with respect to abdominal body contouring and reconstructive surgical procedures. The rectus muscle originates from the pubic crest and the interpubic ligament and inserts into the costal arch, primarily into the cartilaginous portions of the fifth, sixth, and seventh ribs and the xiphoid process. Typically, the tendinous inscriptions divide the muscle belly transversely into three divisions. They firmly attach the rectus muscle to the anterior rectus sheath. These inscriptions are not necessarily symmetric in their location from one rectus muscle to the other. One of them is usually found at the level of the umbilicus and another close to the costal margin. The third usually exists midway between these two. Often another can be present as an incomplete tendinous insertion between the umbilicus and the pubis.[2,3,5,9]

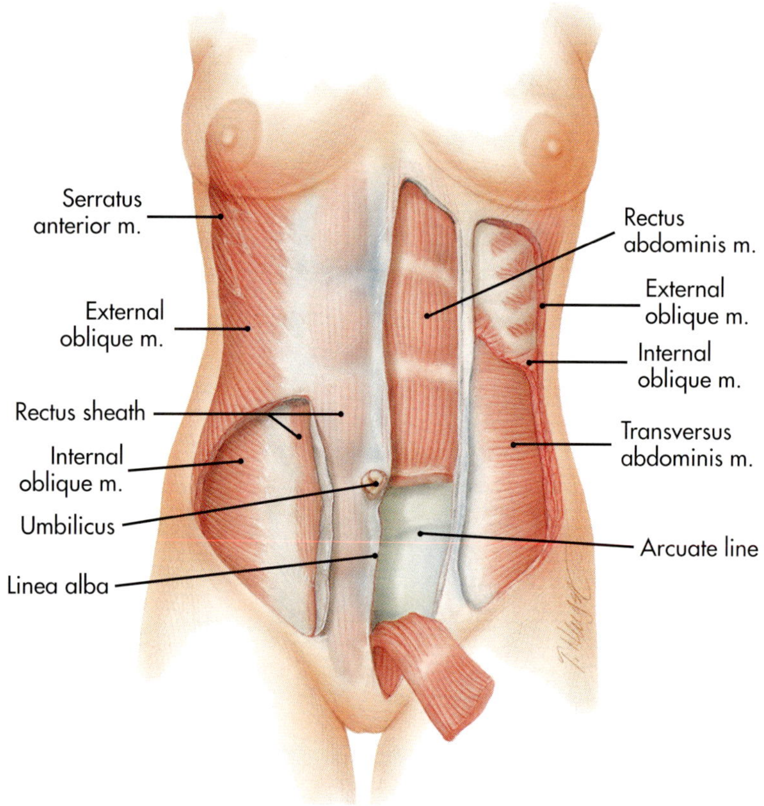

FIGURE 7-12
The abdominal wall musculature is shown. The paired rectus abdominis, external oblique, internal oblique, and transversus abdominis muscles represent the major muscle groups of the abdominal wall. Tendinous inscriptions divide the rectus muscle into discrete bulges. The external oblique, internal oblique, and transversus abdominis muscles converge to form the anterior and posterior rectus sheaths. These join in the midline to form the linea alba. The linea semilunaris represents the line at which the three abdominal muscles combine to form the anterior and posterior rectus sheaths. The arcuate line (line of Douglas) exists in an infraumbilical location that depicts the transformation of the posterior sheath from one composed of the internal oblique and transversus abdominis muscles superiorly to one composed only of transversalis fascia inferiorly.

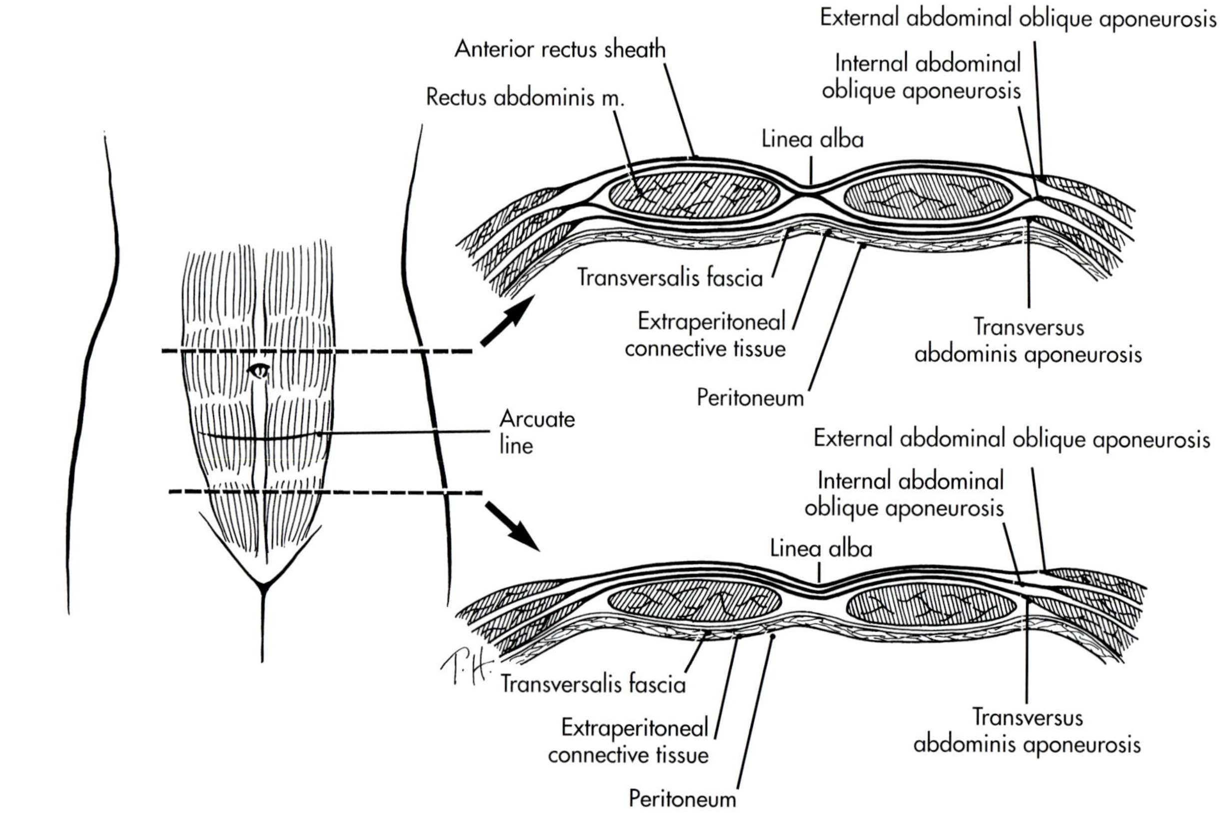

FIGURE 7-13
The rectus sheath superior and inferior to the arcuate line is shown. The top drawing demonstrates the anatomy of the rectus sheath superior to the arcuate line. The anterior rectus sheath is composed of contributions from the external oblique and internal oblique aponeurosis. The posterior rectus sheath is composed of contributions from the internal oblique muscle and transversus abdominis aponeurosis. Inferior to the line of Douglas the external oblique and internal oblique muscles and transversus abdominis aponeurosis combine to form the anterior rectus sheath. The posterior rectus sheath is composed of transversalis fascia only.

Lateral to the rectus abdominis, the abdominal wall is composed of three muscle layers: external oblique, internal oblique, and transversus abdominis. The tendinous portions of these muscles, as they course medially, converge and then divide again to form the anterior and posterior rectus sheaths (Figure 7-13). Their configuration is quite distinct above and below the arcuate line, also known as the semicircular line of Douglas. The arcuate line is approximately at the level of the anterior superior iliac spines. Above the level of the semicircular line the anterior rectus sheath is composed of contributions from the external and internal oblique muscles. Superiorly, the posterior rectus sheath is formed by contributions from the internal oblique muscle and transversus abdominis muscle, which itself is lined by the transversalis fascia. Below the arcuate line, however, the posterior rectus sheath is formed only by the transversalis fascia. In the same area (inferior to the arcuate line), the anterior rectus sheath is formed by tendinous contributions from all three muscle layers.[2,3,5,6] This is significant because disruption of the rectus muscle below the arcuate line can lead to weakness and potential hernia formation of the abdominal wall. As mentioned earlier, the linea semilunaris is defined as the lateral border of the rectus abdominis muscle. This is the line at which the external oblique and other muscles change from their muscular to their tendinous portions.

MOTOR INNERVATION

The motor nerve supply of the abdominal musculature is also segmental and is derived from intercostal nerves T7 to T12 (Figure 7-14). The anterior cutaneous intercostal nerves are accompanied by the intercostal arteries as they course through the abdominal wall.

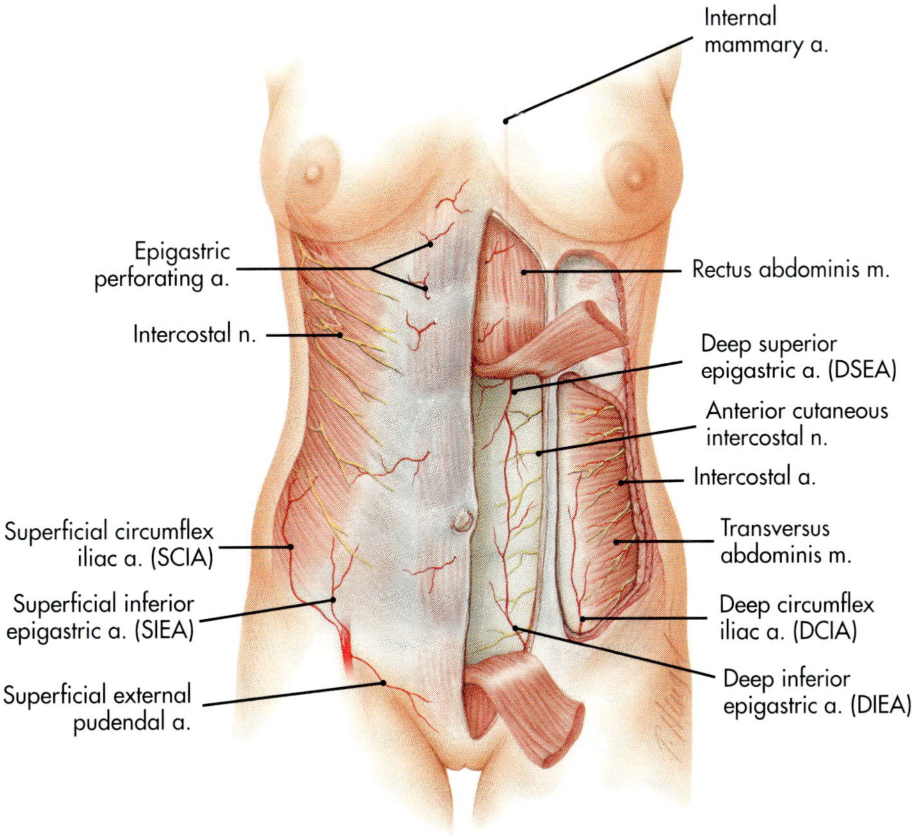

FIGURE 7-14
The motor innervation of the abdominal wall is segmental. The neurovascular structures enter through the posterior aspect of the rectus sheath to supply the rectus muscle segmentally. Before entering the rectus sheath the segmental motor nerves innervate the three layers of the abdominal wall: the external oblique, the internal oblique, and the transversus abdominis muscles.

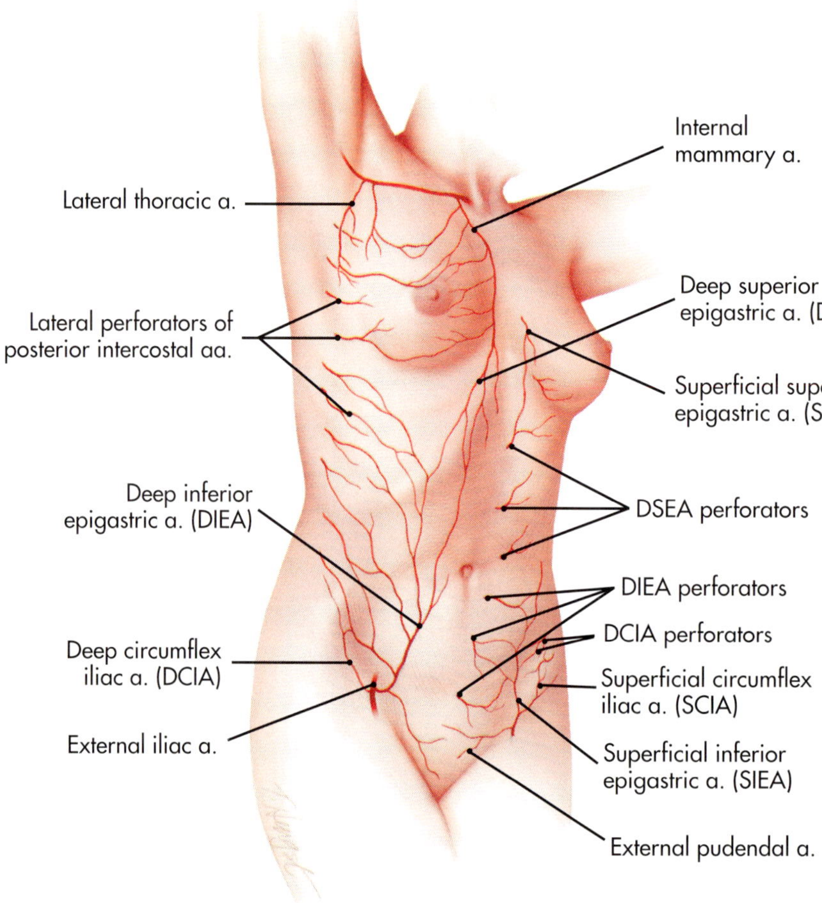

FIGURE 7-15

Vascular supply of the abdominal wall is shown. The vascular supply of the skin, subcutaneous tissue, and deeper structures is composed of both a superficial and a deep system. The deep system arises from the internal mammary artery that continues inferiorly as the deep superior epigastric artery *(DSEA)* and from the external iliac artery that sends forth the deep inferior epigastric artery *(DIEA)*. These anastomose freely within the rectus abdominis muscle. The deep circumflex iliac artery *(DCIA)* arises from the external iliac artery as well. The superficial system is composed of centrally located DSEA and DIEA perforator branches. The superficial superior epigastric artery *(SSEA)* arises beneath the costal margin in the region of the xiphoid process. The superior lateral vascular supply comes from the lateral perforator branches of the posterior intercostal arteries. The superficial inferior epigastric artery *(SIEA)* and superficial circumflex iliac artery *(SCIA)* course in a superior lateral manner to anastomose freely with the many perforating vessels of the abdominal wall.

BLOOD SUPPLY

The blood supply of the abdominal wall and its overlying integument consists of a complex network of interconnecting vessels from a number of distinct major sources (Figure 7-15). These important vascular arcades liberally link the aorta and its main branches in the neck (the subclavian artery) with the groin (external iliac artery). This rich vascular plexus is created by a number of longitudinal anastomoses between the major vessels, which demonstrate significant overlap, thus allowing abdominal contouring procedures to be performed without much danger of vascular compromise.

The main longitudinal anastomoses occur between the deep superior and deep inferior epigastric arteries. This anastomosis takes place within the rectus muscle itself at about the level of the umbilicus. The deep superior epigastric artery (DSEA) is a continuation of the internal mammary artery that originates directly from the subclavian artery. The deep inferior epigastric artery (DIEA) is a major branch of the external iliac artery and is the dominant vascular supply to the abdominal wall. From this rich vascular axis, multiple muscular perforator branches course, which are particularly prominent and of large diameter in the periumbilical region. These perforating vessels supply the overlying subcutaneous tissue and dermis. They anastomose liberally with the lateral segmental vessels, which course in an inferomedial direction, and are contributions from the intercostal arteries.[10,16-18]

These intercostal arteries arise from the dorsal aorta and course anteriorly into the ventral trunk to anastomose with the perforating vessels from the deep epigastric system. In addition, the intercostal vessels also anastomose longitudinally with branches ascending from the deep circumflex iliac artery (DCIA) in the inferior lateral trunk. The DCIA arises from the external iliac artery. These segmental vessels course between the middle and innermost layers of the abdominal musculature and provide vascular supply to each layer of the abdominal musculature and, in essence, perfuse all layers of the abdominal wall from the peritoneum to the overlying skin. The intercostal segmental arteries course medially into the ventral torso between the internal oblique and the transversus abdominis muscles. As already mentioned, they accompany the lowermost six intercostal nerves. The uppermost vessels course upward, paralleling the costal margin. The middle vessels take a more transverse course, and the inferior vessels course in an inferomedial direction. As noted, these vessels anastomose with the large perforator branches from the deep epigastric system. The most inferior intercostal arteries directly anastomose with branches of the DCIA, particularly its ascending branch, as noted by Taylor.[10,19]

The deep epigastric vessels, superior and inferior (DSEA and DIEA), approach and enter the rectus muscle from its deep surface. The DIEA arises from the external iliac artery and courses medially to enter the deep surface of the rectus muscle below the level of the umbilicus. The DSEA enters the muscle inferior to the costal margin. Small branches of both the DIEA and DSEA fan out laterally to anastomose with the intercostal vessels entering the rectus sheath posteriorly.[16-18]

Major superficial vessels also have important anastomoses. These include the superficial inferior epigastric artery (SIEA), which arises from the external iliac artery. It courses superiorly from the groin to anastomose with branches from the medial perforating vessels of the DIEA as well as the inferior lateral perforator branches of the posterior intercostal vessels and also with perforator branches from the DCIA. In addition, the superficial superior epigastric artery (SSEA) arises below the costal margin as a very large cutaneous branch, from the DSEA.[18-20]

Of clinical significance are the large muscle perforator branches coursing from the DIEA and the DSEA and the anastomoses between them (Figure 7-16). These large perforating vessels are important in transverse rectus abdominis muscle (TRAM) flap breast reconstructive procedures. They supply the cutaneous paddle of the rectus muscle used either as a pedicle flap or as a free tissue transfer. As they emerge from the anterior surface of the rectus sheath, they supply not only the sheath but, more importantly, the overlying subcutaneous tissues and skin. The largest of these perforators are usually found in the periumbilical area.[16,17,19] In abdominoplasty, or in other abdominal operations during which these vessels are divided, the vitality of the abdominal skin and subcutaneous tissue is maintained only by lateral vascular branches, which arise segmentally from the intercostal arteries. These course in an inferomedial direction (Figure 7-17).[21]

It is evident that the cutaneous and subcutaneous arteries of the abdomen are many and varied, providing a rich vascular supply to the region (Figure 7-15). The central and inferior abdominal area is supplied by branches from the SSEA, DSEA, SIEA, superficial circumflex iliac artery (SCIA), and most inferiorly by the external pudendal artery. These vessels anastomose freely with branches from the lateral perforator branches of the posterior intercostal arteries that course around the ventral trunk in an inferomedial direction to provide the vascular supply to the skin and subcutaneous tissues over the thorax, the flank, and the inguinal region. The lateral cutaneous perforators of the posterior intercostal arteries exit the muscle and enter the subcutaneous tissue in the midaxillary line. The location of the large perforating branches from the DSEA and DIEA arcade exit through the anterior rectus sheath in a paramedian distribution.[16,19] Again, these are most numerous and are of largest caliber in the periumbilical area. If they need to be divided care should be taken to surgically control these vessels because they have a tendency to retract beneath the anterior rectus sheath.

The venous drainage of the abdomen parallels the arterial supply (Figure 7-17). The veins are not

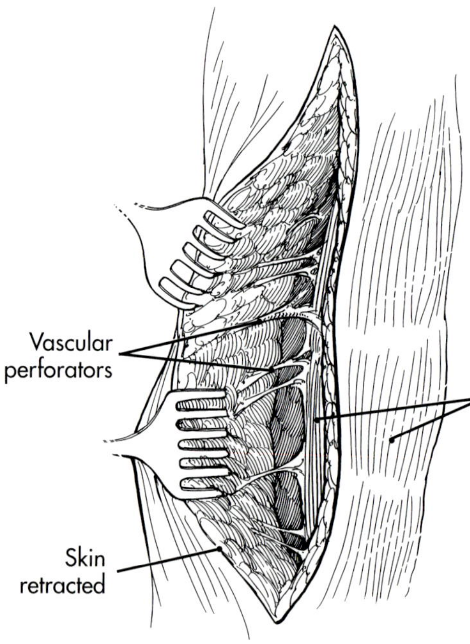

FIGURE 7-16
The vascular perforator branches from the rectus sheath are shown. Important perforating vessels from both the deep inferior epigastric artery *(DIEA)* and deep superior epigastric artery *(DSEA)* are found to be most numerous in the periumbilical region.

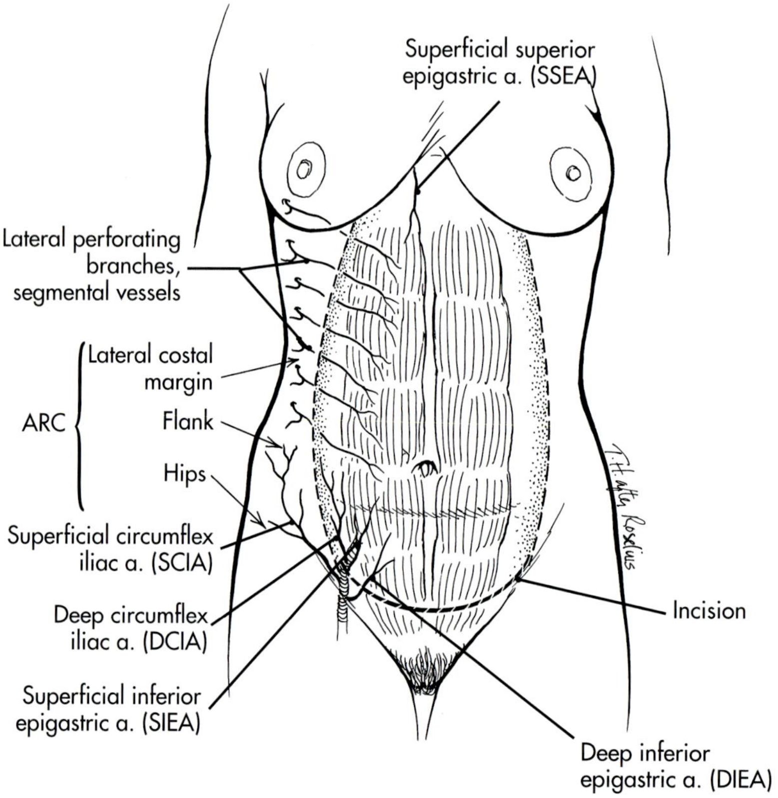

FIGURE 7-17
The vascular supply to the abdomen following abdominoplasty is significantly altered because of the division of all the important rectus perforating vessels. The central abdomen becomes completely dependent on the anterior branches of the lateral perforating segmental vessels. The inferior lateral aspect of the abdomen remains perfused by the superficial circumflex iliac artery *(SCIA)* and deep circumflex iliac artery *(DCIA)*.

necessarily immediately adjacent to but course in near proximity to the subcutaneous arteries. This relationship is maintained until the vessels approach the deep fascia, where they become intimately associated.

SUMMARY

In addition to all the important new perspectives given by the endoscopic technique in plastic surgery, there is an aspect worth mentioning that adds excitement and even new scientific interest—paradoxical as this may seem in conjunction with a discipline as established and devoid of surprises as anatomy. Through its intrinsic approach of visualization from the inside, endoscopy affords the surgeon an unprecedented view of anatomic structures from the depth to the surface, from the inside to the outside, and from below upward. This completely new perspective has the effect of the endowing this visualization—even for the experienced surgeon—with an excitingly fresh perception and sense of rediscovery.

REFERENCES

1. Bostwick J: *Anatomy and physiology in plastic and reconstructive breast surgery,* St Louis, 1990, Quality Medical Publishing.
2. Gardner E, Gray DJ, O'Rahilly R: *Anatomy of regional study of human structure,* ed 4, Philadelphia, 1975, WB Saunders.
3. Hollinshead WH: *Textbook of anatomy,* ed 3, New York, 1974, Harper and Rowe.
4. Little JW III, Spear SC, Romm S: *Reduction mammoplasty and mastopexy.* In Smith JW, Aston SJ, editors: *Grabb & Smith's plastic surgery,* ed 4, Boston, 1991, Little, Brown.
5. Woodburne RT: *Essentials of human anatomy,* ed 6, New York, 1978, Oxford University Press.
6. Anderson JE: *Grant's atlas of anatomy,* ed 7, Baltimore, 1978, Williams & Wilkins.
7. Clemente CD: *Anatomy: a regional atlas of the human body,* Philadelphia, 1975, Lea and Febiger.
8. Pansky B: *Review of gross anatomy,* New York, 1979, Macmillan.
9. Spalteholz W: *Hand atlas of human anatomy,* vols 2 and 3, ed 2, Philadelphia, 1906, JB Lippincott.
10. Taylor GI: In discussion of RamastrySS, Tucker JB, Swart WM, et al. The internal oblique muscle flap: an anatomical and clinical study, *Plast Reconstr Surg* 73:731, 1984.
11. Lockwood T: Superficial fascia system (SFS) of the trunk and extremities: a new concept, *Plast Reconstr Surg* 87(6):1009, 1991.
12. McMinn RMH, Hutchings RT: *Color atlas of human anatomy,* Chicago, 1977, Year Book Medical Publishers.
13. Anson BJ, Wright RR: Blood supply of the mammary gland, *Surg Gynecol Obstet* 26:468, 1939.
14. Lockwood T: Transverse flank, thigh, buttock lift with superficial fascial suspension, *Plast Reconstr Surg* 187(6): 1019, 1991.
15. Fodor PB: From the panniculus carnosus (PC) to the superficial fascia system (SFS) (editorial), *Aesth Plast Surg* 17:179, 1993.
16. Boyd JB, Taylor GI, Corlett RJ: The vascular territory of the superficial epigastric and the deep inferior epigastric arteries, *Plast Reconstr Surg* 73:1, 1984.
17. Taylor GI, Watterson PA, Zelt RG: *The vascular anatomy of the anterior abdominal wall: the basis for flap design.* In Bostwick J, Drukker S, editors: *Perspectives of plastic surgery,* vol 5, St. Louis, 1991, Quality Medical Publishing.
18. Watterson PA, Bostwick J III, Hester TR Jr: Analysis of the complications of the TRAM flap. Presented at the Annual Meeting of the American Association of Plastic Surgeons, Hot Springs, VA, April 1990.
19. Moon HK, Taylor IG: The vascular anatomy of rectus abdominis musculocutaneous flaps based on the deep superior epigastric system, *Plast Reconstr Surg* 82(5):815, 1988.
20. Taylor GI, Corlett RJ, Boyd JB: The extended deep inferior epigastric flap: a clinical technique, *Plast Reconstr Surg* 72:751, 1983.
21. Matarasso A: Abdominoplasty, *Clin Plast Surg* 16:2, 1989.

CHAPTER 8

Evaluation of Breast Prosthesis Integrity

Gustavo A. Colon

Mammoscopy or endoscopic evaluation of breast implants is only part of the total evaluation of patients who are concerned about the condition of their breast implants. The patients seen in our office practice are usually our own or those of other physicians who wish to have their implants evaluated.

Because of the increased anxiety levels in these patients the physician must show a great deal of personal concern. Many of these patients have no problems and are seeking evaluation of their breast prostheses. The concerns of these patients can usually be handled very easily by routine mammograms, and they do not need to have further evaluation if there is no symptomatology, no physical problems, and no evidence either clinically or radiographically of ruptured implants.

Patients who have perceived problems either because of local conditions, such as capsular contracture or pain, or even fibrocystic changes in the breasts may need further evaluation, with the possibility of having further imaging studies done, such as echograms, xeromammograms, and magnetic resonance imaging (MRI).[1,2] Many of these patients may have ruptured implants with symptomatology that they may anecdotally relate to the breast implants. Patients who have a questionable mammogram or other imaging study that reveals the possibility of a ruptured implant must be evaluated for the possibility of implant exchange or must have endoscopic evaluation for the condition of the breast implants.[3,4] It is important that these patients be made aware that these are invasive procedures of the breast and that rupture of the implant could occur during either procedure. If an implant is found to be broken at the time of endoscopic evaluation, then explantation and implant exchange with or without capsulectomy is performed immediately. In patients who are candidates for breast implant evaluation, therefore, a complete history and physical examination must be done prior to considering endoscopic evaluation to assess the condition of the implants. An appropriate noninvasive imaging workup should be done as indicated,[5] and there should be multiple detailed and documented consultations to establish the appropriate treatment or surgical program for these patients. Obviously, none of these operative procedures are emergency measures, even if an implant has ruptured. Of course, appropriate informed consent and releases must be obtained from the patient when any operative procedure is contemplated.

The equipment used is a 5-mm, 25-degree angle, modified arthroscope with a videocamera fiberoptic light attached (Figure 8-1). It is best to perform the procedure with minimal fluid irrigation, which is used primarily to clear blood and for debridement at the tip of the endoscope. A small periareolar incision is made and blunt dissection is gently performed through the subcutaneous and breast tissue down to the capsule (Figures 8-2 and 8-3). An insulated electrocautery is used to incise the capsular tissue. The endoscope is then inserted with the blunt obturator, and with gentle probing the instrument is placed between the prosthesis and the capsule (Figure 8-4). The image is then seen on the video and recorded for future reference.

The examination of an intact mammary prosthesis reveals a domelike shape that can easily be noticed as the instrument glides over the implant. The glistening capsule is easily identified (Figures 8-5 and 8-6). If the implant is ruptured the endoscope will go directly into the gel; therefore, the smooth edge of the implant will not be seen (Figures 8-7 and 8-8). In some broken implants the outer envelope can easily be visualized (Figure 8-9).

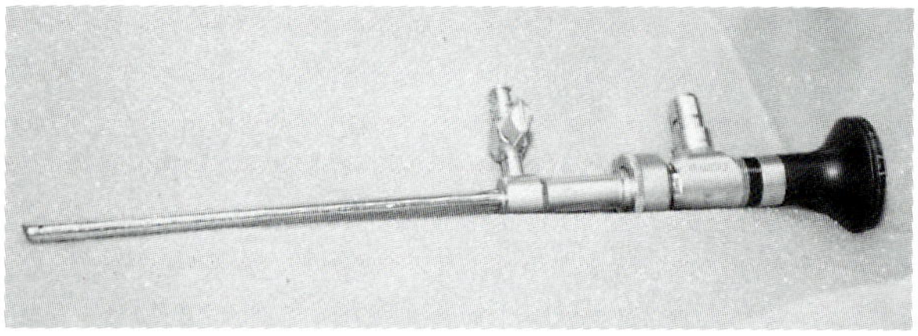

FIGURE 8-1
A 5-mm, 25-degree angle endoscope is shown.

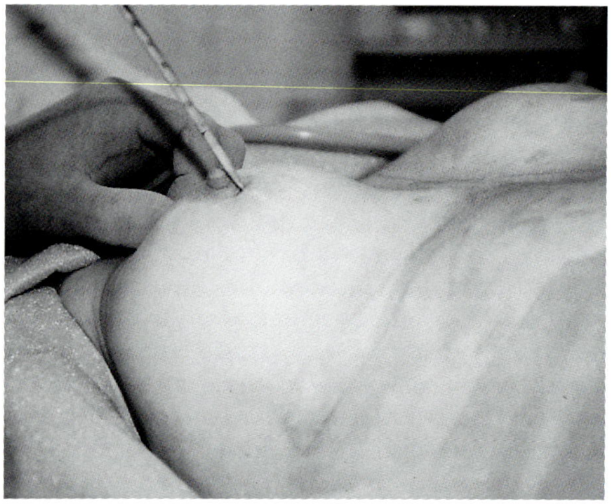

FIGURE 8-2
A blunt instrument used for dissection down to the capsule is shown.

In polyurethane implants the irregular surface of the gel's outer envelope is seen after the polyurethane has separated (Figure 8-10).

The surgical procedures of endoscopy and possible explantation are usually performed on an outpatient basis and can be done with local anesthesia and sedation or general anesthesia. The endoscopic procedure is videotaped to evaluate the intracapsular condition of the breast implants. Once the evaluation is done the appropriate surgical procedure can be performed. If the implant is found to be intact and no further surgery is indicated, the procedure is terminated. However, if the patient wishes to have the implant exchanged the procedure is then continued by doing either a capsulotomy or a capsulectomy after removal of the implant. I prefer to do a capsulotomy in nonruptured implants and a capsulectomy in implants that have any type of silicone extravasation or leak. A saline implant, textured or smooth, is then used for the reconstruction. I prefer to insert the implants below the pectoralis and serratus muscles as a complete sheath if this can be achieved, particularly in the implants that have previously been placed in a prepectoral plane. The use of a textured implant is preferred for this submuscular approach; should the implant need to be placed anterior to the pectoralis fascia in the prepectoral plane, a smooth-shelled saline implant is used. These implants are overinflated to minimize the wrinkling effect that might be felt from the implant shell. It is best to explain to these patients that in all these saline implants, particularly those that are placed in the prepectoral plane, some wrinkling and irregularity may be felt. The operative procedure is continued in the surgeon's usual technique. The removed implants are set aside, and the implants and the capsule are videotaped and photographed for documentation purposes. Should there be evidence of other pathologic areas in the breast tissue, the capsule, or the surrounding tissue, a biopsy should be performed and sent for pathologic examination.

Because of Occupational Safety and Health Administration (OSHA) regulations the implants are soaked in sterilizing solution for 24 hours and then sent to a pathologist for independent evaluation. Again, after appropriate sterilization, the implants may be returned to the patient, or to whomever the patient designates, or they may be destroyed.

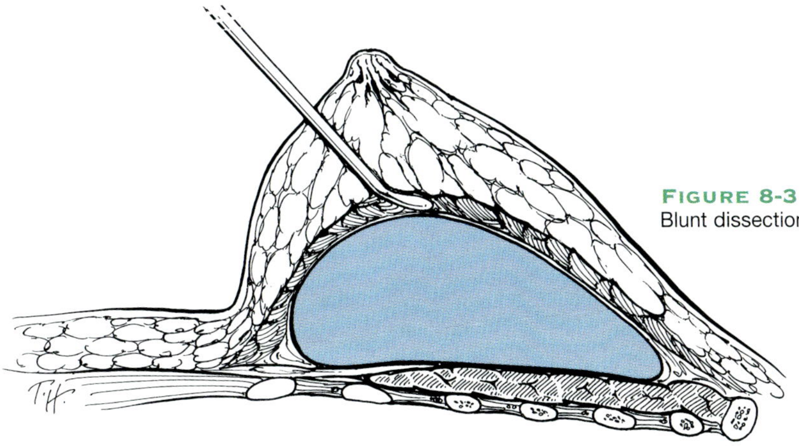

FIGURE 8-3
Blunt dissection to the capsule is shown.

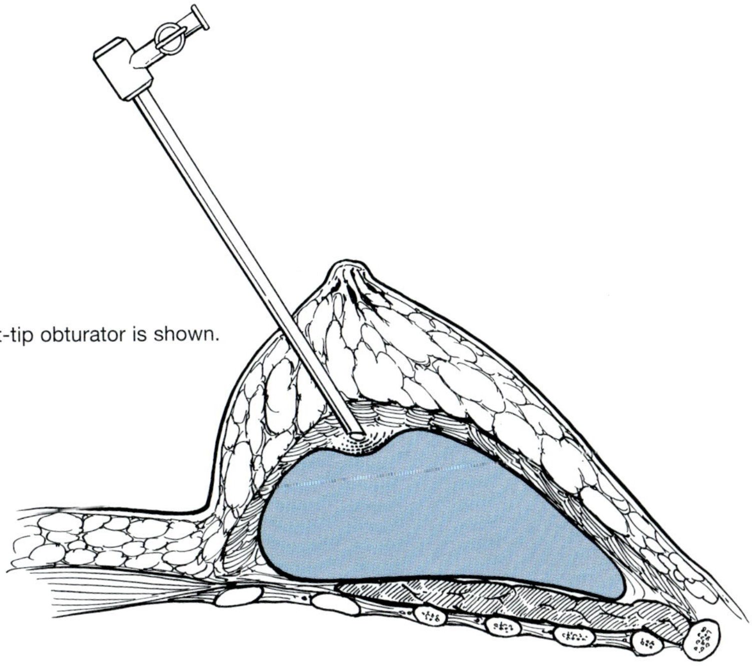

FIGURE 8-4
Insertion of an endoscope with a blunt-tip obturator is shown.

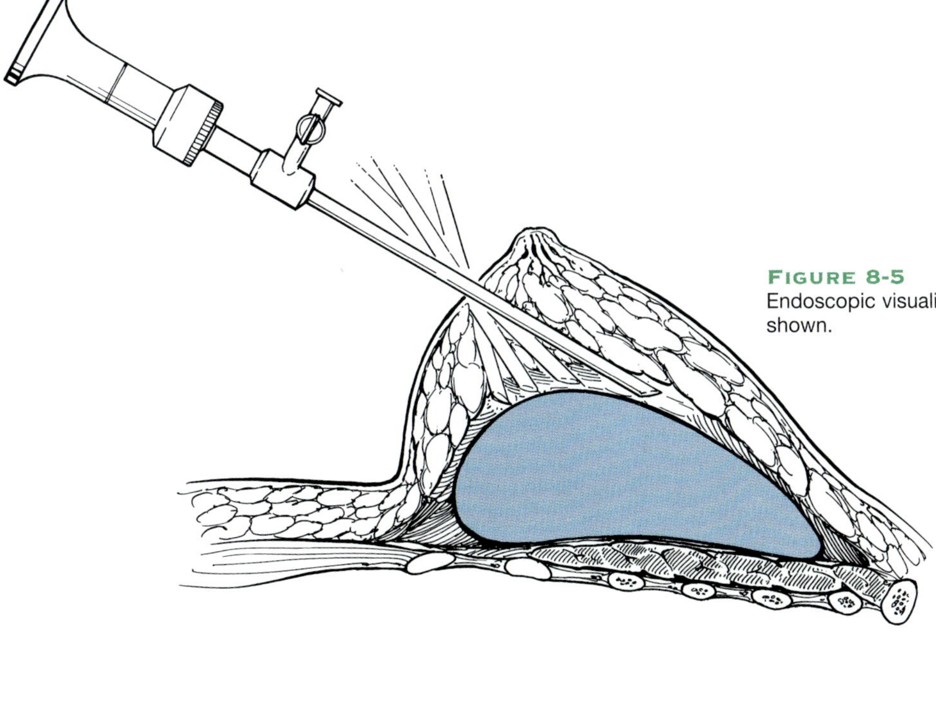

FIGURE 8-5
Endoscopic visualization of the intracapsular contents is shown.

Breast implants come under the heading of "Other Potential Infectious Material" in OSHA regulations (Federal Register, Vol. 26, No. 235, December 6, 1991) and thus are considered to be contaminated hazardous waste. They are regulated as hazardous waste and must be decontaminated and sterilized before they can be returned to the patient with instructions for the care and disposal of biohazardous material. The implants must also be in a leak-proof container that is appropriately labeled when returned. In 1991 OSHA placed in the Federal Register appropriate guidelines for disposal of potentially infectious material.

Under the Food and Drug Administration's (FDA) Safe Medical Devices Act of 1990, breast implants are considered to be a medical device that needs to be reported. The Safe Medical Devices Act regulates any facility, hospital, ambulatory surgical facility, nursing home, and outpatient treatment facility in which there is any type of adverse occurrence and where there is information that reasonably suggests that there is a probability that the

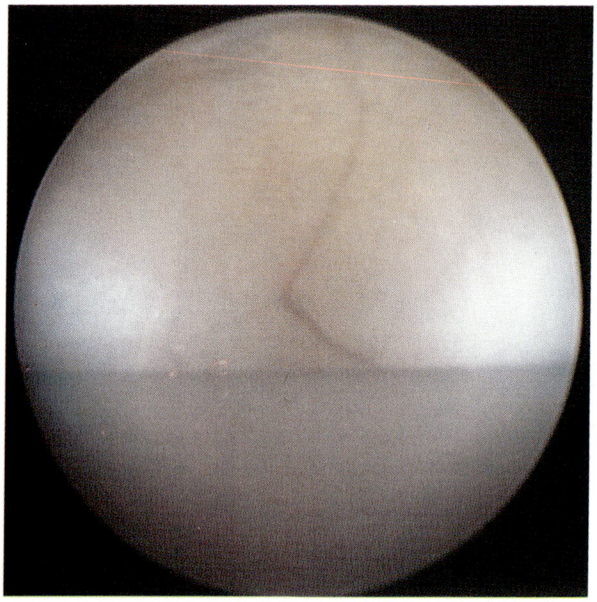

FIGURE 8-6
The implant edge can be seen inferiorly in the capsule with its vascularity shown superiorly.

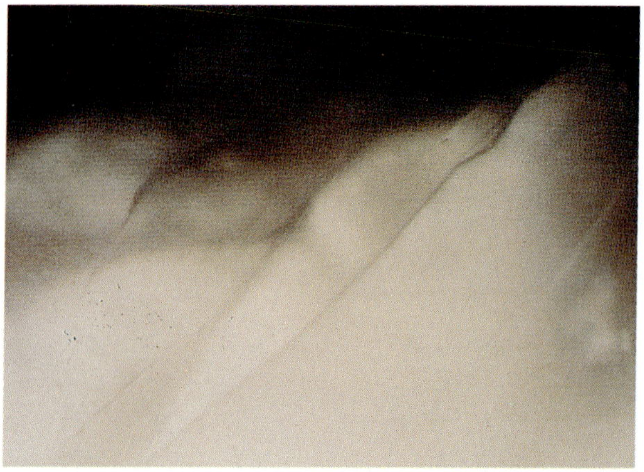

FIGURE 8-7
Free flowing gel in a ruptured implant is shown.

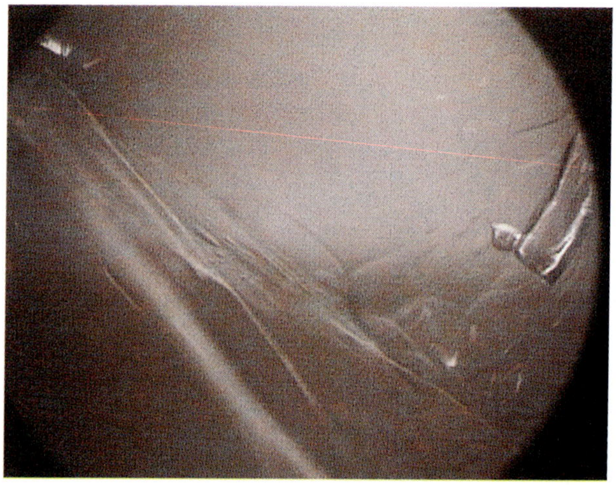

FIGURE 8-8
Free flowing gel in a ruptured implant and particles of the implant envelope are shown.

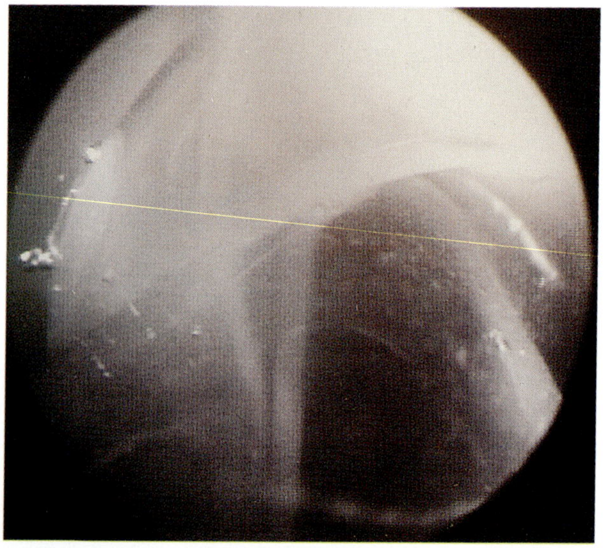

FIGURE 8-9
The folded outer envelope of an implant (Linguini's sign) is shown.

device may have contributed to death, serious injury, or illness. Therefore, under FDA regulations, ruptured implants must be reported to the FDA under this act through the implant tracking program that went into effect in 1993. This is usually done through the implant manufacturer or through a voluntary Med Watch program of the FDA (Federal Registry, Vol. 27, No. 104, May 29, 1993), which is a voluntary tracking program of medical devices that fall under the act.

All patients with concerns about their breast implants must be seen expediently and spoken to very honestly regarding the controversy over breast implants and the scientific evidence in hopes of allaying their fears and anxieties.

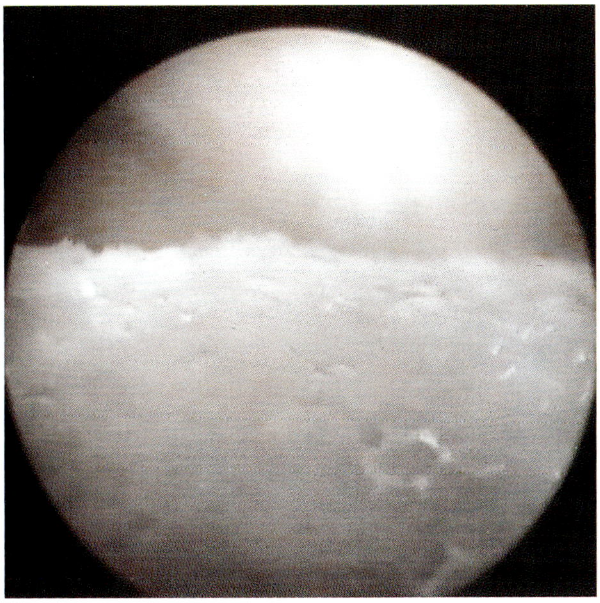

FIGURE 8-10
A polyurethane implant's irregular outer covering of silicone envelope is shown.

Mammoscopy seems to be a very promising technique because it allows evaluation of implant integrity and documentation of the condition of the implant in situ. Possible applications are diagnosis and evacuation of hematomas, and one has to consider intracapsular surgical procedures through a different port. However, because of the tightness and firmness of the capsule it is very difficult to do multiple manipulations because rupture of the implant can occur with excessive instrumentation. I have found that it is best to use the endoscope for visualization and documentation and to minimize the amount of manipulation that must be done through either the same or a separate port with another instrument. Mammoscopy is a definite useful adjunct for the evaluation and treatment of intracapsular conditions arising in the augmented or reconstructed breast.

REFERENCES

1. Scott IR, Muller NL, Firzpatrick DG, Burkenne LJW: Ruptured breast implant: computed tomographic and mammographic findings, *J Can Assoc Radiol* 39:152, 1988.
2. Burg WA, Caskey CI: Diagnosing breast implant rupture with MR imaging, ultrasound, and mammography radiographics, *Radiographics* 13(6):1323, 1998.
3. Colon GA, D'Amore TF: Mammoscopy, the endoscopic intracapsular evaluation of mammary prosthesis, *J Plast Reconstr Surg* 91(2):382, 1993.
4. Dowden RV, Nain S: Endoscopic implant evaluation and capsulotomy, *J Plast Reconstr Surg* 91(2):283, 1993.
5. Silicone breast implant ruptures in an animal model: comparison of mammography, and MR imaging, ultrasound, and CT, *Radiology* 190:227, 1993.

CHAPTER 9

Evaluation of Breast Prosthesis Integrity

Shirley A. Anain
Richard V. Dowden

Silicone gel breast implants have come under close scrutiny since 1990 and the involvement of the Food and Drug Administration (FDA).[1-6] Prior to this, we were studying endoscopy of the breast as a technique for capsulotomy while leaving the implant in situ.[7] Because of the recent interest in evaluating implants, our focus has been on utilizing breast endoscopy as a diagnostic tool to assess implants for ruptures or leaks by examining the surface through a small "window" in the capsule.

A leak is defined as a small hole in an implant that allows a minute amount of gel to escape while the shell otherwise remains intact. In the leaks we have seen, both with the endoscope and after explantation, the silicone forms a gel film over the entire implant. It certainly must start as a small localized area just around the small hole, but it apparently creates a circumferential coating fairly quickly. This allows us to make a small window at any one point in the capsule to survey the adjacent implant surface and determine the integrity of the entire implant, without having to examine the entire implant surface. We feel confident in assuming that if there is a leak, the silicone will have spread to cover the entire implant surface. This seems to be the case from our own studies in patients and from laboratory work done long ago on the behavior of silicone, as will be discussed below.

Gross ruptures allow silicone to freely fill the capsule space. Any small window in the capsule will allow direct inspection of the gel, which will protrude or flow through the window.

We all have seen in consultations many patients with concerns about their breast implants. These patients certainly should have a routine mammogram, but this is a notoriously poor technique for assessing the integrity of an implant, except in those cases where silicone has extruded beyond the capsule. Xeromammograms are somewhat better in detecting ruptures; however, the accuracy rate is only about 50% for leaks and 80% for ruptures.[8] In addition, there are many areas of the United States in which these kinds of mammograms are no longer available.

Ultrasonography has recently received attention as a potential diagnostic tool for implant leaks. However, it appears to be only about 70% accurate in detecting large ruptures and totally inadequate for leaks.[9]

Magnetic resonance imaging (MRI) is probably the best noninvasive diagnostic tool for implant inspection. A ruptured implant can be diagnosed with some confidence—about 90%. However, again, fine leak detection is not yet possible with MRI.[10]

The only method currently available for accurately diagnosing leaks in implants is direct viewing. Breast implant endoscopy allows us to directly visualize the implant with a tiny incision and local anesthesia, while keeping the implant in place and in no danger of rupture.

INDICATIONS

Initially, implants were endoscopically inspected only if the patient's history raised suspicion of implant rupture, that is, trauma, noninvasive test results, change in breast shape or breast mass that was suspicious for silicone, or suspicious findings on examination.

As the implant issue has unfolded, the indications for endoscopy have changed. We use endoscopy for diagnosis in patients who have negative findings for leak or rupture on examination or noninvasive testing if they have strong concerns about knowing the status of the implants or if they have the older type of implant that has fixation patches. Endoscopy can also be used prior to any explantation for diagnosis, to assist in management and for legal documentation. With endoscopy, a videotape can be made of the state of the implant in vivo prior to any manipulation.

Prior to the endoscopic procedure, it is critical to have a detailed consultation with the patient, who is likely to be anxious about the outcome of the test.[11] The possible results of the endoscopy should be discussed as should what the patient wishes to do if the implants are intact, if both are ruptured, or if one is ruptured and one is intact. Doing so before the operation allows adequate preparations to be made.

PROCEDURE

The equipment needed is easily obtainable. A short (6-cm) end-on, 0-degree-angle, 4-mm-diameter endoscope is preferred, with television monitor, video recorder, camera, and light source. The magnification using this technique is approximately × 100. A trocar is not used, to avoid damaging the implant, but a sleeve is necessary to keep the tissue away from the scope's lens. Having tried a variety of instruments, we have found that a simple sleeve can be fashioned from a tuberculin (TB) syringe barrel. The plunger is removed and the end is cut 1 mm longer than the scope. Also needed is a hand-controlled electrocautery with a long, flat blade (uncoated). Very hot water is used for fog prevention (not antifog, which contains silicone or detergent and can alter the findings). Cotton-tipped applicators and a basic instrument set with scalpel and blunt scissors complete the essential supplies.

Because the procedure takes only 10 to 15 minutes and is not particularly uncomfortable, local anesthesia is usually used.

A 1-cm incision is made in the old incision in an area with close access to the implant and capsule. Blunt dissection is used to dissect to the capsule (Figure 9-1). The sleeve (the cut-off syringe) is then inserted as far as the capsule's surface (Figure 9-2), followed by the scope. If fogging occurs during the procedure, warm the end of the scope in hot water. The capsule appears bluish-white under direct visualization, fat appears yellow, muscle is pink, and breast tissue is yellow-white. Once the capsule has been reached, the scope is removed and the electrocautery is inserted. Back the cautery tip off the surface of the capsule, turn on the cutting power, and advance the cautery quickly and smoothly through the capsule about 0.5 cm (it may be felt to give) (Figure 9-3). Do not forcefully jab the capsule or let the cautery become hot, because either will damage the implant. Turn off the power as soon as the capsule gives way. If the tip is already touching the capsule when the power is turned on, it will coagulate the surface and will not allow the opening to be made.

Once through the capsule, the cautery is removed, a cotton-tipped applicator is inserted gently and rotated to clear any serous fluid from the implant surface, then withdrawn, and the warmed scope is reinserted to visually inspect the field (no gas or fluid is inserted). The implant appears to be black when the capsule is opened. A second small burst of cautery may be needed to further open the capsule. The opening is approximately 3 mm and the implant can now be inspected. We feel it is unnecessary, and unwise, to insert the scope inside the capsule, as others have described.[12]

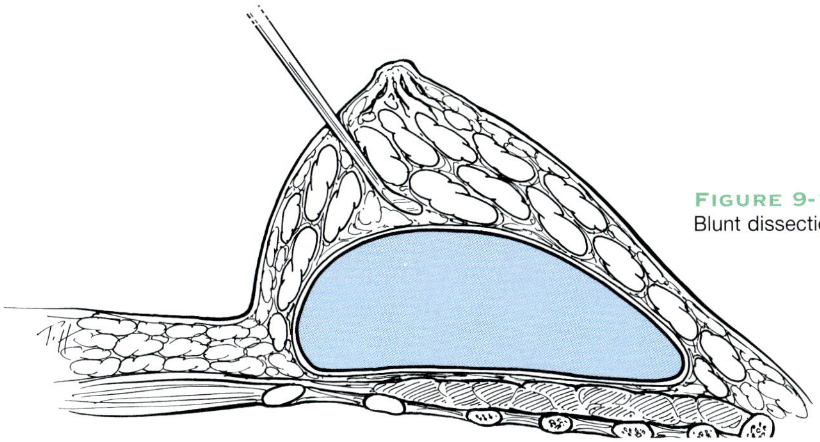

FIGURE 9-1
Blunt dissection to the capsule is shown.

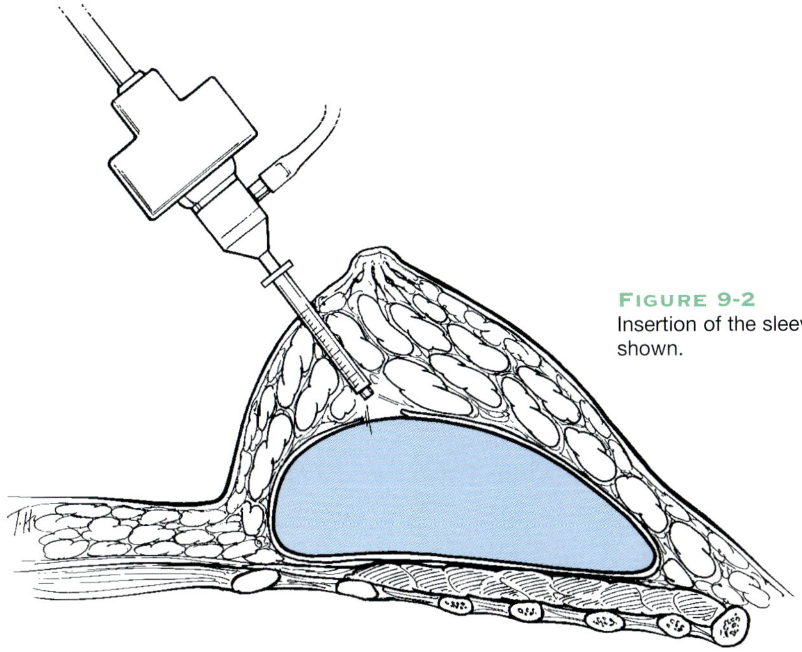

FIGURE 9-2
Insertion of the sleeve (cut-off syringe) to the capsule surface is shown.

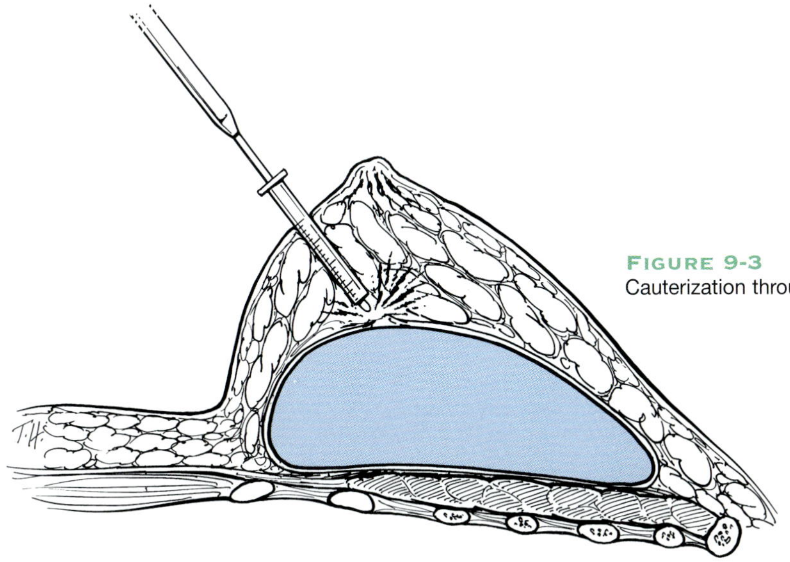

FIGURE 9-3
Cauterization through the capsule is shown.

ENDOSCOPIC FINDINGS

A clear black image of an intact, smooth-walled implant is quite distinct (Figure 9-4). There is a sharp light reflex, and no streaks, ridges, or sticky strands of silicone are seen (Figures 9-5 to 9-9).

Grossly ruptured implants immediately ooze silicone from the small capsular opening. The silicone often wells up into the sleeve and is quite obvious (Figures 9-10 to 9-12).

It takes more practice to identify small leaks of silicone. By moving the implant externally while directly viewing through the scope, the silicone can often be seen as streaks, viscous strands, and ridges along the edges of the capsule. If it is still difficult to determine if there is a leak (which is the case in extremely thin films) the scope can be removed and an applicator stick inserted. The cotton end is touched to the implant surface, removed, and rubbed on a clean glove. When free silicone is present, doing this will create a shiny streak that will remain after any moisture has dried (Figures 9-13 to 9-16).

Once the status of the implant is determined the next step depends on the choices made in the preoperative consultation with the patient. If explantation is done, we routinely excise the inspection tract in cases of implant leakage or rupture.

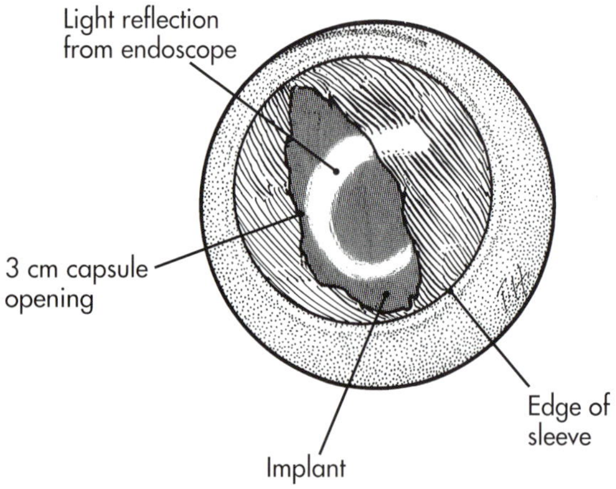

FIGURE 9-4
This is the clear image of an intact, smooth-walled implant.

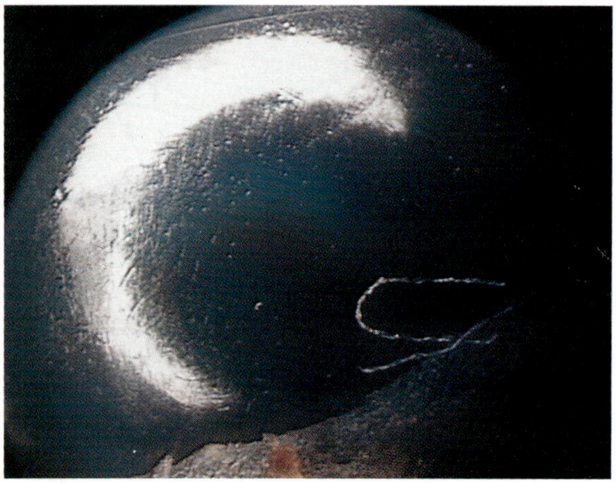

FIGURE 9-5
An intact, nonleaking implant is shown in which the edge of the capsular window can be seen in the lower right, with a curled cotton thread visible. The crescent-shaped white area is the reflection of the light of the endoscope from the dark blue–black surface of the implant. At this magnification, the surface of the implant may appear somewhat irregular, as seen here. That this is not a silicone gel film is demonstrated by the fact that the pattern does not change when swabbed or moved past the window.

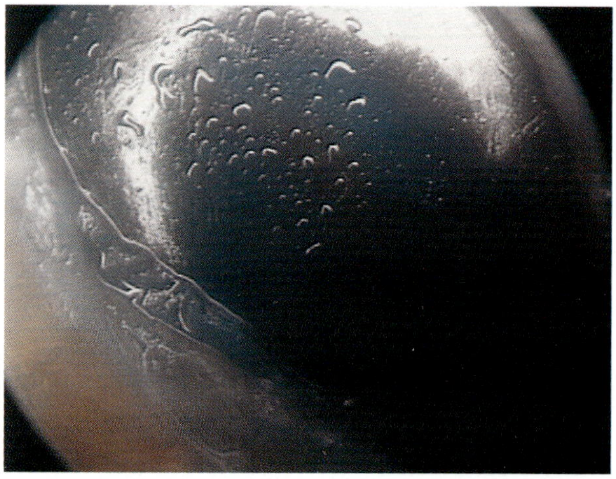

FIGURE 9-6
Another intact implant is shown in which the edge of the capsular window is to the lower left. This implant is similar to the one in Figure 9-5; however, here there are small beads, which are droplets of water, on the surface. Silicone gel from a leaking implant does not bead up in this manner. Both this implant and the one in Figure 9-5 were removed, minutely examined as is the routine, and found to be intact.

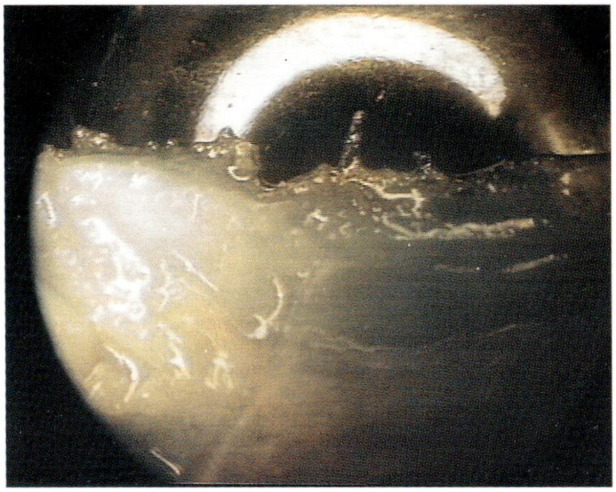

FIGURE 9-7
An intact implant is shown, with the crescent-shaped reflection of the endoscopic light clearly seen. Note the sharp cut-off where the light reflex stops at the edge of the capsule, in contrast to the picture of ruptured implants as described below.

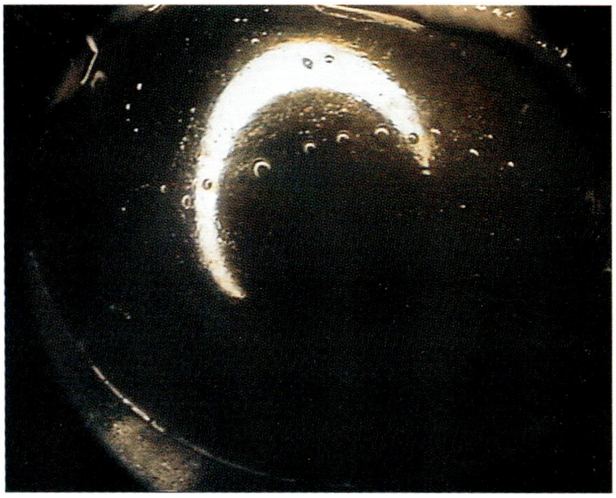

FIGURE 9-9
Another intact implant is shown, with the crescent-shaped light reflex clearly seen. Again, the water droplets are a normal finding as long as they do not grow rapidly during observation.

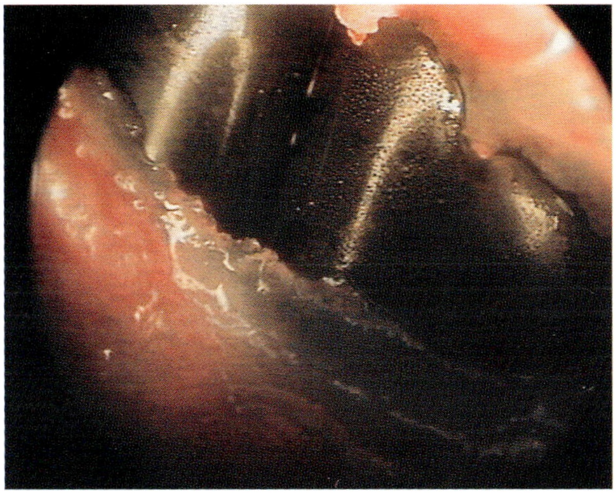

FIGURE 9-8
An intact implant is shown, in which the site of the capsular window happens to overlie a fold in the implant shell. The small beads of water on the implant were static and are not the "rapidly coalescing droplets" described previously. That phenomenon is an action process that does not lend itself to still photography. Basically, the picture changes from something like that in Figure 9-5 to something like in that Figure 9-6 over the course of about 30 seconds, with the droplets growing before one's eyes. It is a sign of an extremely thin coating of silicone gel from a tiny leak.

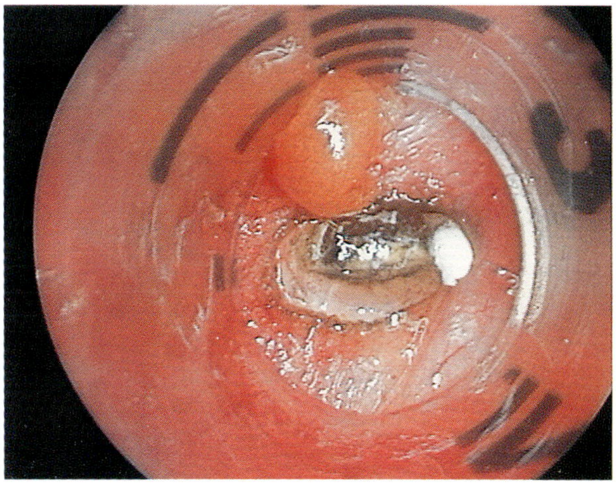

FIGURE 9-10
A ruptured implant diagnosed endoscopically is shown. The view here shows the end of the barrel of the clear plastic tuberculin (TB) syringe, with its visible markings. In the center is the oval-shaped capsular window, from which is extruding a droplet of silicone gel, overlapping the edge of the window and exhibiting a distorted reflection of the endoscope's light. The white dot to the right of the droplet is probably a calcium deposit from within the capsule, and the pink-orange object above the silicone is a small fat globule.

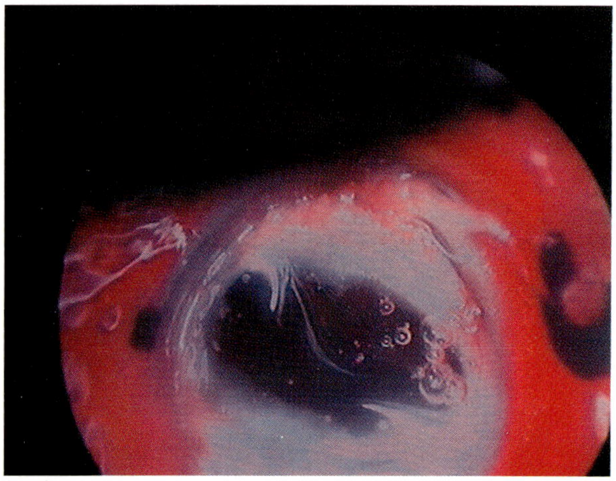

FIGURE 9-11
This is another implant found to have ruptured. The surrounding red circular area is some bloody tissue held back by the TB syringe barrel. Silicone gel has welled up 1 or 2 mm out of the window in the capsule and displays distorted light reflexes extending beyond the border of the window, as well as highly refractile stable bubbles in the silicone gel.

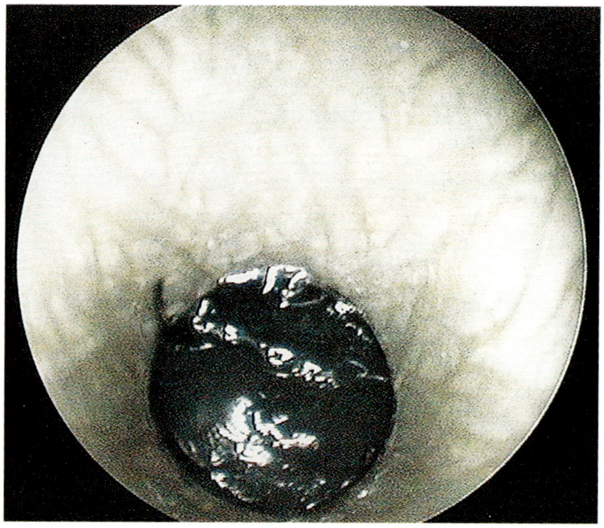

FIGURE 9-13
This is an implant with a small leak, exhibiting an external coating of silicone gel about 0.5 mm thick. In this case, the sleeve, which is light gray, was touching the implant surface, which we do not recommend. The multiplicity of irregular small light reflections is one hallmark of a leak. The leak in this case was found to be on the opposite side of the implant, in a chronic fold fault.

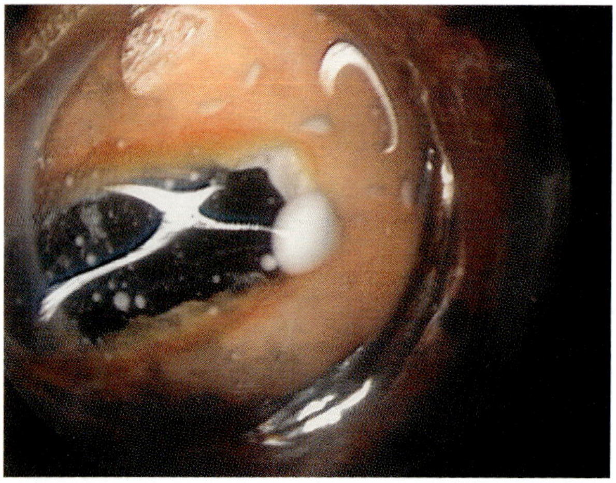

FIGURE 9-12
Free gel within the capsule from a ruptured implant is shown. Note the distorted light reflection extending beyond the confines of the capsular window. There are several white droplets visible within the silicone gel, believed to be calcium deposits.

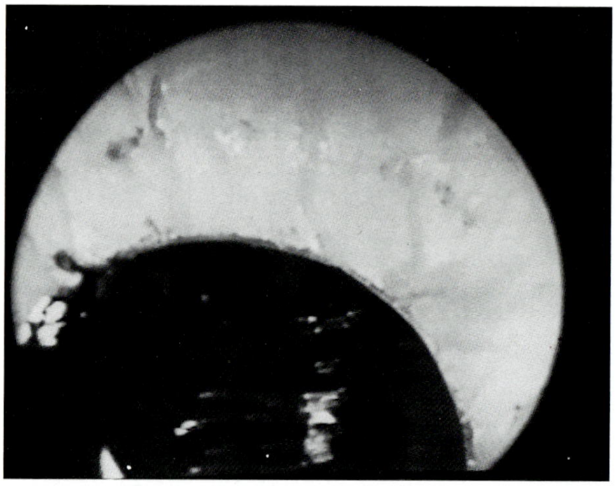

FIGURE 9-14
The same technique as in Figure 9-13 was used here in this leaking implant. The dark implant surface is clearly seen, but with horizontal ridges and streaks—another hallmark of leak. The leak point was about 1 mm in diameter, between two fixation patches on the posterior aspect of the implant.

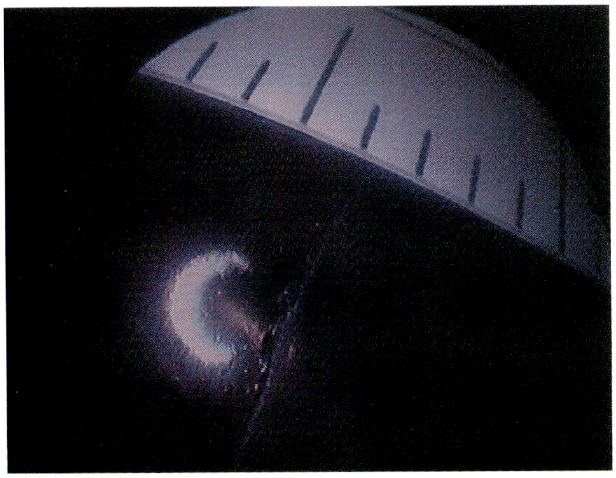

FIGURE 9-15
Shown is the leak point in a case that showed the rapidly coalescing droplet sign. In the upper right is a millimeter scale. To the right of the crescent-shaped light reflection can be discerned the seam of a posterior manufacturing seal, running from 1 o'clock to 7 o'clock. In that seam, near the lower tip of the crescent, can be seen a tiny separation, about 0.3 by 0.1 mm, which was the source of the leakage detected endoscopically. This illustrates the need to meticulously inspect under magnification the entire surface of the implant after explantation of any implant found to have external gel on its surface. Such a small leak can easily be overlooked and mistaken as an indication of gel bleed.

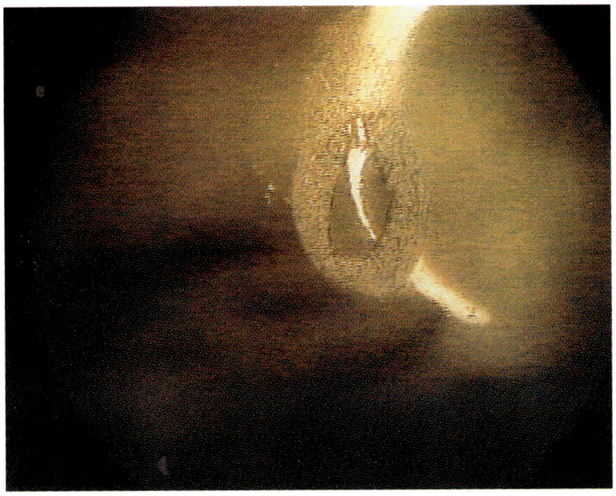

FIGURE 9-16
Highly magnified endoscopic in vitro view of an irregularity 1 mm in diameter on the surface of an implant, the significance of which is not known.

RESULTS

We have performed a total of 142 endoscopic breast implant examinations to date, most of them in patients considered to have a high probability of having failed implants. Therefore our findings (Table 9-1) cannot be extrapolated to all patients with gel implants, because this group of patients is not representative of the whole population of women with breast implants. No implants were injured iatrogenically using the technique described here.

All but five implants were immediately removed and inspected in an open manner. There have been no false positives or false negatives so far using this technique, although they could potentially occur. In all the implants identified with leaks, the silicone coated the entire implant and was never seen localized around the hole. From these results, it appears that the silicone spreads quickly over the entire surface, but the exact timeframe is unknown. It has long been known that silicone gel is remarkable in its ability to rapidly creep along the surface of silicone, a property that is considered to be partly related to the very low intermolecular forces and flexibility of the silicone molecules.[13] In the laboratory the spontaneous spreading of heterogeneous polydimethylsilicone liquid on a compatible quiescent surface has been measured at 0.07 cm in 43 minutes.[14] This suggests that it can spread about 2 cm per day in a quiescent situation. It is not known how this might apply to the human situation, but it would not be surprising if silicone gel from a leak could cover an implant in a matter of months.

TABLE 9-1 IMPLANT CONDITION AND OUTCOME IN 142 ENDOSCOPIC EVALUATIONS

	INTACT	LEAKING	RUPTURED
Replaced	34*	15	18
Removed	40*	20	7
Left in	8	0	0
Total	82	35	25

*These patients decided in advance to have their implants replaced or removed, regardless of the findings, and endoscopy was done to document the condition of the implant at the start of the procedure. In addition, many of the implants that were removed intact represent the second side in cases where the first side required replacement or removal because of leakage or rupture.

Much has been written about silicone "bleed" through an intact shell, which laboratory testing indicates amounts to about 1 ml per 5 years.[15] This no doubt occurs in vivo, but at the magnification used for endoscopy, we did not identify this in any patients. We speculate that this is because the low molecular weight silicone capable of bleeding through the implant shell also passes on through the capsule. In no patient was a coating of silicone present on the capsular surface without an identified source.

In two patients with minute leaks in implants we saw an interesting phenomenon. Leaving the scope to watch the surface for approximately 30 seconds, beads of moisture formed and coalesced rapidly on the implant's surface. A very tiny hole was identified in these implants as the source of the leak. We do not understand the mechanism of this phenomenon.

Without inserting the scope into the capsule, this technique is limited in the identification of the location of the leak. It may be from a hole, a valve leak in a double-lumen implant, or a prior ruptured implant or sizer in the same capsule. If the scope were placed within the capsule more information could be obtained; however, this is not only dangerous to the implant, but is, moreover, unnecessary because most patients in our practices opt for explantation if external silicone is identified, regardless of the source. Silicone can be seen in the depths of *folds* from gel bleed, but not on the capsular surface.

COMPLICATIONS

Fortunately, we have not seen any complications from breast implant endoscopy. The patient is informed preoperatively that there is a small theoretic risk of infection or iatrogenic implant rupture that must be considered. Our laboratory investigation has shown that the risk of implant puncture is extremely small if the procedure is done properly, as described, and if laboratory practice is done prior to attempts in vivo.

OTHER APPLICATIONS

This technique was developed for use in assessing smooth, single-lumen, silicone gel–filled implants. It has been used for other types of gel-filled implants, but based on our experiences there are limitations in other such situations. The endoscope has been used for detection of complete rupture in textured implants, but the subtle signs of a small leak may be obscured by the texturing. Moreover, if the textured implant surface happens to be tightly adherent to the capsule, theoretically, there would be a risk of perforating the implant. Polyurethane-covered implants, early after implantation, may pose a problem for the same reason. However, with time the polyurethane covering dissipates, leaving a relatively smooth surface. Diagnosing complete rupture is straightforward, but again, diagnosing subtle leaks may be more difficult.

Our experience includes several double-lumen implants that were either completely intact or completely ruptured, both of which were easy to diagnose. However, some types of double-lumen, implants show evidence of external silicone gel despite being intact. For example, in permanent expanders with an inner saline lumen and an outer silicone lumen, the saline-filling tube is withdrawn through the silicone compartment. Laboratory testing has shown that a tiny amount of silicone gel reaches the outer surface, where it is spread around, hence giving a false positive for a leak. Similarly, some manufacturers of standard double-lumen implants injected a droplet of silicone gel into the valve site to aid in sealing, which has resulted in a thin, visible, external silicone gel coating. Thus, in these situations, the endoscope is presently limited to diagnosing only major ruptures.

Prior to the implant controversy, the endoscope was used for capsulotomies. By making several ports and inserting the endoscope and endoscopic instruments directly intracapsule, the capsule can be incised with the electrocautery without removing the implant. The same technique can be used for biopsies, cultures, and placement of drains. However, these other procedures do put the implant at risk for puncture, while having minimal advantages in most cases, and we no longer use endoscopy for them.

LABORATORY STUDY

Prior to any attempt at breast endoscopy clinically, this procedure was studied extensively in the laboratory setting for patient and implant safety. The exercises will prove useful for obtaining technical skill in this procedure. The first exercise is to create an artificial "capsule" as follows: tightly wrap an implant in a wet, strong, paper towel and place it on a cautery pad, which is then immersed in a basin of saline. The cautery is then used to make openings in the "capsule," as described above. It will become quite obvious that if the cautery tip is neither allowed to become hot nor forcefully jabbed, it is nearly impossible to breach an intact implant.

The second step is to take an explanted silicone gel implant, with the capsule intact or resutured, to a back table. Again, place it on a cautery pad, and use the cautery to practice entering the capsule under direct view. The scope can then be inserted to practice assessing implants endoscopically and a thin layer of silicone gel from another implant spread across the surface. Intentionally try to rupture an implant by forcefully jabbing the cautery into it, to view an iatrogenic hole. The edges of such a hole are sharp and jagged and occur directly under the opening in the capsule, and they would not be mistaken for anything else.

SUMMARY

As the breast implant controversy continues, our patients are looking to us to identify better ways of diagnosing failure of gel implants. Noninvasive techniques have no more than a 70% to 80% accuracy rate in diagnosing leaks and ruptures, with both false positives and false negatives. By using endoscopy, we can offer a straightforward, safe, accurate method of diagnosing the status of silicone gel implants.

REFERENCES

1. Woods JE, Arnold PG: Fiction obscures the facts of breast implants, *Wall Street Journal* April 7, 1992.
2. Huber P: A woman's right to choose, *Forbes* February 17, 1992.
3. Image of perfection once the goal: now some women just seek damages (editorial), *JAMA* 267:2439, 1992.
4. Council on Scientific Affairs, Silicone Gel Breast Implants, *JAMA* 270:2602, 1993.
5. Kessler DA: A call for higher standards for breast implants, *JAMA* 270:2607, 1993.
6. Brody GS: Silicone gel breast implants (letter), *JAMA* 272:271, 1994.
7. Dowden RV, Anain S: Endoscopic implant inspection and capsulotomy, *Plast Reconstr Surg* 91:283, 1993.
8. McNamara M, Feng L: Xeromammography of breast implants. Presented at the Annual Meeting of the Radiological Society of North America, Chicago, November 1992.
9. Chilcote WA, Dowden RV, Paushter DM, et al: Ultrasound detection of silicone gel breast implant leaks and ruptures: a prospective analysis (presented at the Radiological Society of North America annual meeting, Chicago, December, 1993), *Breast Dis* 7:307, 1994.
10. Ahn CY, Shaw WW, Narayanan K, et al: Definitive diagnosis of breast implant rupture using MRI, *Plast Reconstr Surg* 92:681, 1993.
11. Stone JS, Dowden RV: Breast implant endoscopy: detecting leaks in silicone-gel breast implants, *AORN J* 59:1007, 1994.
12. Colon GA, D'Amore TF: Mammoscopy: the endoscopic intracapsular evaluation of mammary prostheses (letter), *Plast Reconstr Surg* 91:382, 1993.
13. Owen MJ: *Siloxane surface activity.* In Zeigler JM, Fearon FWG, editors: *Silicone-based polymer science: a comprehensive resource,* Washington, DC, 1990, American Chemical Society.
14. Bascom WD, Cottington RL, Singleterry CR: *Dynamic surface phenomena in the spontaneous spreading of oils on solids.* In Fowkes FM, editor: *Contact angle, wettability, and adhesion,* Washington, DC, 1964, American Chemical Society.
15. Yu LT, Latorre G, Marotta J, et al: In vitro measurement of silicone bleed from breast implants. Presented at the 27th Annual Meeting of the Aesthetic Society, Dallas, TX, April 15, 1994.

CHAPTER 10

Evaluation and Proposed Classification of Breast Prosthesis Integrity

Paul H. Rosenberg

Recent controversies surrounding the possible risks associated with silicone breast implants have led to growing concern among many patients. Between 500,000 and 2.5 million women currently have silicone gel–filled breast implants in place, and many of these patients are expressing increased concern over the integrity of these implants.

In recent decades our colleagues in gynecology, orthopedics, general surgery, and other specialties have been performing minimally invasive surgery with increasing frequency. Use of the endoscope in the plastic surgical specialty is a relatively new phenomenon, and its potential as a diagnostic and therapeutic tool is currently under investigation. This chapter serves as a brief introduction to yet another possible use of videoendoscopy—that is, to evaluate silicone gel–filled breast prostheses, diagnose implant rupture, and classify the extent of the silicone leakage.

There are currently several modalities being used routinely to diagnose implant rupture, and some debate exists as to which technique offers the best diagnostic accuracy and the earliest detection of leakage. Ranging from the least to the most invasive techniques for evaluation of silicone gel–filled implants, current modalities include clinical examination, radiologic studies such as mammography,[1,2] magnetic resonance imaging (MRI) with and without breast coil signal amplification,[3,4] computed tomography (CT) scan[5] and ultrasonography,[6-10] endoscopic implant examination,[11,12] and direct implant examination via an open surgical technique.

Possible causes of free silicone in the implant cavity include "silicone gel bleed," shell fatigue, base plate separation, microperforations, and blunt trauma to the implant secondary to chest wall injury or closed capsulotomy.[13,14] The reported incidence of implant rupture following closed capsulotomy is as high as 16%.[15]

Regardless of the cause or whether the perforation occurs on the anterior or posterior wall of the implant, the disruption in shell integrity leads to escape of the gel contents from the prosthesis. In the author's modest experience with endoscopic implant examination, all but a few relatively new implants have shown at least traces of silicone gel on the external surface of the prosthesis, even when no specific point of implant perforation could be found endoscopically. This finding is shared by others who have examined intact implants after removal.[16] In the case of significant shell rupture or base plate separation, the leakage may be extensive and is easily identified. In cases such as frank rupture and silicone spillage, the foreknowledge afforded by the endoscopic implant evaluation may be quite useful when planning an "open" procedure for implant removal or exchange.

Several researchers, such as Dowden and Anain, who have pioneered endoscopic implant inspection and have the largest patient sample size have questioned the existence in vivo of what has been called *silicone gel bleed*.[16] In their experience, none of the intact implants showed any gel on the surface, and all the implants with silicone gel on the exterior surface of the implant shell had a localizable perforation.[17]

Previously, the only means by which to definitively diagnose implant rupture was an open approach. Recent advances in radiographic and ultrasonographic evaluation of these implants have facilitated earlier detection of large silicone leaks. Caskey, Berg, and co-workers found a sensitivity of 58% (11 of 19 detected) and specificity of 88% (28 of 32) for detection of breast implant rupture using MRI.[18] Gorczyca and co-workers independently noted a highly significant finding that they have called the *linguini sign* and have reported a 76% sensitivity and 97% specificity for implant wall disruption when this sign is present (Figure 10-1).[3] Their use of surface coils for some of their patients almost certainly accounts for their higher accuracy.

Radiologists using the new MRI scanner with local antenna claim to be able to achieve a pixel resolution of 1 mm and the ability to clearly see the back wall of the implant. The medical cost for this study is not insignificant, currently ranging between $750 and $1000. Recent advances in radiographic and ultrasonographic evaluation of breast

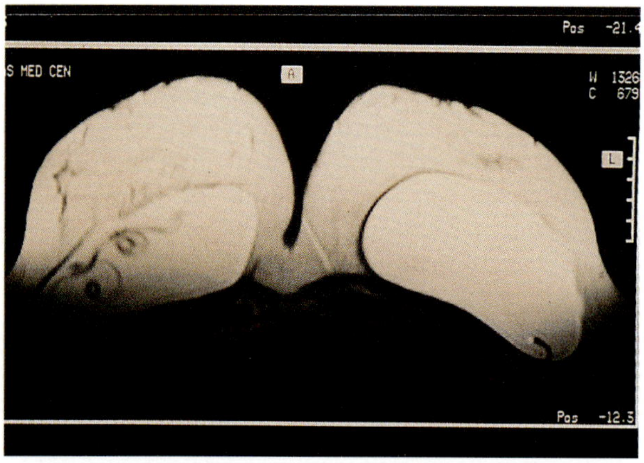

FIGURE 10-1
The linguini sign of implant rupture on magnetic resonance imaging study is shown.

implants have facilitated earlier detection of large silicone leaks, but smaller leaks are not discernible by these methods. In addition, techniques such as ultrasonography may achieve diagnostic sensitivity as high as 87%, but the data on which the diagnosis of implant integrity is made are based on inferential findings. These findings include increased echogenicity, abnormal contents, free fluid, marked redundancy in the shell, and presence of abnormal silicone.[8] Although correlation rates between some radiologic "signs" and clinical implant status with ultrasonography[8,19,20] and MRI[3] may be high, these inferential data are difficult to quantify unless each radiologic study is followed by an open examination of the implant. In a recent study performed at Emory University,[20a] preoperative MRI was followed by explantation and examination of 38 implants in 28 patients. The sensitivity for detection of leakage using a silicone-sensitive magnetic pulse sequence was 94% and the specificity was 100%. Categorization was based on the presence or absence of silicone leakage at surgery, with no subclassification for degree of silicone spillage or mention of gel bleed.

Direct implant inspection, despite the increased attendant invasiveness and cost, permits clear visualization of the implant shell as well as additional tactile data based on manual implant manipulation. Under these advantageous conditions, it would appear that it is far less likely to miss seeing even a minute implant perforation in an open or endoscopic inspection than in a radiologic one.

Endoscopic inspection of silicone gel–filled breast implants is a new technique, first introduced by Dowden and Anain in 1993.[11] As noted in this landmark paper, under the right conditions, a complete rupture may be detectable by physical examination alone or by an inferential radiologic examination; however, the detection of a pinpoint leak that results in a very thin (less than 1 mm) coating of silicone gel adherent to the surface of the implant is beyond the resolution of these methods. Inspection of breast implants using the endoscopic technique combines the advantages of "seeing with one's own eyes" with the minimal invasiveness of a radiologic test.

Although the physiologic sequelae of free silicone are largely unknown at the present time, multiple conflicting reports of health risks due to free silicone may be found in the literature.[21,22] Various independent subjective studies have confirmed the correlation between silicone leakage (gel bleed and ruptures) and capsule formation.[8,23,24]

An additional benefit of endoscopic inspection of silicone gel implants is the ability to more closely quantify the degree to which silicone gel has escaped from the hard silicone envelope. These data could then be used to more precisely identify the cause-and-effect relationship, if one exists, between silicone gel bleed, frank silicone leakage, and the various purported clinical findings such as capsule firmness and systemic complaints collectively referred to as "human adjuvant" symptoms.

Just as with the Baker classification of periprosthetic capsules, it might be advantageous to grade the status of a breast implant itself as well. Classification allows better communication of findings and correlation of this data with clinical and radiologic information obtained by our colleagues.

The proposed endoscopic grading system is based on the presence or absence of silicone leakage, degree of silicone escape from the implant, and containment of the silicone.[25]

A grade I implant is completely intact, with a sharp light reflection, implant transparency, brilliance at the reflected edges, and free separation from the adjacent capsule (Figures 10-2 to 10-4). This connotes a prosthesis whose integrity is undisrupted, with full containment of gel within the implant interior.

A grade II implant has lost the sharp light reflection and transparency. There may or may not be a thin film of silicone visible on the surface, but no obvious perforations are seen. A grade II implant is consistent with silicone gel bleed (Figure 10-5). In

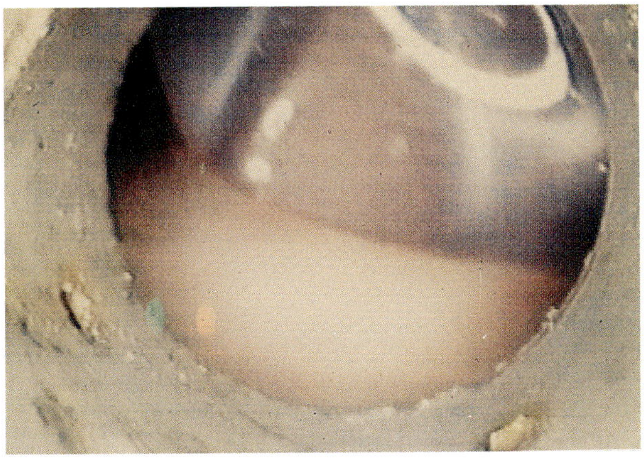

Figure 10-2
A grade I implant is shown: sharp light reflection, well-defined contour, and implant transparency.

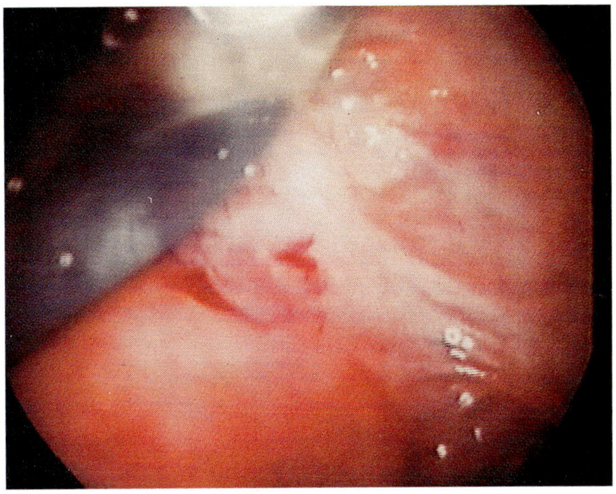

Figure 10-4
A grade I implant is shown.

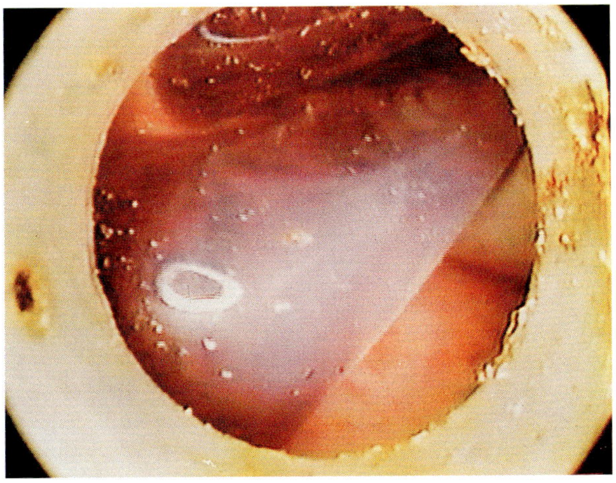

Figure 10-3
A grade I implant is shown.

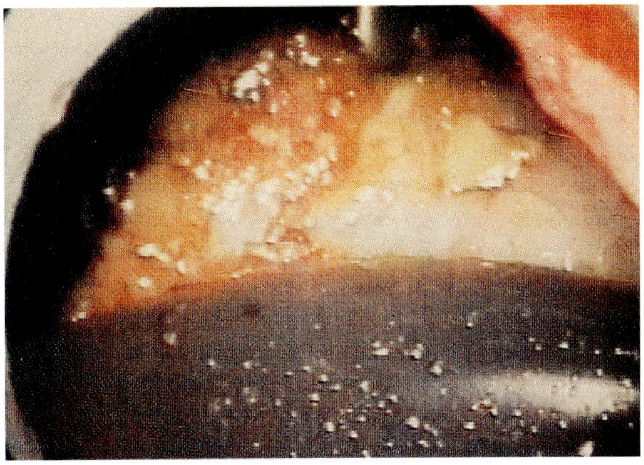

Figure 10-5
A grade II implant is shown: silicone gel bleed.

open examination of implants placed prior to 1980, while 25% to 30% were found to have discrete ruptures, virtually all the intact implants demonstrated some degree of silicone gel bleed, even in the absence of a frank perforation.[26] Since this phenomenon, although disputed, is clinically observed, it warrants special classification until further studies clarify the issue.

A grade IIIa implant has a small rupture that can be found by careful gross examination or under loupe magnification once the implant has been removed from the body.[27] Free silicone is obvious on the exterior surface of the implant shell, and the surface is generally hazy (Figures 10-6 and 10-7). A grade IIIb implant has a gross perforation with significant amounts of free silicone contained within the capsule. This is often seen with Baker grade III or IV capsules, and in the author's experience it correlates highly with a positive linguini sign on MRI (Figures 10-8 and 10-9). Grade IIIb ruptures also are seen with base plate separations and in patients with a history of closed capsulotomies.

A grade IV implant status denotes a gross perforation or a disintegrated implant, often with extrusion of silicone into the adjacent tissues. Grade IV classification connotes shell disintegration, history of compression capsulotomy, and breast asymmetry and deformity. Arrival at this classification may rely on combined visual data from endoscopic and open

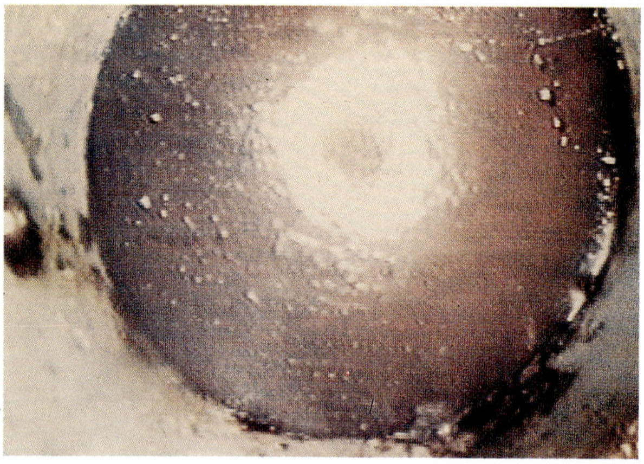

FIGURE 10-6
A grade IIIa implant is shown: microperforation.

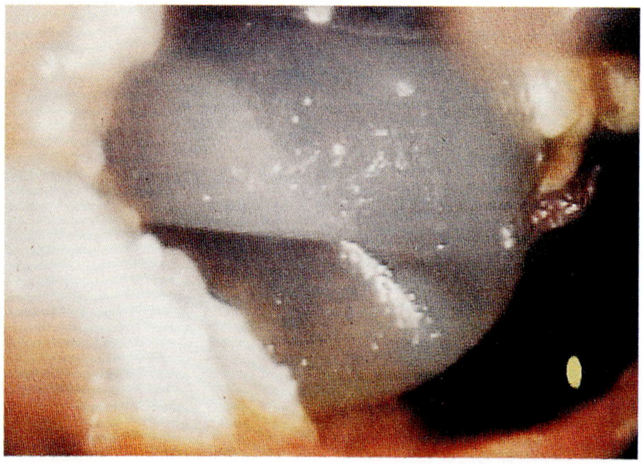

FIGURE 10-7
A grade IIIa implant is shown.

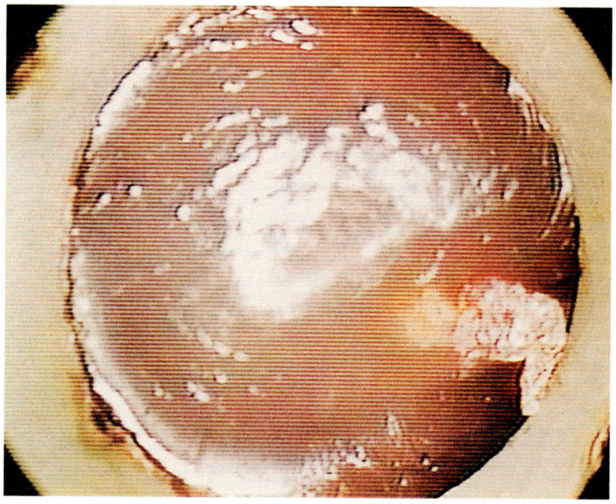

FIGURE 10-8
A grade IIIb implant is shown: loss of sharp light reflection and free silicone gel outside the implant.

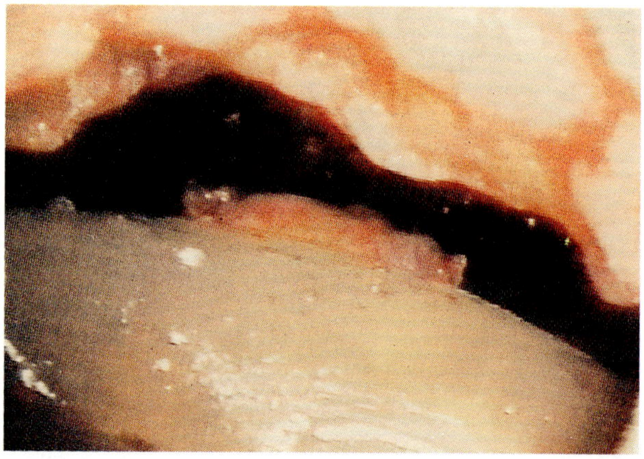

FIGURE 10-9
A grade IIIb implant is shown: note the silicone spillage and thick overlying capsule.

surgical views at the time of implant removal. Additionally, preoperative data based on physical examination, patient symptoms, and radiographic data correlate well with grade IV status.

Although the concept of endoscopic implant inspection is new and this is the first classification system based on endoscopic examination, the general idea of classifying severity of disease processes is a well established one. In the case of silicone breast implants, a classification system using minimally invasive techniques may help clinicians and researchers gain clarity and correlation between the clinical data, endoscopic data, radiologic studies, and serologic data we are now in the process of accumulating.

REFERENCES

1. Basset WB, Brenner RJ: Considerations when imaging women with breast implants, *AJR Am J Roentgenol* 159:979, 1992.
2. Destouet JM, Monsees BS, Oser RF, Nemecek JR, Young VL, Pilgram TK: Screening mammography in 350 women with breast implants: prevalence and findings of implant complications, *AJR Am J Roentgenol* 159:973, 1992.
3. Gorczyca DP, Sinha S, Ahn CY, et al: Silicone breast implants in vivo: MR imaging, *Radiology* 185:407, 1992.
4. Mukundan S, Dixon WT, Kruse BD, Monticciolo DL, Nelson RC: MR imaging of silicone gel–filled breast implants in vivo using a novel method to visualize silicone selectively, *J Magnet Reson Imag* 3:713, 1993.
5. Brem RF, Tempany CMC, Zerhouni EA: MR detection of breast implant rupture, *J Comput Assist Tomogr* 16:157, 1992.
6. Wingerden JJ, Staden MM: Ultrasound mammography in prosthesis-related augmentation complications, *Ann Plast Surg* 22:32, 1989.
7. Harris KM, Ganott MA, Shestak K, et al: Detection of silicone implant leaks: a new sonographic sign, *Radiology* 181:134, 1991.
8. Petro JA, Klein SA, Niazi Z, Salzberg CA, Byrne D: Evaluation of ultrasound as a tool in the follow-up of patients with breast implants: a preliminary, prospective study, *Ann Plast Surg* 32:580, 1994.
9. Levine RA,Collins TL: Definitive diagnosis of breast implant rupture by ultrasonography, *Plast Reconstr Surg* 87:1126, 1991.
10. Rosculet KA, Ikeda DM, Forrest ME, et al: Ruptured gel-filled silicone breast implants: sonographic findings in 19 cases, *AJR Am J Roentgenol* 159:711, 1992.
11. Dowden R, Anain S: Endoscopic implant evaluation and capsulotomy, *Plast Reconstr Surg* 91:283, 1993.
12. Colon GA, D'Amore TF: Mammoscopy: the endoscopic intracapsular evaluation of mammary prostheses, *Plast Reconstr Surg* 91(2):382, 1993.
13. Laughlin RA, Raynor AC, Habal MB: Complications of closed capsulotomies after augmentation mammoplasty, *Plast Reconstr Surg* 60:362, 1977.
14. Nelson GD: Complications from the treatment of fibrous capsular contracture of the breast, *Plast Reconstr Surg* 68:969, 1981.
15. Derman GH, Argenta LC, Grabb WC: Delayed extrusion of inflatable breast prosthesis, *Ann Plast Surg* 10:154, 1983.
16. Caputy GG, Flowers RS: Endoscopic implant evaluation and capsulotomy (letter), *Plast Reconstr Surg* 93(5):1103, 1994.
17. Dowden R: Reply to editorial "Endoscopic implant evaluation and capsulotomy," *Plast Reconstr Surg* 93(5):1103, 1994.
18. Caskey CI, Berg WA, Anderson N, Sheth S, Chang B, Hamper UM: Breast implant rupture; diagnosis by ultrasonography, *Radiology* in press.
19. Ganott MA, Harris KM, Ilkhanipour ZS, Costa-Greco MA: Augmentation mammoplasty: normal and abnormal findings with ultrasound, *Radiographics* 12:281, 1992.
20. DeBruhl ND, Gorczyca DP, Ahn CY, Shaw WW, Bassett LW: Sonographic evaluation of silicone breast implants, *Radiology* 189:95, 1993.

20a. Monticciolo DL, Nelson RC, Dixon WT, et al: MR detection of leakage from silicone breast implants: value of a silicone-selective pulse sequence, *Am J Roentgenol* 163(1):51, 1994.

21. Gabriel SE, O'Fallon WM, et al: Risk of connective-tissue diseases and other disorders after breast implantation, *N Engl J Med* 24(330):1697, 1994.
22. Domanskis EJ, Owsley JQ: Histological investigation of the etiology of capsular contracture following augmentation mammoplasty, *Plast Reconstr Surg* 58:689, 1976.
23. Barket DE, Retsky MI, Shultz S: Bleeding of silicone from bag-gel implants, and its clinical relation to fibrous capsule reaction, *Plast Reconstr Surg* 61:836, 1978.
24. Rotatori DS, Hathaway CL, Steinbach BG, Caffee HH: Non-invasive assessment of implant capsule, *Plast Reconstr Surg* 87:703, 1990.
25. Rosenberg P: LSNA Forum on Endoscopic Surgery, Dallas, TX, April 3-4, 1994.
26. Hester TR: Personal communication, 1994.
27. Dowden R: Personal communication; also presented during a panel discussion at the LSNA Forum on Endoscopic Surgery, Dallas, TX, 1994.

CHAPTER 11

BREAST AUGMENTATION: TRANSUMBILICAL RETROGLANDULAR APPROACH

Gerald W. Johnson
Richard V. Dowden

The routes of breast implant insertion can be divided into local,[1,2] regional,[3] and remote.[4,5] Local insertion is carried out through incisions on the breast skin, either inframammary, periareolar, or through existing suitable breast scars. The regional route of insertion is the axillary approach. The third route of insertion is through an incision remote from the breast, axilla, or chest. An example of remote breast implant insertion reported on previously is through an abdominoplasty incision.[4,5]

The main advantage of the inflatable saline implant is that it can be inserted noninflated through a small incision. In 1991, when Christ and I[6] first introduced the idea of insertion of inflatable saline breast implants through an umbilical incision, the initial response of patients was disbelief. Patients are conversant with the idea of "band-aid surgery" for other purposes, and quickly grasp the concept when discussed in those terms.

The initial response from our plastic surgery colleagues was quite skeptical, including such questions as "How can you cut to create the pocket from so far away?," "How can you control the bleeding?," and "How can you control symmetry?" The key concept of this procedure is blunt creation of the pocket by controlled intraoperative expansion from a remote location. Breast augmentation through an umbilical incision is based on a combination of established techniques of suction-assisted lipectomy, operative endoscopy, and tissue expansion with inflatable tissue expanders. The transumbilical approach produces results that are not different from other methods of placement of prepectoral saline-filled implants, but it does have other advantages, as discussed further. The disadvantages are simply those associated with prepectoral saline implants, in particular that of superior pole wrinkling in the thin women.

Because these implants are the only type currently available in the United States, they will become more popular as the request for this surgery returns to previous levels. With this will come a renewed discovery of the flexibility of insertion of the inflatable implants through small and remote incisions. Rediscovery of the lower incidence of capsular contractures in saline implants versus silicone gel implants will benefit the patients.

PREREQUISITES OF REMOTE INCISION

The endoscope is essential to the safe performance of remote incision breast augmentation. The early pioneers in endoscopic plastic and reconstructive surgery include Aiache, Anain, Colon, Core, Dowden, Ellenbogen,[7] Faris-Correa, Gerow, Isse, Johnson,[6] Liang, Narayanan, Ramirez,[8] Rosenberg, Teimourian, and Vasconez.

Although the umbilical incision for the transumbilical route was the initial incision, and remains today the most commonly used incision for our remote or endoscopic approach to breast augmentation, there are other approaches. One example is that when (1) doing a mastopexy on one breast and an augmentation on the opposite breast (as in unilateral micromastia), (2) doing a submuscular reconstruction of a modified mastectomy on one side and an augmentation on the contralateral breast, or (3) doing a bilateral augmentation mammoplasty for a patient with a mass in one breast that the surgeon plans to biopsy, the incision can be made on the "primary" breast first, performing all necessary surgical procedures on that breast, then using the incision on the primary breast the endotube can be passed trans-sternally for augmentation of the contralateral breast. We have also done endoscopic augmentations through scars in epigastric, subcostal, right lower quadrant (McBurney), and paramedian locations. The limiting factors for the remote location are the length and rigidity of the endoscope. In a very short patient it would be possible to utilize a pubic incision.

We use a 10 mm × 30 cm long, rigid, zero-degree angle view endoscope of the type commonly used in gynecology and general surgery. Most of the necessary instrumentation can be found in any set of plastic surgery instruments, but some items are particular to the procedure. An endotube with obturator is essential for creation of the correct plane of dissection, for insertion of the implant, and for visualization via the endoscope of each step of the procedure. As with any surgical technique, familiarity with the local anatomy and currently available instrumentation are necessary for success. The local anatomy is not reviewed here except to note that the lower end of the lateral edge of the pectoralis muscle is usually lateral to a line drawn tangential to the inner border of the areola to the umbilicus.

PREOPERATIVE EVALUATION AND INFORMED CONSENT

We believe that the preoperative assessment is as important as the surgical procedure itself. Our patients are all fully informed regarding the surgery, implants, long-term results, and postoperative course by means of video, actual implants, and preoperative and postoperative photographs of other patients. Patients are given printed information available from the Food and Drug Administration (FDA), the implant manufacturers, The American Society of Plastic and Reconstructive Surgeons, and the State of Maryland. We do a thorough clinical history and breast and chest examination, including multiple measurements of the breasts and nipples in relation to the torso. The patient is interviewed in the standard fashion, and after the expectations of the patient have been evaluated and found to be realistic and acceptable for augmentation mammoplasty, the methods of breast augmentation are explained. A choice is given in the methods available for insertion of the inflatable saline-filled implants. Informed consent is given by the patient for transumbilical or remote incision for placement of the implant if that is the method to which both surgeon and patient agree.

An understanding between patient and surgeon must be established that conversion of insertion from transumbilical to an "open" breast incision may be necessary if any technical difficulties arise that could adversely affect the final result, such as bleeding.

A careful examination and evaluation of the patient's breasts and careful communication with the patient are necessary to select the proper size implant for each patient. We use the "Johnson/Spira Method of Analysis of Volumetric and Linear Measurements of the Female Breast," as described further. Knowing the relationship between the linear and volumetric measurements of the breast allows the surgeon to make an accurate preoperative estimate of the volume the patient needs to obtain the desired postoperative breast size. The ability to accurately select the volume of the implant before operation obviates the use of a sizer to determine that volume intraoperatively, at a considerable savings of operating room time.

The surgeon performing aesthetic and reconstructive breast surgery should understand differences in **band** size (32, 34, 36, and so on) as well as differences in **cup** size (A, B, C, D, and so on). These are both relatively imprecise measurements used by the garment industry. The **band** measurement denotes the **pectoral circumference** of the person; however, the **cup** size denotes the **proportion between the circumference and size** of the breasts. The band size is determined by measuring around the chest, just under the axilla (Figure 11-

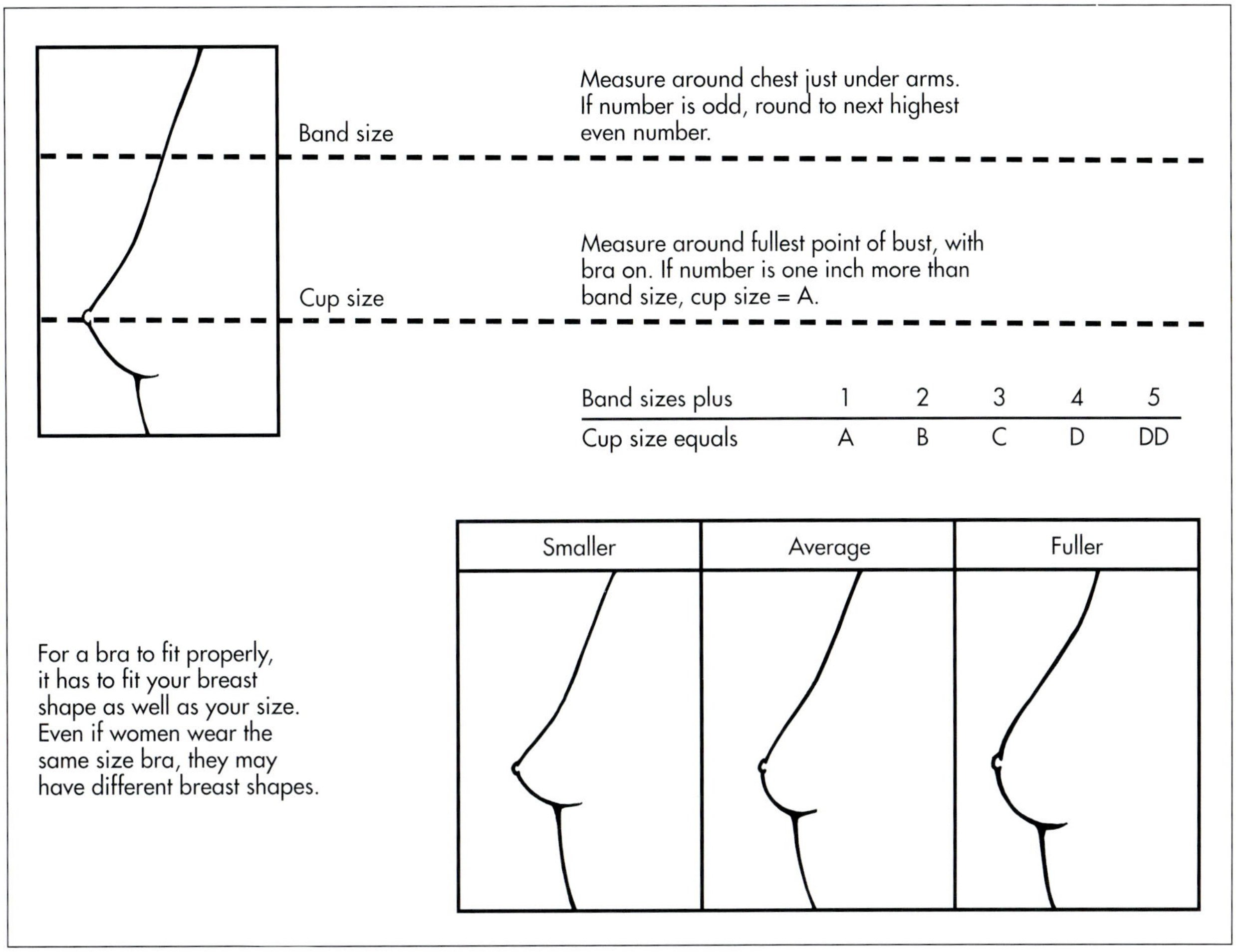

FIGURE 11-1
How to determine your bra size is shown.

1). The measurement is in inches. If the number is odd, it should be rounded to the next highest even number. The bra cup size is determined by measuring around the fullest point of the bust, with the patient wearing a bra. If the number is 1 inch more than band size, the cup size is A; if the number is 2 inches more than band size, the cup size is B; the progression is linear by unit. Of the chest and breast measurements we (GWJ) have made in 6000 patients over the past 17 years, we have found the most common band size to be 34 and the most common postoperative cup size to be a C. For discussion and evaluation, therefore, we have selected the 34C measurement as the benchmark.

Most women have little idea how to determine their true bra size, instead selecting their bras by what feels comfortable. The key to understanding this is that a nominal cup size varies in volume as the band size changes. For example, a C cup in a 34 band size is about 400 ml in volume, a C cup in a 36 is about 550 ml, and a C cup in a 32 is about 280 ml volume. As a corollary, a woman who is a true 34C size would have to go to a D cup if she prefers the snug fit of a 32 band or to a B cup if she prefers the looser fit of a 36 band. This has been described by Regnault and Daniel.[9] The volumes we have determined to be appropriate differ somewhat from this text; however, the basic concepts are the same.

THE PREOPERATIVE EXAMINATION

Initial and important information requested (Figure 11-2) includes such questions as the following: What size bra does the patient wear?, Does she always wear a bra?, Does she think her breasts droop too much?, What type of surgery does she

Date: ____________

NAME: ______________________________ AGE: ________ NUMBER: ____________

HT. ______ WT. ______ Office Use ________

Age of onset of menses: ____________

Age breast development began: __________

Number of pregnancies: ______________ Number to full term delivery: __________

Size bra you presently wear: __________ Padded?: ________

Do you always wear a bra: ____________

Have you ever gone without a bra for several months or years: __________

Do you routinely sleep in a bra: ________

Do you feel your breasts droop too much: ______________

Have you ever had breast surgery: ________ If so explain: ______________

Do you have any blood relatives with breast disease or cancer: ______________

If so, relation: ____________________________________

Do you have any breast pain: __________

Have you had a recent mammogram: _____ Results: ____________________

Do you want to be: ______ Enlarged ______ Reduced in size

______ "Brought up" ______ Enlarged and "brought up"

______ Reduced and "brought up" ______ Have all breast tissue removed and replaced with implants

Medicine is an art, not a science, so nothing "exact" can be promised; however what size breasts would you ideally like to have: __________

OFFICE USE ONLY:

Exam: __________

____

____

__________ ______________________________

Signature Date

Photos preop: _____

Photos post op: _____

Implants: Type _____

Size _____

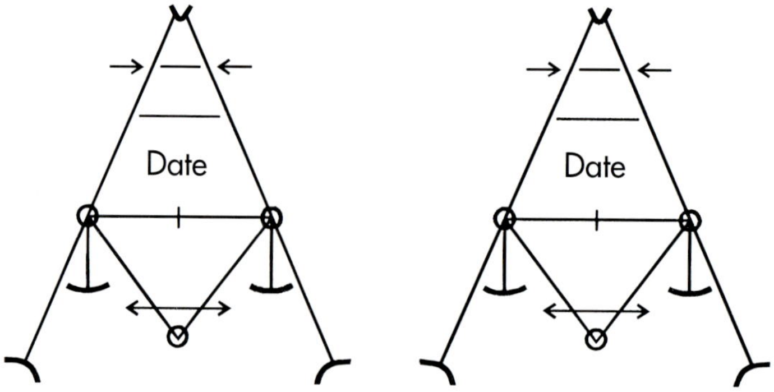

FIGURE 11-2
The Johnson Breast Surgery Questionnaire is shown.

want?, Does she want to wear a larger size bra, meaning she is seeking breast augmentation, or does she just not want her breasts to droop?, Does she think she needs both augmentation and elevation?, and finally, What does she want her final breast size to be? Frequently, the patient really does not know how to explain what breast size she wants to attain, and it is not unusual for the discussion of size to take up a significant part of the interview and examination. One can use an album put together from photographs of women from lingerie magazines as an aid in helping the patient choose a size. The album should contain photographs of women with B, C, D, and DD cups, with small, medium, and large of each cup size. The patient is advised as follows: "Try not to let the form of the breast influence your choice, but pick the model who has the proportion of breast to body that you like." If the patient chooses two sizes she likes, for example a medium C and a full C, always select the larger size. Another method is to have the patient try on bras with larger cup sizes (with the same band size) with some cotton stuffing until she achieves the look she wants, then measure the difference using a water-filled expander in the bra. Patients almost never request reoperation for a decrease in size. In our series, 94% of reoperations to alter the breast size were for an increase in size.[10] Note that it does not matter if a patient wears a 32 or 42 bra, the **proportion** of the size of her breasts to the size of her chest creates the cup size. At this point you are not yet concerned about the band size (i.e., 32, 34, 36, and so on). At some point, you should also make it clear that you do not represent to her that you can or will make her breasts the exact size she describes. Your objective is to determine the volume or size she thinks is ideal.

Note that the patient is not queried as to what **shape** breast she desires. Depending on the operative plan (augmentation versus mastopexy with augmentation), discussion could include desired nipple size and location, nipple point direction, fullness in the upper part of the breast, slope of the upper part of the breast, and the appearance of "cleavage." The garment industry also recognizes the problem of shape related to size (Figure 11-1) and breaks down the sizes further into smaller, average, and full. We also refer to the small, average, or full cup in our discussion with the patient. Each third of a cup is equal to approximately 50 ml. Therefore, a small cup plus 50 ml equals an average cup, an average cup plus 50 ml equals a full cup.

The actual examination of the patient is recorded on the form shown in Figure 11-3, which is an enlargement of part of the form actually used in the office, the Breast Surgery Questionnaire (Figure 11-2). You may decide that you do not need all these measurements, but we believe that at a minimum you need A through F, which are outlined below.

Measurement A, the distance from the suprasternal notch to the nipple, is important because even though the "accepted" method of judging ptosis of the nipple is the profile evaluation of the nipple in relation to the inframammary fold, if the nipple is farther than 22 cm from the suprasternal notch in the woman with an average bra size of 34 who is of average height, you must evaluate and discuss with her the alternative of mastopexy plus augmentation to give her the shape she wants at the size she has chosen. If she refuses to accept the scars of a mastopexy, she will have been properly informed when she signs her consent.

Measurement B is the distance from the midsternal line to each nipple (e.g., 9 cm in the woman with an average 34 bra size) and varies between 16 and 20 cm from nipple to nipple (Figure 11-4). If a patient with average 34 bra size measures 11 or 12 cm on each side, she will have nipples that point more laterally than normal. The surgeon needs to explain to her how and why the augmentation will

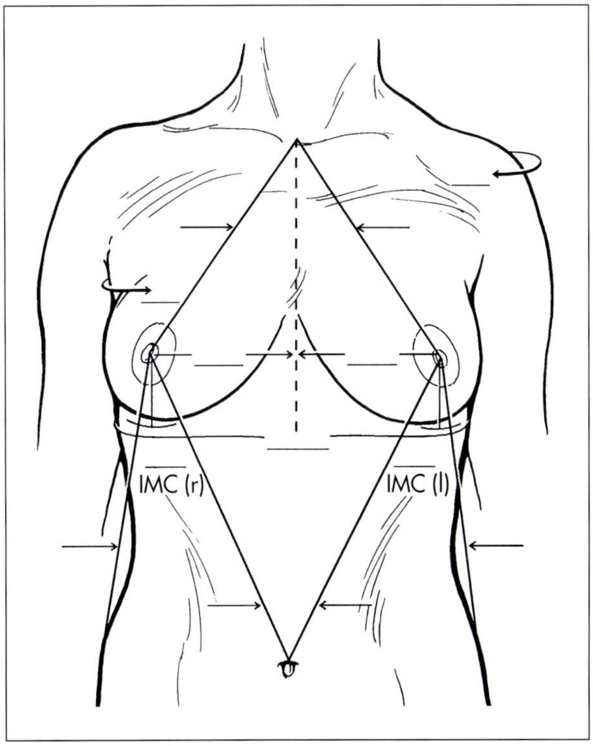

FIGURE 11-3
Record measurement E in cm (inframammary crease [R] inframammary crease [L]).

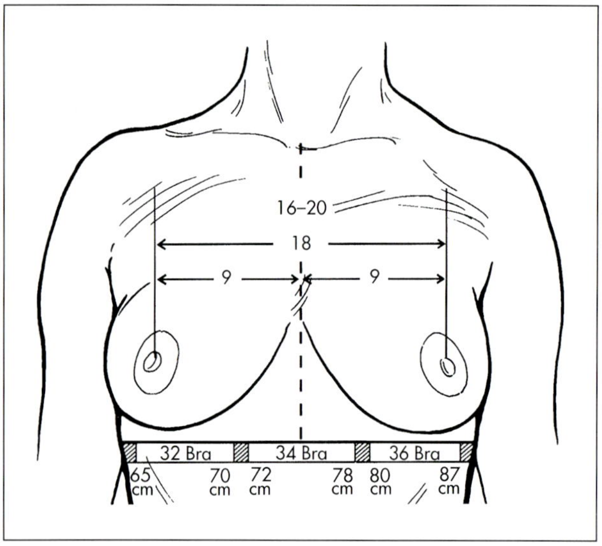

FIGURE 11-4
Measurement B is the distance from the midsternal line to each nipple (32 bra, 34 bra, 36 bra).

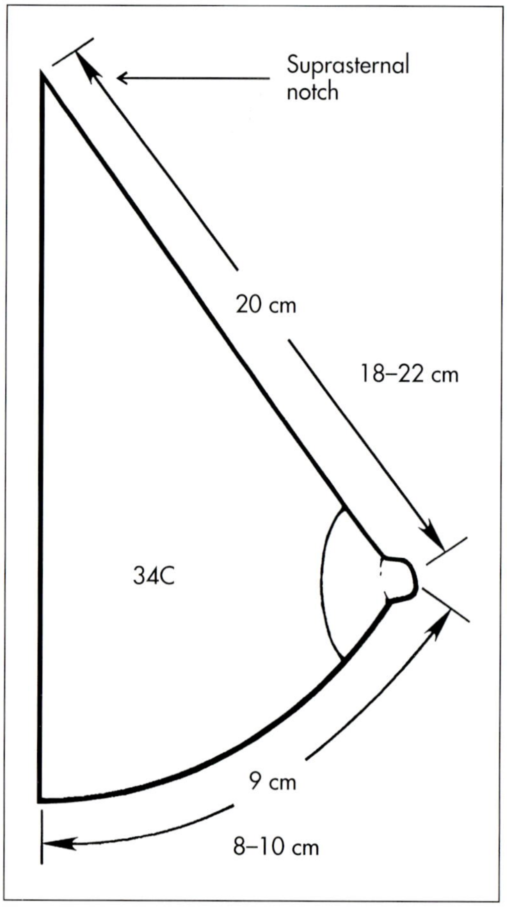

FIGURE 11-5
Measurements A and C are shown.

not change the "point" of her nipple unless additional surgery around the nipple is done.

Measurement C, the distance from the nipple to the inframammary crease (IMC), is important (Figure 11-5). (Due to variation in the diameter of the areola, we do not use the areola-to-IMC measurement.) In our idea of an ideal 34C cup size breast the ideal distance from nipple to crease is 8 to 9 cm. In a D cup that distance is about 9 to 10 cm. If the preoperative length of measurement C is already 8 cm (which means the patient may have a somewhat ptotic breast mass with a normally positioned nipple), then it is not necessary to plan lowering of the IMC. However, if the patient has a 5-cm C distance, then lowering the crease and stretching the inframammary skin to some extent must be done to obtain a "normal" 8 to 9 cm distance for measurement C.

Measurement D is not very important other than to note and record the breadth of the patient's shoulders (the distance between her shoulders).

Measurement E (in inches) indicates band size (Figure 11-1). We record measurement E in cm on our records (Figures 11-3 and 11-4).

Measurement F is used to determine the true band size of the patient, which enables us to determine the volume of breast needed to approximate the size of the augmented breast desired (Figure 11-4). An F measurement of 65 to 70 cm indicates a true 32 bra size. A measurement of 70 to 72 cm is a transition zone, and if the patient normally wears a 32 bra, the size is a 32; if she normally wears a 34 bra, the size is a 34. A measurement of 72 to 78 cm is a true 34 bra size. Again, 78 to 80 cm is a transition size, and the true bra size is based on what the patient normally wears. A measurement of 80 to 86 cm is a true 36 bra size. Again, 86 to 88 cm is the transition zone between 36 and 38 bra sizes. Measurements of 88 to 94 cm generally correspond to a 38 bra. Any measurement of F that exceeds 95 cm makes it difficult to determine which bra size the patient should be wearing, and in fact most of the women have difficulty finding a properly fitting, comfortable bra.

Once the true bra band size of the patient has been determined, one more determination must be made before choosing the implant size and volume needed. An estimate of the volume of the breast is necessary. This can be accomplished by putting a sizer or prosthesis of known volume that, along

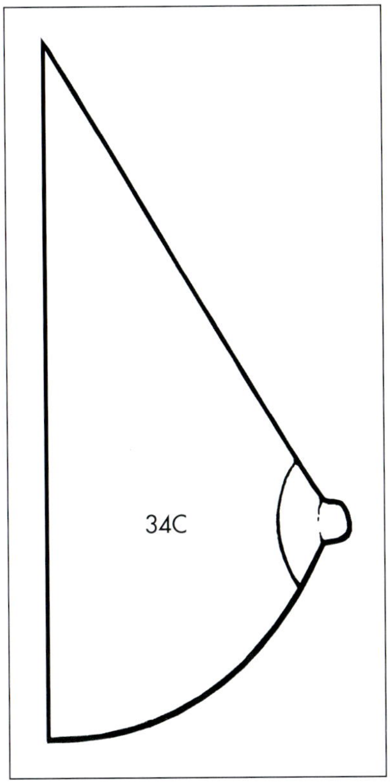

FIGURE 11-6
The volume of an average-size breast is shown: 400 ml (350 to 400 ml).

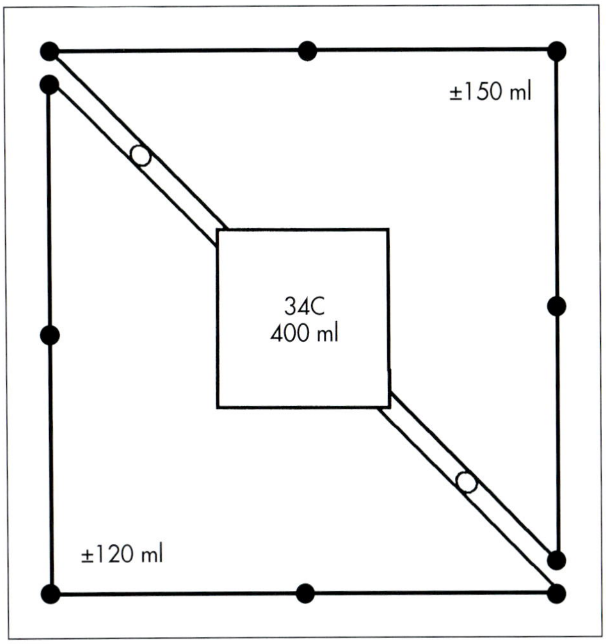

FIGURE 11-7
The center square is shown (34C, 400 ml), upper right triangle (150 ml), lower left triangle (120 ml).

with her natural breast, fills a bra of the cup size the patient seeks. Alternatively, an estimate of how much the breast specimen would weigh if the breasts were removed can be made based on the surgeon's past experience. Weight and volume are treated as essentially the same for the purposes of these measurements.

Knowing the estimated volume of each breast, the surgeon need not be concerned with any size discrepancy between the breasts, unless it seems to exceed a 20 ml volume. If so, appropriate adjustments for differential volume of the implants should be planned. Most women experience some degree of postpartum breast atrophy, with resultant loss in breast volume. Many plastic surgeons believe that all patients experience some degree of postoperative atrophy after any major breast surgery, which may be as high as 20% to 25% of the preoperative volume. Therefore 20% to 25% of the volume should be subtracted from the figure of the preoperative breast volume.

For the purpose of exemplification we will use the average 34C as our benchmark. The volume of such a breast is 400 ml (Figure 11-6). The upper right triangle says ±150 ml (Figure 11-7). This means that to increase the breast by one cup size, to 34D, or to go up one band size, to 36C, approximately 150 ml must be added. The lower left triangle says ±120 ml. This means that to decrease the breast by one cup size, to 34B, or to go down one band size, to 32C, approximately 120 ml must be subtracted.

The arrows and numbers in Figure 11-8 indicate the volumes to be used to change cup sizes and how these changes in volume correlate with different band sizes. If the "true band size" measurements do not correspond to the band size the patient is wearing, the surgeon should explain the significance of this discrepancy so that her postoperative expectations are in agreement with those of the surgeon.

In conclusion, the bra size the patient customarily wears is not very important in the surgeon's decision making. Only her true band size as determined by measurements and the cup size desired by the patient are important parameters. However, it is important that the patient be educated as to the relationship between band size, cup size, and volume because the patient must understand how the surgeon reached his decision on the size of the implant required to achieve the desired result. It is also important to allow an additional amount to

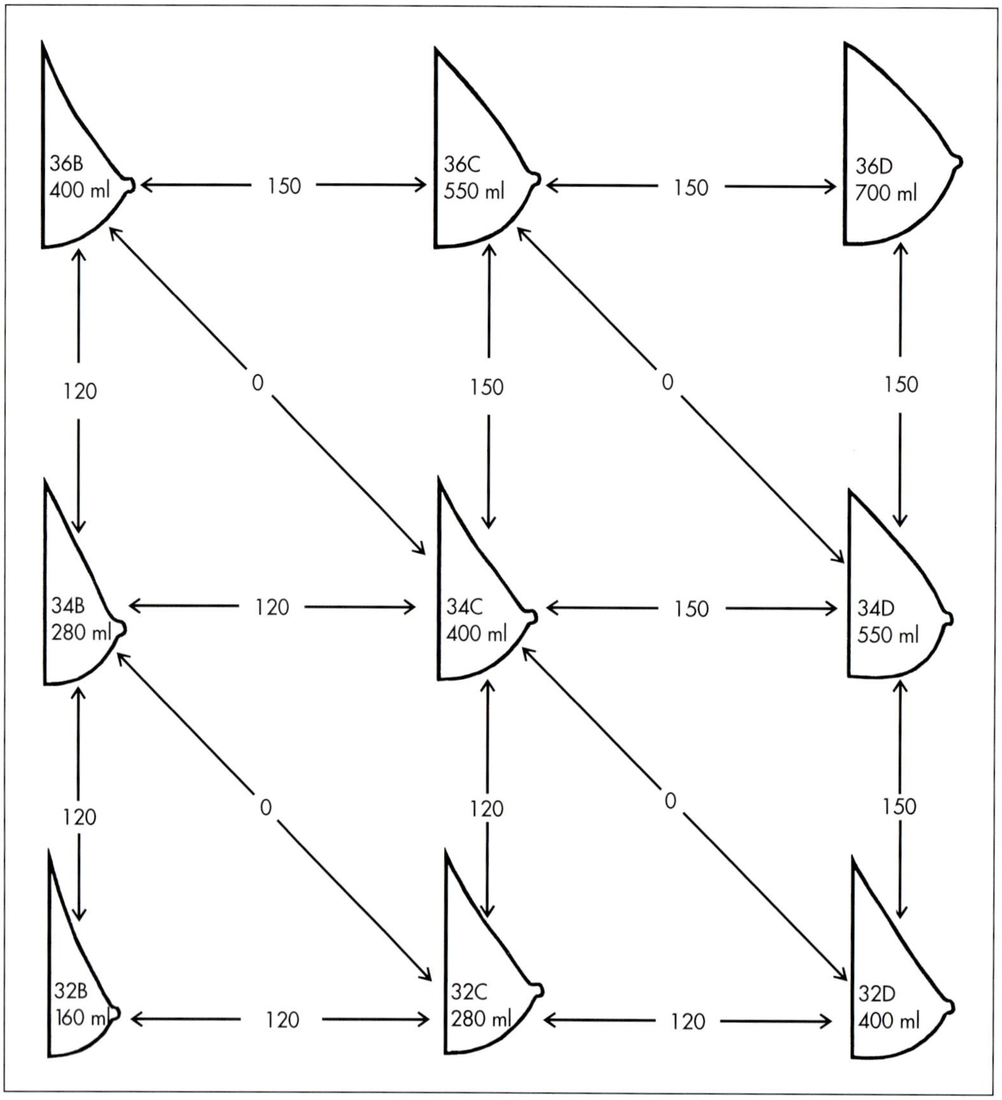

FIGURE 11-8
Nine breast drawings marked from left to right, top to bottom: 36B/400 ml, 36C/550 ml, 36D/700 ml, 34B/280 ml, 34C/400 ml, 34D/550 ml, 32B/160 ml, 32C/280 ml, 32D/400 ml.

compensate for customary atrophy, which experience leads us to expect, as discussed earlier.

After the desired implant volume has been determined, the final step is to decide which size implant to fill and with what volume to fill it. It is widely appreciated that the manufacturer's suggested fill ranges are too low to prevent upper pole wrinkling and indentations. For this reason, many plastic surgeons routinely overfill by 10% to 20% (going even farther can distend the implant unacceptably, producing edge scalloping and visible demarcation of the upper pole). Manufacturers are in the process of revising their limits upward.

Obtaining the measurements and performing the calculations as described enables the surgeon to approach the procedure with confidence about the size of the implant to be inserted, the type of implant, and the volume with which it is to be filled to produce the final result desired by both surgeon and patient, fully achieved 3 to 6 months postoperatively.

OPERATIVE TECHNIQUE

In the operating room the patient is positioned in the supine position, with arms extended 90

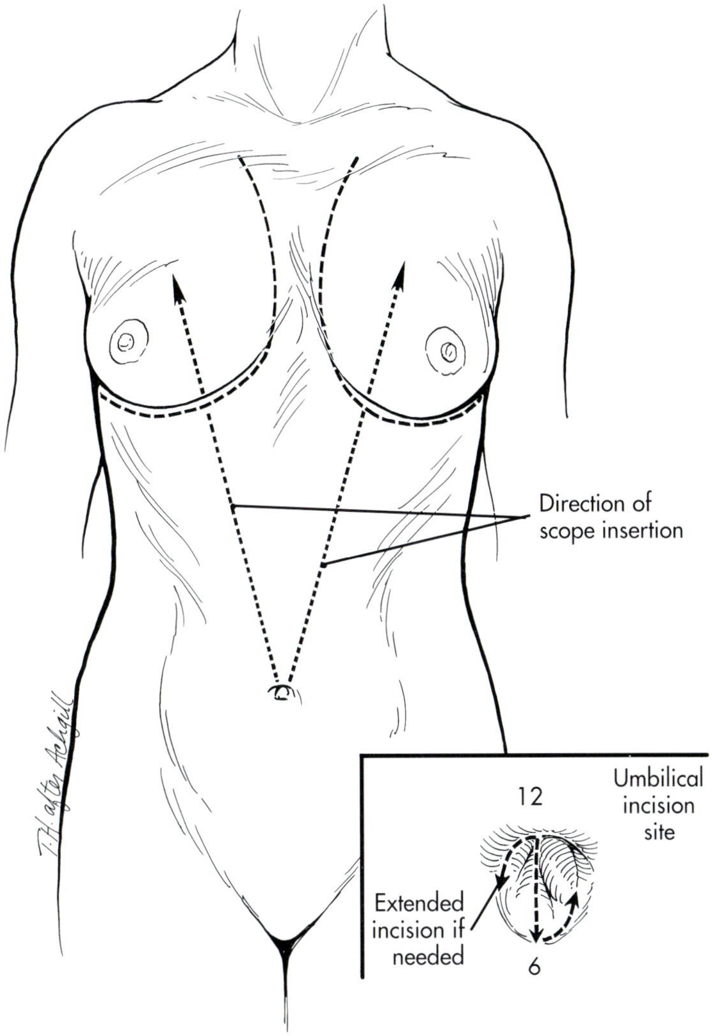

FIGURE 11-9
The umbilicus incision site is shown.

degrees. General endotracheal anesthesia is administered. An antibiotic is given intravenously. The patient is prepared and draped in the standard fashion, leaving exposed the entire chest and anterior abdominal surface. The breasts are marked in the same manner used for the standard augmentation mammoplasty to delineate the extent of the pockets to be created by the expander dissection. The midline is also marked from sternal notch to umbilicus. On each side a line is traced from the umbilicus just medial to the medial border of the areola (Figure 11-9).

The assistant elevates the umbilical ring with skin hooks placed at 12 o'clock and 6 o'clock positions. An incision is made in the umbilicus (Figure 11-9). The incision must be large enough to allow insertion of the index finger with no resistance. The Mayo scissors are then used to dissect superiorly onto the abdominal fascia (Figure 11-10).

Then the tip of the endotube with obturator in place is inserted through the umbilical incision. With the skin and subcutaneous tissue "tented" and supported with the opposite hand, the endotube is advanced in the plane between the fascia and subcutaneous tissue. Unlike suction-assisted lipectomy, one continuous steady forward push is used, because multiple strokes can make small dead-end tunnels that will cause difficulty in introduction of the tissue expander and implant. The endotube is advanced on the muscle fascia over the costal mar-

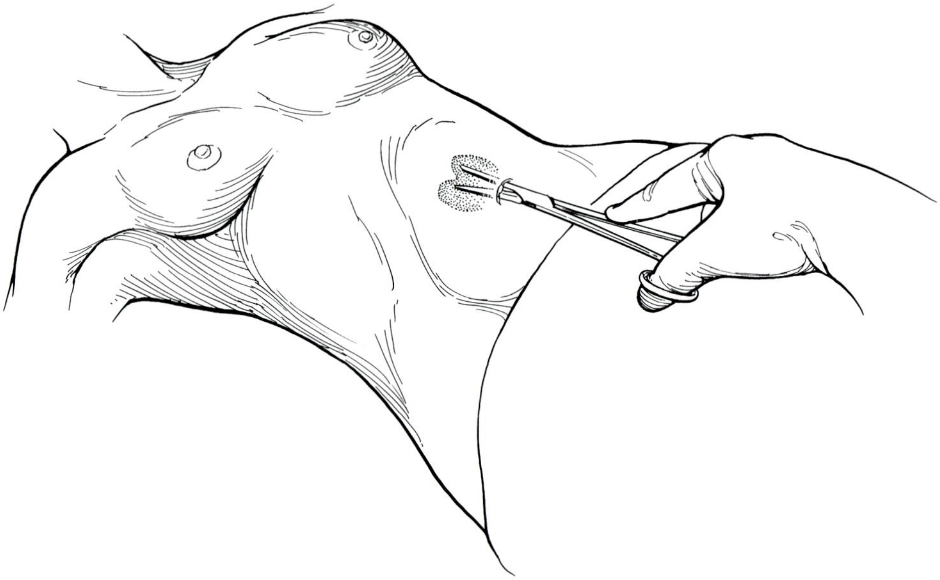

FIGURE 11-10
Initial undermining is shown.

gin. The opposite hand maintains constant countertraction on the skin surface to help keep the tip of the endotube in the correct plane (Figure 11-11). Care should be taken not to lift up on the breast, as this increases the likelihood of subpectoral passage. A notable decrease in resistance in the advancement of the endotube signals passage through the denser tissue at the inframammary crease. The endotube is then advanced to a position superior (cephalad) to the nipple (Figure 11-12), taking care that the vertical extent of passage is identical on both sides. The internal obturator is then removed, and the endoscope is inserted to check for the proper plane of insertion and to confirm that the field is bloodless (Figure 11-13), which is usually the case. The undersurface of the breast will appear as a glistening white to yellow-white color; the pectoralis major muscle appears a mahogany or reddish-brown color. The endoscope and endotube are then slowly withdrawn, while inspecting the entire passageway.

One extremely important change in our technique not reflected in an earlier article is that we no longer use the implant itself as the expander.[10] Instead, we use a tissue expander in an extra step. We still overexpand the pocket by 50% above the final volume of the implant. In preparation for insertion the expander is connected to an extension tube and one-way valve and is evacuated of air

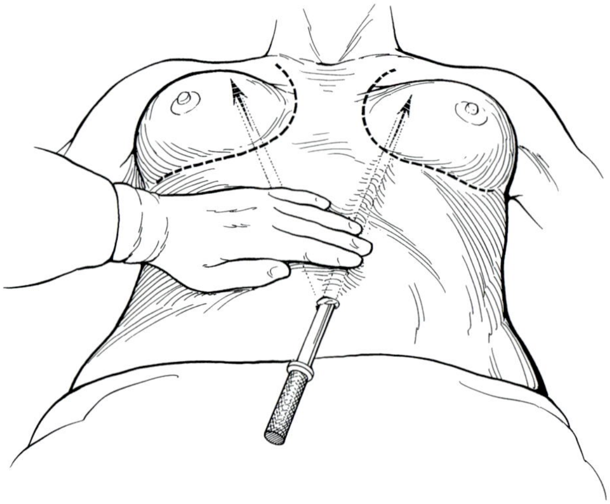

FIGURE 11-11
Creating the tunnel is shown.

(Figure 11-14). The expander edges are rolled in a cigarlike fashion from each side to cover the fill-tube insertion site (Figure 11-15), and the tubing is passed through the endotube. The inferior end of the rolled expander is gently lodged a few centimeters into the open end of the endotube. With an Army–Navy retractor in the umbilical incision, the

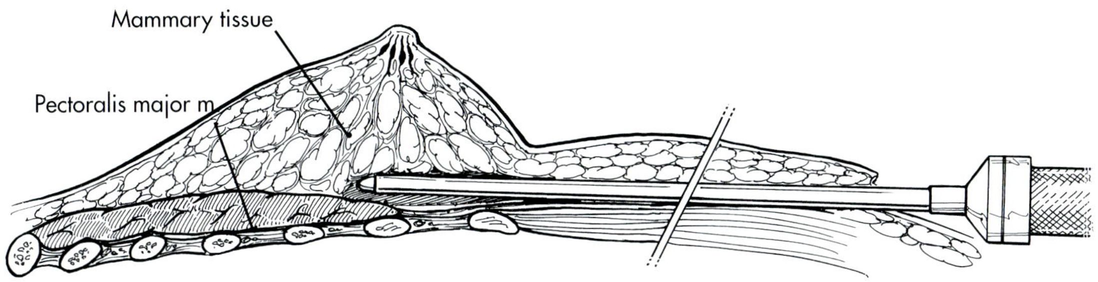

FIGURE 11-12
Mammary tissue, umbilicus, and the pectoralis major muscle are shown.

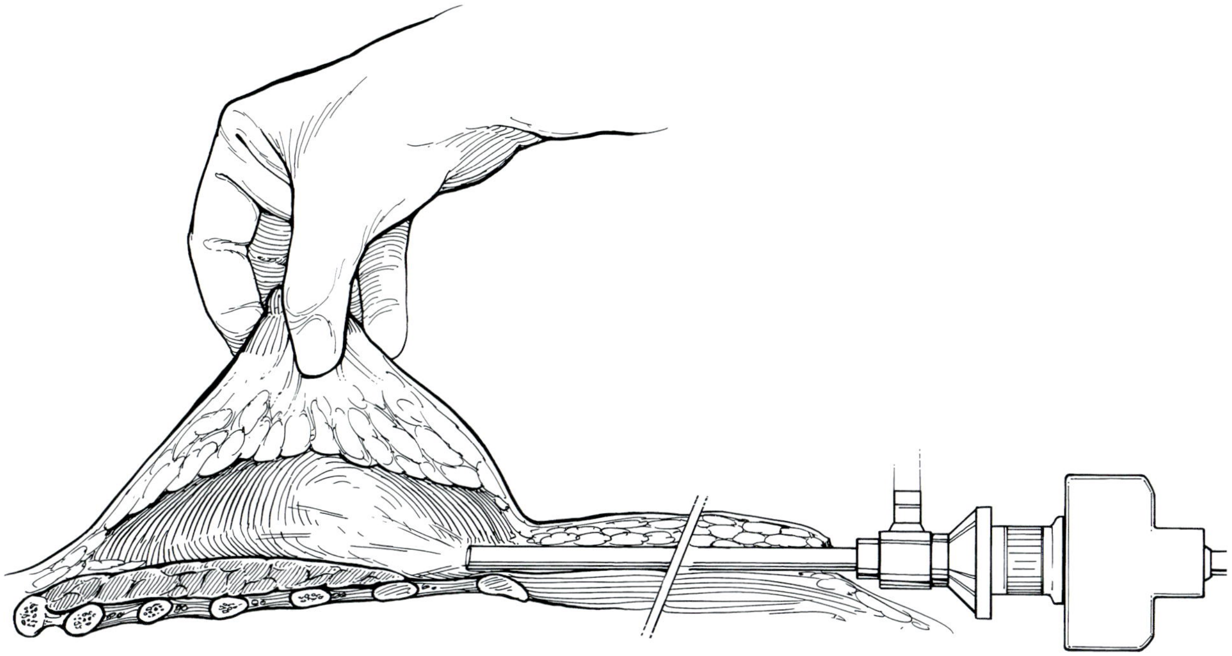

FIGURE 11-13
Mammary tissue *(above)* and the pectoralis major muscle *(below)* are shown.

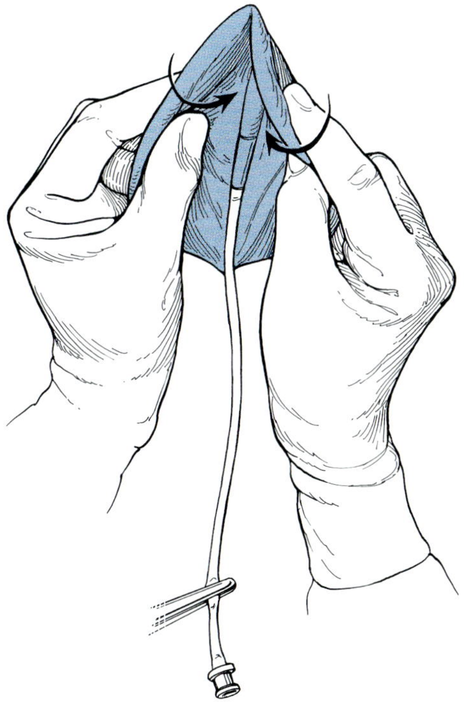

FIGURE 11-14
Two gloved hands showing expander edges rolled from each side to cover the fill-tube insertion site.

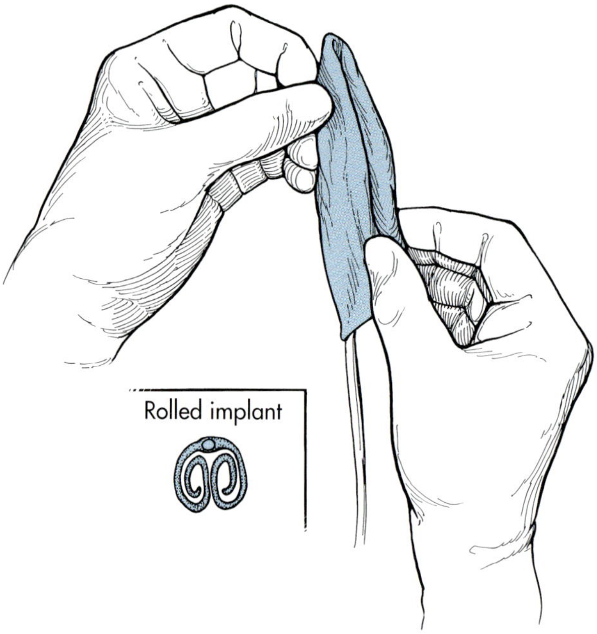

FIGURE 11-15
A rolled implant is shown.

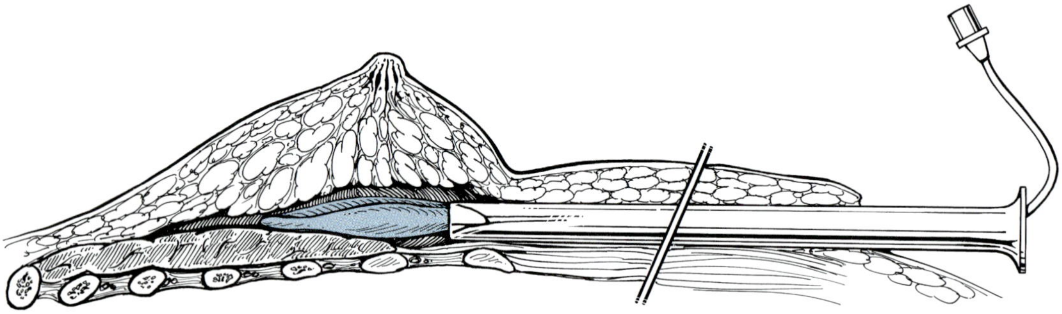

FIGURE 11-16
The expander is advanced into the retromammary plane, with its fill-tube insertion site facing posteriorly.

superior end of the expander is introduced into the umbilical incision and advanced through the tissue tunnel. Note that neither the expander nor, later, the implant is passed through the endotube. Once the expander and tip of the endotube are fully inserted the expander is advanced into the retromammary plane with its fill-tube insertion site facing posteriorly (Figure 11-16). While the opposite hand is palpating and securing the expander, the endotube is withdrawn.

Because the volume put into the expander does not require extreme precision, we use an inflation pump (the same pump we use to inject saline during liposuction). With a sterile, calibrated, metal container on the Mayo stand, we can rapidly fill the expander to the 50% overexpanded volume, compress or manipulate it as required to create the pocket, then reverse the tubing and suction out the saline (Figure 11-17). Traction on the filling tube is then sufficient to withdraw the expander. The implant itself is then prepared. We always submerge the air-inflated implants as soon as their sterile package is opened to be certain there is no leak. The implants are rolled and inserted in the

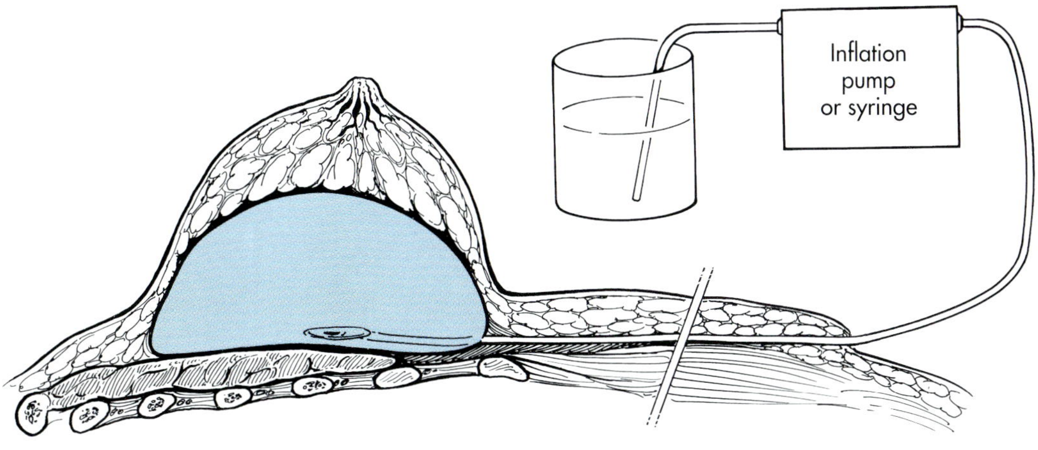

FIGURE 11-17
Expander, or implant inflation, is shown.

same manner as the expander, advanced into position, and inflated with syringes to the specified volume (Figures 11-18, *A* and *B*). It is our preference to use low-dose steroids, and we add Solumedrol (4 mg for each 100 ml of saline) to a maximum of 15 mg. We understand the hesitation of some surgeons to use steroids intraluminally; however, the primary author (GWJ) has done so since the 1970s and believes that, when used judiciously in low doses, they allow some suppression of capsule formation in the first few weeks of healing. This gives the patient a head start toward obtaining a good aesthetic result.[11,12] After inflation the fill tube is removed by pulling on the end while holding back on the implant with the other hand (Figure 11-19).

The next step is to reintroduce the endotube and obturator behind the implant, remove the obturator, and use the endoscope to visually inspect the implant valves to verify that there is no leak. The implant is compressed while visualizing the valve to be certain there is no leak even when the implant is put under pressure. Since we began inspecting the implant valves with the endoscope, we have found one leaking anterior diaphragm valve and one torn edge of a posterior leaf-valve, which we replaced even though it was not leaking. These were the only two implants we found to be questionable out of approximately 196 implants used in 98 patients. This inspection is an excellent opportunity to visualize the implant cavity to verify that there is no excessive bleeding. In approximately 400 patients operated on since October 1991, we have not had one case of hematoma or excessive bleeding using this technique of dissection by intraoperative tissue expansion. We have had two cases of a postoperative hematoma, which are reported on in this chapter. One was in a patient for whom we could not adequately expand the inframammary region on one side, and we had to complete the dissection by converting it to an open procedure. The patient had a hematoma the next day that required operation. During surgery an arterial bleeder was found to be in the area where we had opened the pocket by sharp dissection. The second patient had a forceful manual compression done two weeks postoperatively, which produced a hematoma that was evacuated with suction several days later through a small inframammary incision.

After inspection of the pocket, implants, valves, and passageways, the incision is closed, using 4-0 plain gut sutures. This is another minor change in the procedure since our earlier report (Figure 11-20).[6]

Antibiotic ointment and a cotton ball are placed in the umbilicus and taped. Two folded 4 × 4 inch gauze pads are placed over the cotton ball and taped. A large ABD pad is placed over each breast and an elastic bandage is wrapped tightly around the upper chest to compress only the upper hemisphere of the breasts. Part of the elastic bandage can be brought down and wrapped around the upper abdomen to provide some compression over the tunnels, or an abdominal binder can be used.

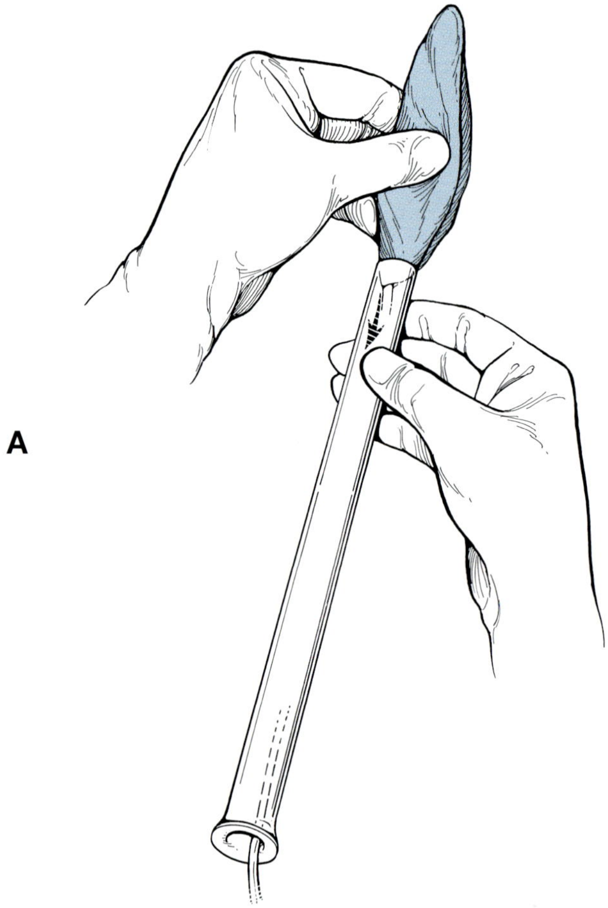

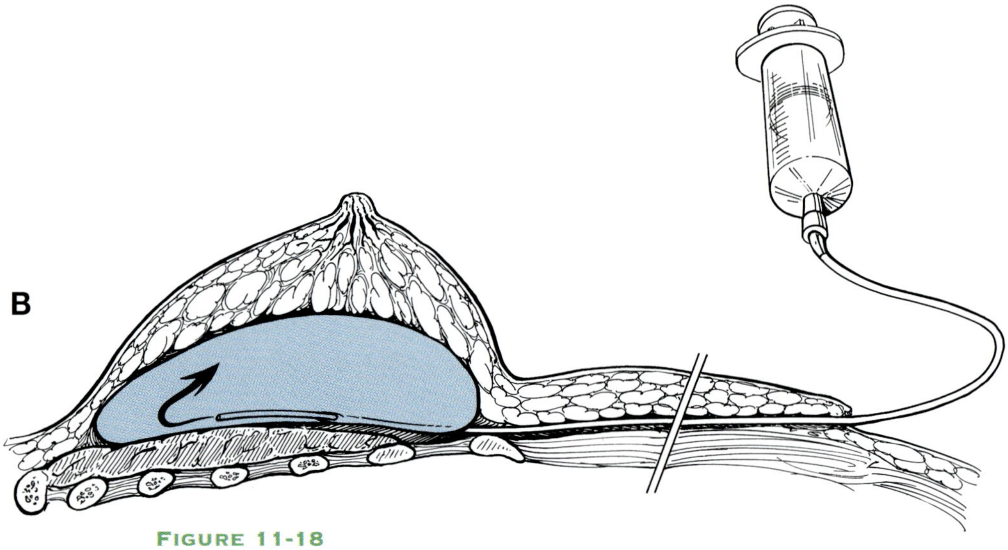

FIGURE 11-18
A and B, The implants inflated with syringes to specified volume are shown.

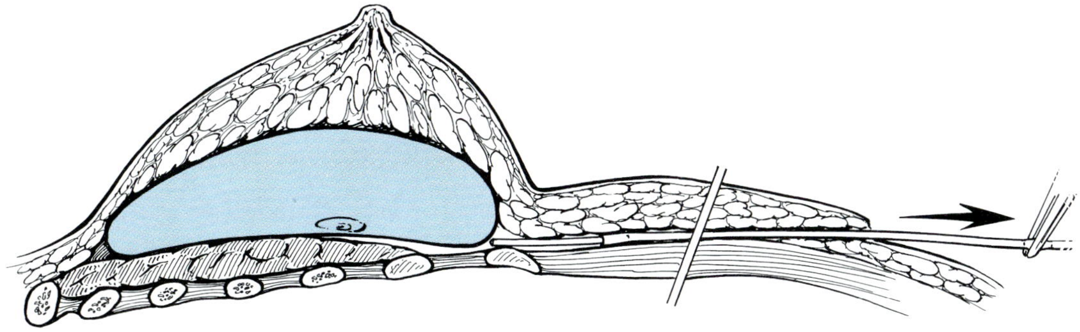

FIGURE 11-19
The fill tube removed from the implant is shown.

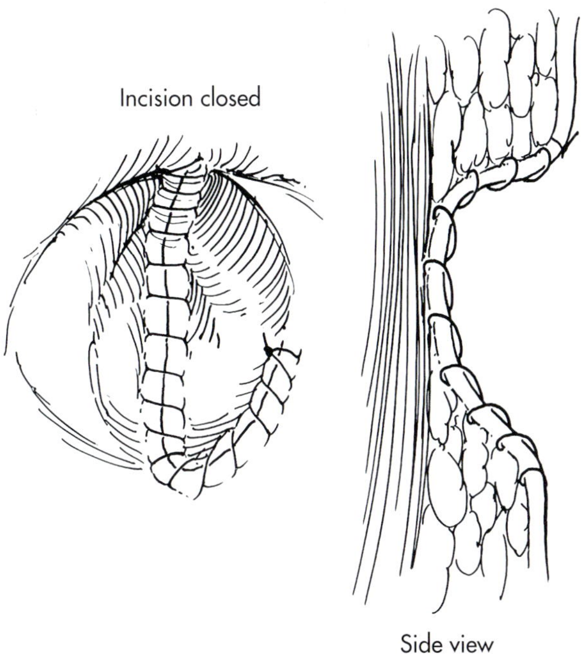

FIGURE 11-20
The closed incision using 4-0 plain catgut sutures and the side view are shown (enlargement of incision).

TECHNICAL CONSIDERATIONS

The transumbilical breast augmentation is a reliable, "patient-safe" procedure; however, there are technical considerations related to the implants available.

Whenever umbilical augmentation is planned, at least one additional backup implant is mandatory. Because of the variation in availability of certain sizes and types of implants, care is necessary in adapting implants from one manufacturer with fill tubes from another, or in mixing one brand or one style implant with another. Please note that at the time of this writing, the Mentor Company, although not objecting to the transumbilical route of insertion, does not permit their implants to contact metal objects during surgery, which can restrict their use for this procedure, requiring introduction of the implants by milking them up the tunnels. The mixing of brands and/or styles of implants in the same patient is very likely to produce visible and palpable asymmetries. Although the endoscopic breast augmentation method appears conceptually simple, technical pitfalls can complicate the execution of the procedure and increase the cost if implants are irreparably damaged.

In more than 80% of the patients the surgery involves no intraoperative difficulties whatsoever, and the rest are minor difficulties with which the surgeon must be prepared to cope. The most frequent minor difficulty is inadvertent penetration of the pectoralis muscle, making the tunnel subpectoral. In our first 150 patients, this was not infrequent, and in fact our inability to correct it required conversion to an open approach in three patients. However, we eventually developed techniques to avoid and correct such subpectoral tunnelling. In the most recent 200 patients we have occasionally obtained a subpectoral tunnel on the initial pass with the endotube, but in none of these cases did we have to convert to an open incision. To avoid subpectoral tunnelling, it is important to avoid lifting up on the breast when the endotube is penetrating the inframammary crease. Diagnosing a subpectoral passage is visually easy to do with the endoscope, through which the muscle fibers can be visualized superficial to the pocket. The best way to correct a subpectoral tunnel is to slowly withdraw the endotube with the endoscope in place, to determine precisely where the muscle penetration occurred, and to mark the corresponding point on the skin. A long, blunt, hockey-stick dissector should be passed first with the tip pointed medially, teasing it into the plane above the muscle and medial to the point of penetration of the muscle. Then the hockey stick must be bluntly and carefully pushed cephalad to above the level of the second rib. Next the tip is rotated up and over so it points laterally. The hockey stick is then pulled downward, and when it reaches the muscle penetration point a tunnel superficial to the muscle has been created. The process may be repeated as needed to make a wide tunnel, which is sometimes necessary in this situation to achieve adequate expansion.

POSTOPERATIVE CARE

If not allergic, all patients are given cephalexin 500 mg orally twice daily and pain medication. Almost without fail the number one postoperative complaint, starting in the recovery room, is the tightness of the bandage. However, if the patient is able to get enough pain relief, we insist that the bandage stay in place, untouched, until the next day. Rarely, we will see a patient who cannot get enough pain relief. Rather than overdose her with narcotics we will allow removal and replacement of the elastic bandage.

The bandages are removed and a lightweight, elastic, nonsupportive bra applied the next day in the office. If there is still excessive upper pole fullness, the elastic wrap or a tight tube-top is reapplied. A sphere will contain the maximum volume with the minimum surface area of any form. When the volume remains constant, as in the breast implant, compression of a sphere increases its surface area. Therefore direct compression of a sphere (breast implant) is the most simple and effective way to keep the pocket expanded. The patient may shower or bathe immediately. Running, aerobics, and heavy lifting are restricted for 1 to 3 weeks, depending on the individual's rate of recovery; after that time, basically unrestricted activity is permitted. Our usual recommendation is "If it hurts, don't do it."

Early manipulation can be encouraged for a minute or two every waking hour for the first 3 weeks, depending on the surgeon's preference. Vitamin E, 1000 to 2000 IU per day, can be used if desired.[13] The use of a bra is based on how the patient looks the first day postoperatively and how she wants to look. If the breasts have excessive superior fullness (i.e., the implants are "riding high," which is the case in most patients) and the patient likes that look, she is given a good supportive underwire bra, with tight nonstretch straps. If she wants the breasts to droop a little (which we prefer), we recommend to her wearing a lightweight stretch bra, as explained above, or electing not to wear a bra. If a patient wants her breasts to droop more than "normal," then we would suggest to her not wearing a bra in addition to direct massage and compression of the upper hemisphere of each breast with elastic wrap to help force the implant downward. All these manipulations are only for the first 3 weeks, when we reevaluate the need to continue them. The 1 week postoperative visit for suture removal has been eliminated with the use of plain gut to close the incision. We normally schedule postoperative visits at 3 weeks, and then 6 to 12 months. If a patient is having a problem or not progressing as expected, we see her as needed.

EXPECTED PHYSICAL FINDINGS POSTOPERATIVELY

The patient will experience chest and upper abdominal discomfort to varying degrees after surgery, which is usually mild or less than that experienced after use of standard incisions. There may be mild upper abdominal distention caused by a reflex relaxation of the rectus muscles, which lasts about a week. Periumbilical bruising and some subcutaneous induration may occur to varying degrees. The sensation to the breast may be altered but should return to normal in a short time. Bleeding is minimal; therefore, characteristically there is little if any ecchymosis over the breast; however, if bleeding occurs, a hematoma should be suspected and drainage performed as needed. The implants initially ride high on the chest wall, causing excess fullness in the upper pole of the breasts. With daily manipulation, manually pushing downward, and compression, the implants settle into place in about 6 weeks. Figures 11-21 and 11-22 (pp. 163 and 164) preoperative and postoperative results.

SUMMARY OF CLINICAL EXPERIENCE

An independent and unbiased survey of our first 2 years of clinical experience (October 1991 through

October 1993) was conducted by James Black, MD (senior Plastic Surgery resident in the Baylor program under the supervision of Melvin Spira, MD, Chief, Baylor College of Medicine, Division of Plastic Surgery, Houston, Texas) and was presented at the Senior Resident's Conference in Baltimore in May of 1994,[10] being awarded first prize. It is from Dr. Black's paper *Endoscopic augmentation mammoplasty* that the following statistics are extracted.

THE SURVEY COVERED 563 IMPLANTS IN 257 PATIENTS:

- Age range, 16 to 56 years
- Mean age, 29 years
- Implant sizes (volume), 200 ml to 800 ml
- Mean implant size, 395 ml
- Follow-up, 1 to 24 months
- Mean follow-up, 5.5 months
- 0 to 6 months follow-up, 173 patients
- 6 to 12 months follow-up, 55 patients
- 12 to 18 months follow-up, 22 patients
- 18 to 24 months follow-up, 7 patients

THE PATIENT DATA WERE EVALUATED for infection, hematoma and seroma, conversion to the open technique, nipple sensation, implant rupture, reoperation, capsular contracture, aesthetic result, and patient satisfaction:

- Operative infection, 1/257 patients (0.4%)
- Postoperative hematoma, 2/257 patients (0.8%)
- Seroma (presents in the tunnels), 4/257 patients (1.6%)
- Decreased sensation, 2/257 patients (0.8%)

THERE WERE 38/257 PATIENTS (15%) REOPERATED ON FOR THE FOLLOWING:

- Implant leakage, 12/174 (6.9%) from October 1991 through March 1993
- Implant leakage, 2/83 (2.4%) from April 1993 through October 1993 (this timeframe represents our conversion to the routine use of the tissue expander to create the pocket)
- Size adjustment, 18/257 (7.0%)
  - Size reduction—1/18 (5.5%)
  - Size increase—17/18 (94.4%)

The above-mentioned procedures were all done with endoscopic assistance from the umbilical or remote incision.

THERE WERE 6/257 (2.3%) PATIENTS WHO UNDERWENT OPEN PROCEDURES LATER:

- Capsulectomy, 4/257 (1.6%)
- Correction inframammary fold height, 2/257 (0.8%)

Satisfaction regarding aesthetic results was good to excellent in 96.2% of the patients; excellent was 210/257 (81.7%); good was 36/257 (14%); and fair 11/257 (4.3%).

THE FIBROUS CAPSULE AND CAPSULAR CONTRACTURE

The Baker classification is the best method in use today to quantify the degree of firmness of capsules around breast implants.[14] However, the Baker classification is not valid for overfilled saline implants placed in a retromammary position. Saline implants have a thicker shell than the silicone or double-lumen implants most frequently used in the past; therefore, saline implants have an inherently firmer feel to the touch than the silicone implants. Combining this inherent feel of firmness with the need to overinflate the saline implants to help prevent wrinkles, we felt that some new criteria were needed, particularly for the class I situation. We have developed the "Johnson Modified Baker Classification for Saline Implants." The attempt to achieve a Baker class I by underfilling a saline implant would result in visible and palpable wrinkles of the upper pole in thin-skinned patients.

CLASS I	
Baker	The breast is absolutely natural; the surgeon cannot tell that the breast was augmented. The patient has no complaints.
Johnson	The surgeon can detect the implant, but the pocket is 25% to 50% larger than the implant and the implant is freely mobile.
CLASS II	
Baker	There is minimal contracture; the surgeon can detect the implant, but the patient has no complaints.
Johnson	Same as class I except that the pocket is smaller; the patient has no complaints.
CLASS III	
Baker	There is moderate contracture; the patient feels some firmness.
Johnson	The implant feels firm and the margins are visible; the patient feels the firmness.

CLASS IV

Baker	There is severe contracture, which is obvious from observation alone.
Johnson	There is firm contracture; the margins are visible; the patient may have pain.

Finally, silicone is a thermal insulator, whereas saline is a good thermal conductor. Because of this, silicone-implanted breasts may be cool, whereas the saline-implanted breasts tend to be normally warm to the touch, a difference most noticeable in contracted breasts. In the class IV cases (Johnson and Baker) there is no difference in the feel of a saline implant versus a silicone implant, subglandular or subpectoral.

The endoscopic method of insertion of saline inflatable breast implants does not in any way claim superior results in shape, size, or long-term softness compared with standard, established procedures placing saline implants prepectorally. This new procedure does, however, offer a single hidden scar (no breast scars) and a decreased chance of permanent loss of sensation to the breast skin and nipple (0.8% versus 15% to 30% with the open technique). The procedure is a safe, repeatable, effective technique with aesthetic results equivalent to the open techniques, and has a high rate of patient acceptance. The disadvantages of this technique are those inherent in the use of prepectoral saline-filled implants in thin patients, namely upper pole wrinkling or visible edge demarcation.

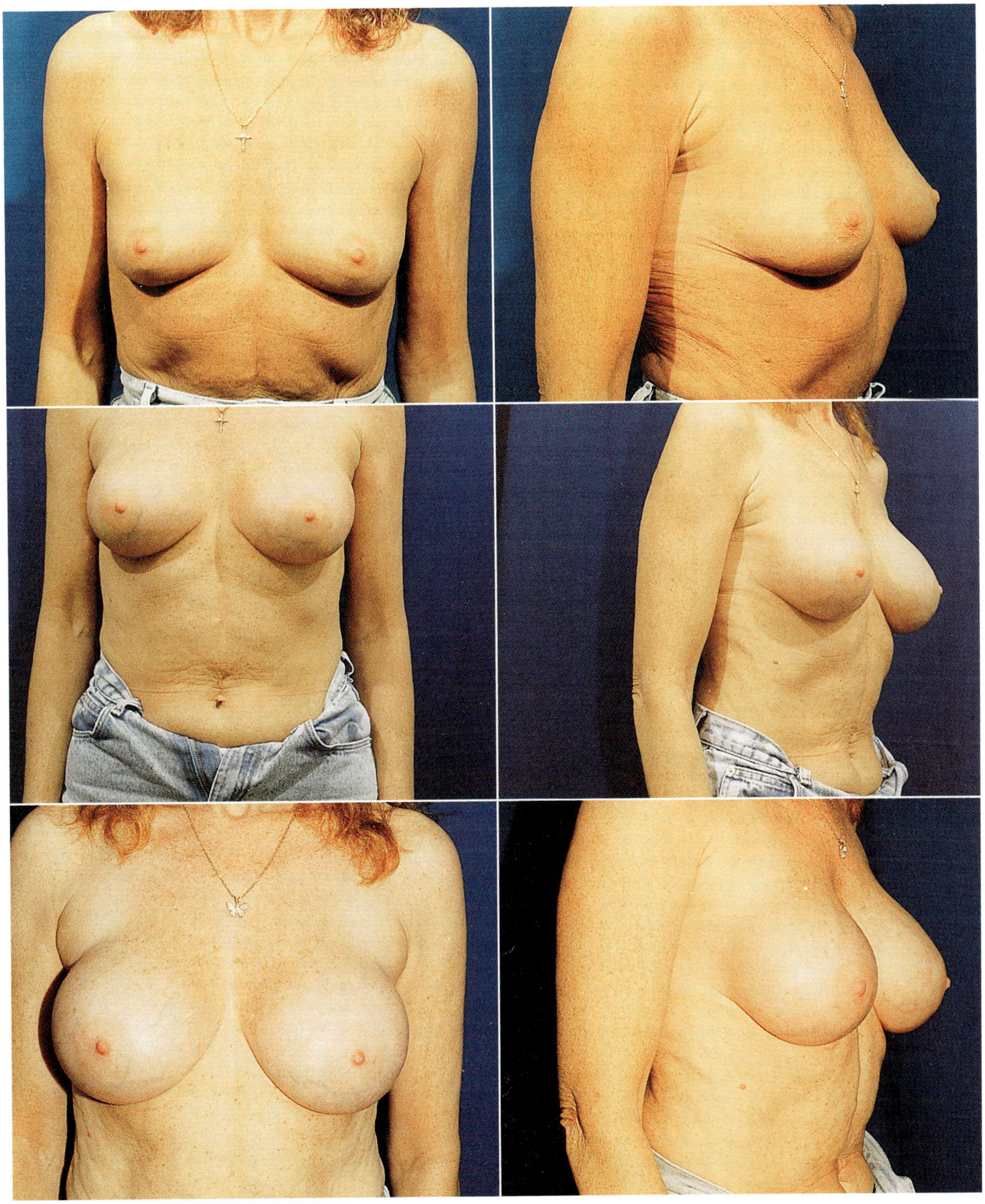

FIGURE 11-21
Case Study 1. **A and B,** Preoperative appearance. **C and D,** Three months following insertion of McGhan 320 ml implants inflated to 350 ml and 20 mg Solu-Medrol added. **E and F,** At 3 months postoperatively, implants were replaced with McGhan 400 ml implants inflated to 470 ml on right and 450 ml on left with 16 mg Solu-Medrol added to each side. Patient shown here at 21 months postoperatively. A leaking right implant was replaced 5 months later.

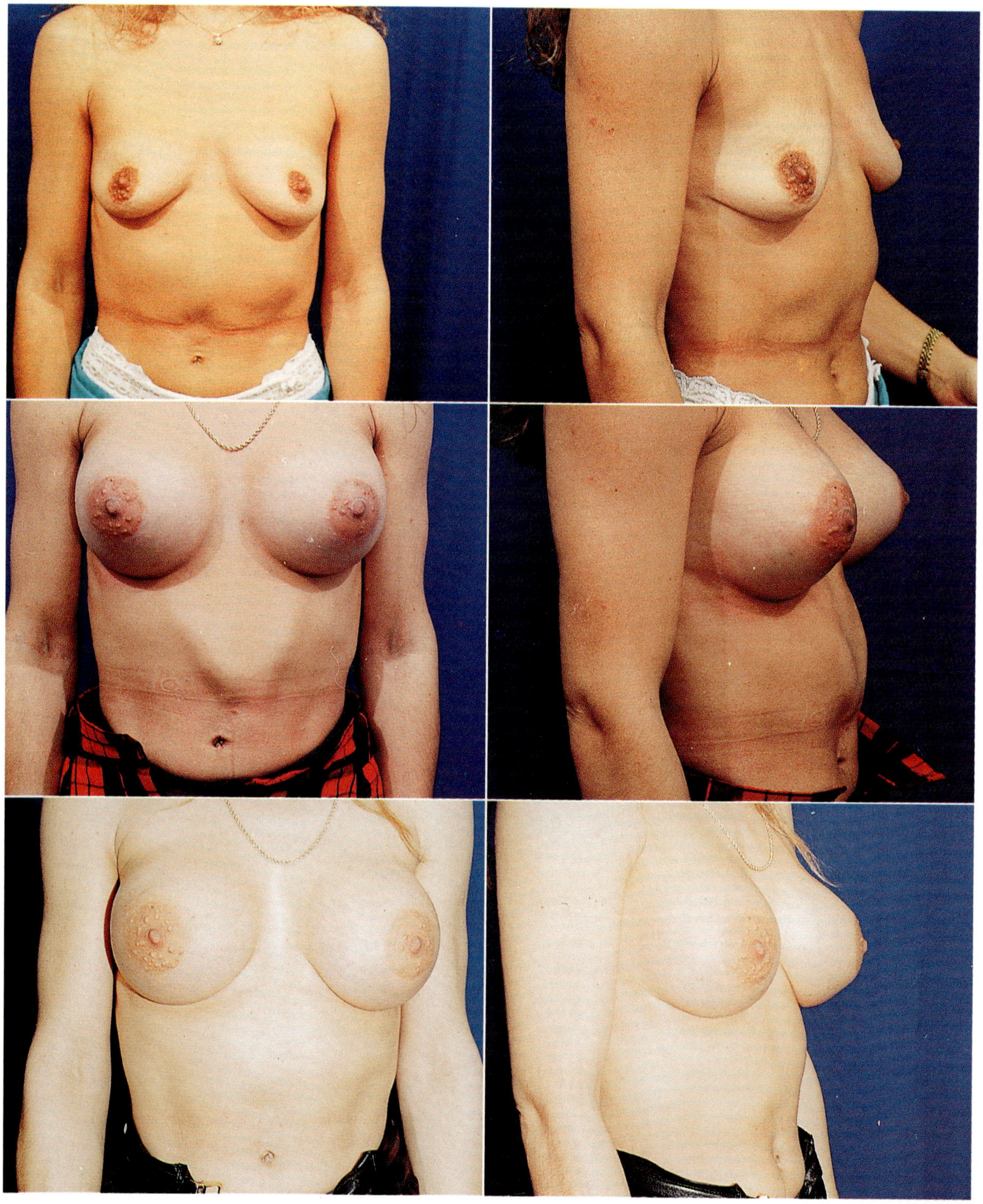

FIGURE 11-22
Case Study 2. **A and B,** Preoperative appearance. **C and D,** One week following insertion of McGhan 400 ml implants inflated to 430 ml and 12 mg Solu-Medrol added to each side. There was a collection of serum in both tunnels. The "V"-shaped seroma above the umbilicus was aspirated and did not recur. **E and F,** One year postoperatively.

REFERENCES

1. Cronin TD, Gerow FJ: *Augmentation mammoplasty: a new "natural feel" prosthesis.* In *Transactions of the Third International Congress of Plastic and Reconstructive Surgery.* (Excerpta Medica International Congress Series No. 66.) Amsterdam, 1974, Excerpta Medica Foundation.
2. Arion H: Presentation d'une prosthese retromammaire, *Soc Fr Gynecol* 35:427, 1965.
3. Hoehler H: Breast augmentation: the axillary approach, *Br J Plast Surg* 26:373, 1973.
4. Planas J: Introduction of breast implants through abdominal route, *Plast Reconstr Surg* 57:434, 1976.
5. Barrett BM Jr: Combined abdominoplasty and augmentation mammoplasty through a transverse suprapubic incision, *Ann Plast Surg* 4:286, 1980.
6. Johnson GW, Christ JE: The endoscopic breast augmentation: the transumbilical insertion of saline-filled breast implants, *Plast Reconstr Surg* 92:801, 1993.
7. Ellenbogen R: Personal communication, June 15, 1994.
8. Rosenberg P: Personal communication.
9. Regnault P, Daniel R., editors: *Aesthetic plastic surgery principles and technique,* Boston, 1984, Little, Brown.
10. Johnson G, Black J, Spira M: Endoscopic Augmentation Mammoplasty, presented by Dr. Black to the 1994 Senior Resident's Conference, Boston, May 27, 1994.
11. Ksander GA: Effects of diffused soluble steroid on capsules around experimental breast prostheses in rats, *Plast Reconstr Surg* 63:708, 1979.
12. Cucin RL, Guthrie RH, Graham M: Rate of diffusion of Solu-Medrol across the Silastic membranes of breast prosthesis: an in vitro study, *Ann Plast Surg* 9:228, 1982.
13. Baker JL: The effectiveness of alpha-tocopherol (vitamin E) in reducing the incidence of spherical contracture around breast implants, *Plast Reconstr Surg* 68:696, 1981.
14. Baker JL Jr: *Augmentation mammoplasty.* In Owsley JQ, Peterson RA, editors: *Symposium on aesthetic surgery of the breast,* St Louis, 1979, Mosby–Year Book.

CHAPTER 12

Breast Augmentation: Periareolar Submuscular Approach

Richard A. Mladick

The endoscope can be a helpful adjunct for the periareolar approach to submuscular breast augmentation. Before discussing the role of the endoscope, a brief review of the periareolar approach is useful.

THE RATIONALE OF THE PERIAREOLAR APPROACH

Are there advantages in the periareolar approach as opposed to the axillary or traditional submammary approach? The periareolar approach is ideally located to provide the most direct and shortest route to the submuscular pocket. The periareolar incision allows easy insertion of the endoscope to all limits of the pocket. This incision also allows easy irrigation and visualization of the entire pocket.

Our experience with almost 3000 periareolar incisions has been such that only two patients have required revision of the scar. The incision is completely covered by all types of clothing, even swimsuits. When the incision is uncovered, it is an excellent scar in a "hidden" area.

There is the ability to directly visualize the entire limits of the pocket with or without an endoscope, which is not possible with the axillary incision. As opposed to the axillary incision, this incision allows direct visualization of the valve closure. The surgeon can easily clean away small particles of fat or blood before removing the filling tube from the superior diaphragm valve. These particles should be cleaned away so that they will not inadvertently disrupt the closing mechanism.

Another important factor is that this incision permits reoperation to be done without damage to the implant (not possible through the axillary approach). It is difficult if not impossible to reoperate through the axillary incision when there is an inflated implant within the pocket. Any attempt to remove an inflated implant through the axillary incision (without first emptying the implant) will cause damage to the implant. Unfortunately, it is not possible to reinsert the filling tube into an inflated implant through the axillary incision. However, minor revisions such as lowering a high pocket or closing off a lateral pocket can easily be done through the periareolar incision. In some cases these revisions can be done without removing the implant.

The inferior periareolar approach can be changed to a superior periareolar approach when necessary. Most often this is when there is a small amount of preoperative sagging that would create a "double-bubble" appearance if a submuscular implant were inserted. For more moderate sagging a total periareolar reduction (donut skin excision) can tighten and provide significant lift.

THE ROLE OF THE ENDOSCOPE

The endoscope can be an excellent tool for better visualization of the limits of the pocket when a small periareolar incision is used. In many cases it is possible to do this procedure through a 2- to 2.5-cm inferior periareolar incision.

Use of the endoscope also provides an excellent view of the precise muscle release, which is a key part of successful submuscular augmentation. The endoscope helps in obtaining good hemostasis.

For didactic and demonstration purposes, the endoscope is an excellent tool and the only way to satisfactorily demonstrate surgery inside the pocket to other professionals. The endoscope was successfully used for this purpose during the breast symposium held at the Center for Cosmetic Plastic Surgery in 1992.[1]

ENDOSCOPIC TECHNIQUE

The operation is done following the basic tenets of the no-touch submuscular augmentation technique, which we reported previously.[2] The no-touch technique is a "super" sterile technique that minimizes or eliminates contamination of the implant to avoid that factor causing capsular contracture.[3-5]

The inferior periareolar incision is made at the junction of the pigmented areolar skin and the inferior breast skin, being careful not to extend past 5 o'clock on the left side and 7 o'clock on the right side. Subcutaneous dissection is carried out inferiorly for approximately 4 cm. A cutting cautery is then used to cut through the breast tissue directly to the pectoralis muscle directly under the areola (Figure 12-1). As soon as the pectoralis fascia is exposed it is opened with a coagulation cautery to keep it from retracting from the pectoralis muscle. Army–Navy retractors then lift up the breast tissue, which pulls up the pectoralis major from the pectoralis minor muscle. The pectoralis major muscle is then entered with a pair of curved Metzenbaum scissors in the superior lateral quadrant. When the surgeon has penetrated underneath the pectoralis major muscle a small amount of areolar tissue can be seen between the major and the minor muscles. It is at this point that the endoscope is inserted. The author prefers a No. 10 straight-sight endoscope. A pushing and sweeping motion easily develops the space between the pectoralis major and the pectoralis minor muscles. As the dissection extends toward the medial and inferior pocket, the blunt dissection will disrupt portions of the medial and inferior insertions of the pectoralis major muscle. The thicker, tougher muscle bundles are severed with a long, insulated, coagulation cautery placed through the wound next to the endoscope (Figure 12-2).

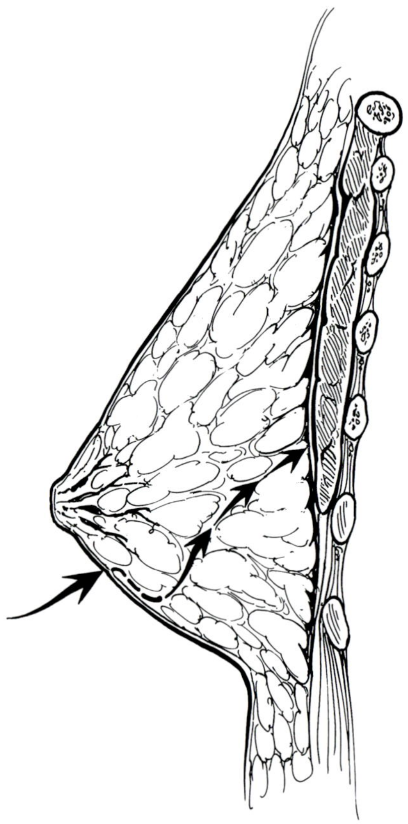

FIGURE 12-1
After infra-areolar incision the dissection is directed subcutaneously 3 to 4 cm, then a cutting cautery cuts through the breast tissue to the pectoralis fascia (muscle).

The initial blunt dissection can also be done with a gloved finger dipped in bacitracin solution. The endoscope is then inserted for the muscle release. The endoscope is directed medially at the level of the third rib and the cautery blade is then used to gently swipe the muscle fibers, layer by layer. The muscle release is carried out from approximately 3 o'clock medially to 6 or 7 o'clock in the inferior pocket (Figure 12-3). The muscle is not totally

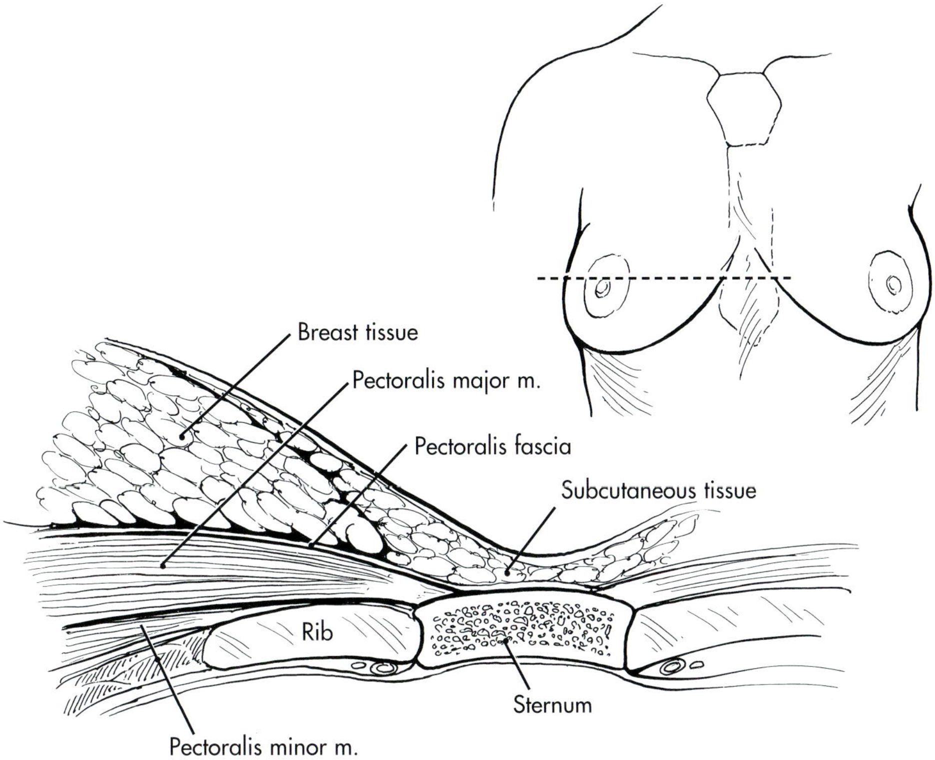

FIGURE 12-2
A diagramatic cross-section of the muscle attachments is shown. Note the overlying pectoralis fascia. The proper muscle release is shown in Figure 12-3.

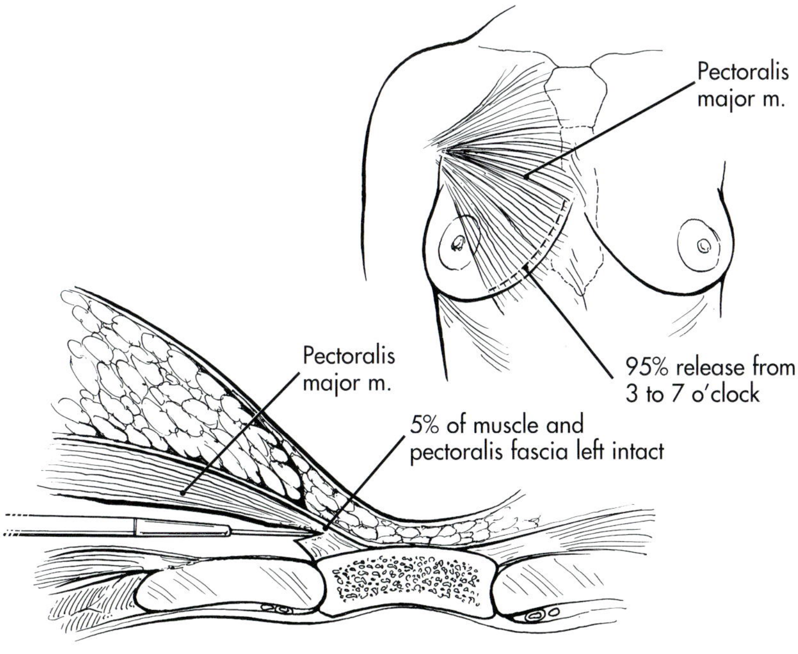

FIGURE 12-3
The pectoralis major muscle is released from 3 o'clock to 7 o'clock. The muscle is not cut all the way through (95%), and the overlying pectoraiis fascia is never released.

released, rather it is cut through 95% of the fibers.[6,7] This dissection is extended to the limits of the preoperatively established pocket, which varies according to the size of the implant.

The precise muscle release is extremely important. The magnified view with the endoscope is extremely helpful in releasing just enough but not too much of the pectoralis major muscle. When the dissection cuts through most of the pectoralis muscle, the pectoralis fascia can be seen as a white layer behind the red muscle fibers. A cutting cautery may release the muscles too quickly. For a more exact, slower release of the last few muscle fibers the surgeon uses the cautery in coagulation mode.

It is essential that the release of the pectoralis major be sufficient to prevent the muscle from forcing the implant into the superior pocket. However, the muscle must not be overreleased, and the surgeon should never release the pectoralis fascia. In rare cases where the inferior pectoralis muscle origin is very high (superior) it may be necessary to totally release the pectoralis muscle and continue the submuscular dissection under the fibers of the superior rectus abdominis and serratus muscle fibers.

When the medial and inferior pectoralis fibers and pectoralis fascia are totally released, distortion will occur whenever the patient contracts the pectoralis muscle. The breast will "jump" laterally toward the shoulder with each contraction. This is especially disturbing to active, athletic women and is a complication that can be avoided by subtotal muscle release.

In addition to the excellent visualization of the muscle release, the endoscope provides excellent visualization for hemostasis in the limits of the pocket (Figure 12-4). Any small bleeders are easily controlled with a long, insulated coagulation blade; long, insulated forceps are used for larger bleeders.

The endoscope is most efficient when there are two monitors. One monitor can be placed on either side of the operating table so that the surgeon is always looking directly at the screen over the endoscope. The correct position of the video screen is important for the highest comfort level when using the endoscope. It is difficult to turn around to look at a monitor behind you when manipulating an endoscope in front (Figures 12-5, *A* and *B*).

Both xenon and the halogen lights have been used and are satisfactory. The xenon provides a brighter field, but the colors are satisfactory with both lights. The amount of light has been totally adequate using the halogen source. The ideal instrument for coagulation is an insulated coagulating blade with a built-in smoke evacuator. If the surgeon does not have a combination smoke evacuator and coagulation blade, smoke can be evacuated by threading a small sterile plastic suction tube into the pocket and keeping it on suction.

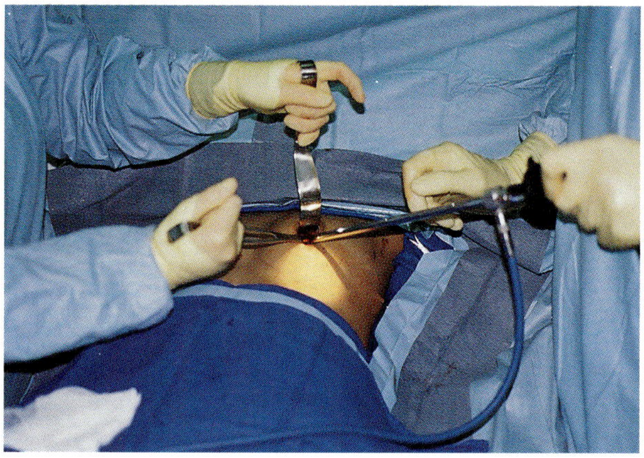

FIGURE 12-4
The breast is retracted so that the endoscope can be inserted under the muscle.

The 4-mm scope may be ideal for facial endoscopy and can be used for breast surgery, but I prefer the 10-mm scope. With the periareolar incision either the straight-view scope or the 30-degree angle scope can be used.

After completing the dissection on one side the endoscope is removed and the pocket irrigated until clear. A drain is inserted and two or three deep muscle sutures are placed and the needles cut off. The surgeon then switches sides and moves the endoscopy feed to the other monitor across the table. If only one monitor is available it can be placed at the foot of the table or simply moved each time to the side opposite the surgeon. The second side is then completed in the same way as the first. Before placing the implants the surgeon returns to the first side and reinspects the pocket for complete hemostasis.

After it is determined that the pockets are of satisfactory size and hemostasis is complete the surgeon changes to new powderless gloves, and the implants are inserted. A sleeve is used during insertion of the implants to conform to the no-touch technique.

Implants are then filled to the maximum using the closed filling system from a 1000-ml intravenous saline bag, which contains 1 g of cefazolin (Keflin) and 36 mg of Solu-Medrol.

The filling tube is then pulled under direct vision to seal the valve securely without trapped particles

FIGURE 12-5
A, When the monitor is behind the surgeon it may be harder to follow and to move the scope into the correct position. **B,** It is easier for the surgeon to have the monitor on the opposite side of the table.

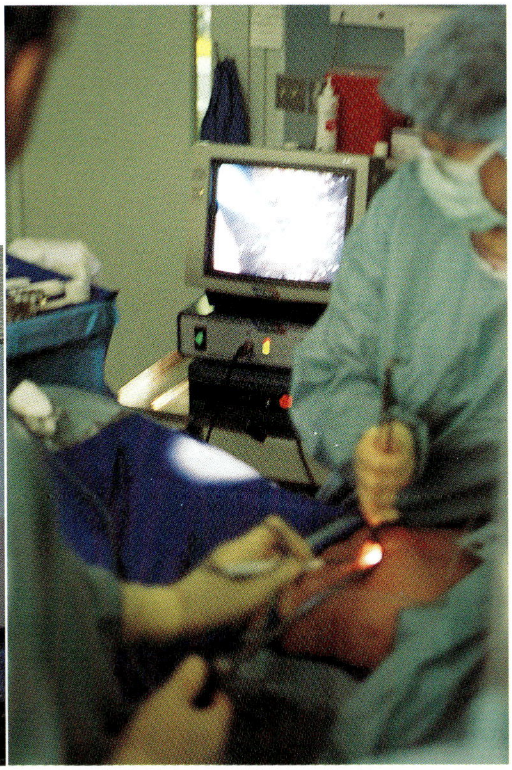

B

A

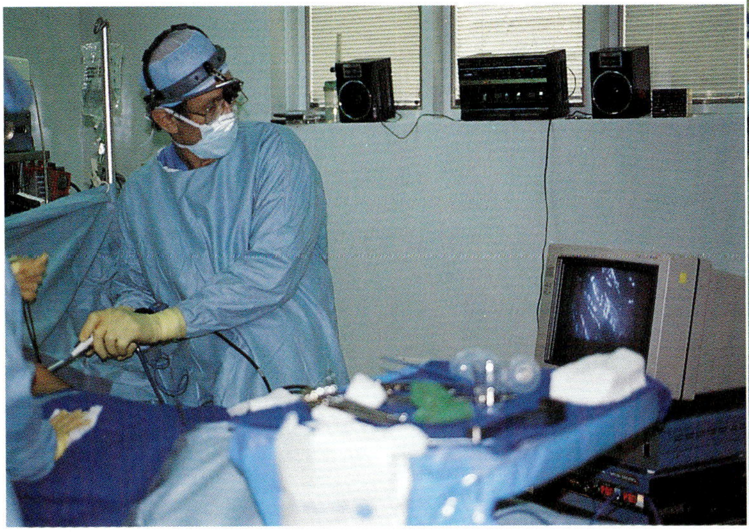

A

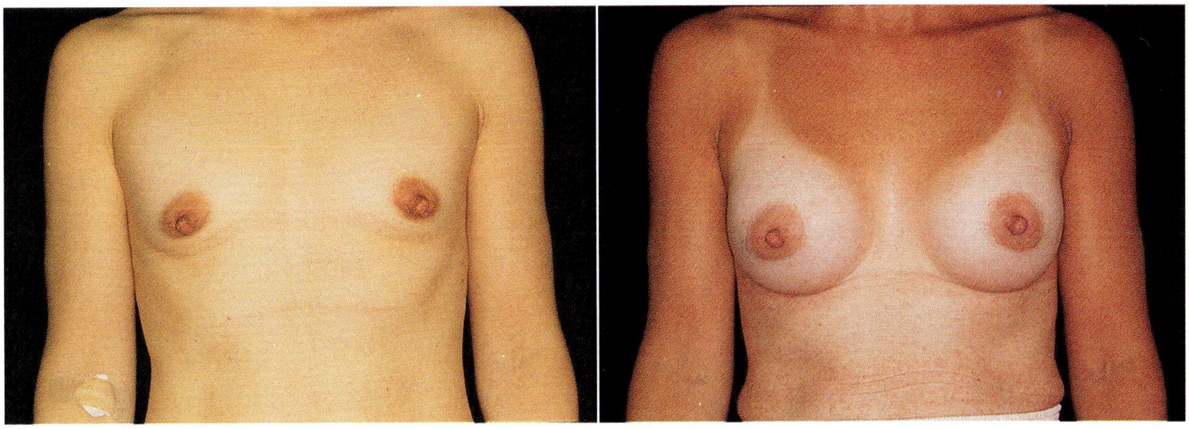

B

FIGURE 12-6
A and B, Typical preoperative and postoperative photographs of endoscopically performed submuscular augmentation are shown. Note that the scar is virtually imperceptible.

of fat or blood. The muscle sutures are tied, then 2-0 absorbable sutures close the breast, and 4-0 absorbable sutures close the subcuticular wound. The final skin closure is then done with 4-0 prolene pull-out sutures. At the end of the procedure the patient is wrapped with an ace bandage across the superior half of the breast, and a solution of bacitracin and bupivacaine (Marcaine) is injected into the drain tubes, to control postoperative pain and infection.

The procedure is best done under general anesthesia but can be done with local anesthesia and IV sedation. This procedure has been done without the endoscope for years, but the endoscope does provide an excellent magnified view as described. Of all the possible incisions, the periareolar incision is an extremely advantageous incision for use of the endoscope (Figures 12-6, *A* and *B*).

CONCLUSION

There are some drawbacks and inconveniences associated with the use of the endoscope. One is the increased operative time, and another is the additional equipment involved. There are some who consider the use of the endoscope superfluous with periareolar incisions because the pocket can be directly visualized. I believe, however, that the real question that remains to be answered is whether the endoscope will ultimately help the surgeon to perform better. As more experience is being gained and information is accumulating, we will be in a better position to answer this question in the future.

References

1. Advanced Symposium, Augmentation Mammaplasty with Saline Implants, held at the Center for Cosmetic Plastic Surgery, Virginia Beach, VA, March 20-21, 1992.
2. Mladick RA: "No-touch submuscular saline breast augmentation technique, *Aesth Plast Surg* 17:183, 1993.
3. Burkhart BR: Capsular contracture: hard breasts, soft data, *Clin Plast Surg* 15:521, 1988.
4. Dubin D: Presented at Annual Meeting of American Society of Aesthetic Plastic Surgeons, Orlando, FL, May 1980.
5. Sanger JR, Sheth NK, Franson TR: Adherence of microorganisms to breast prosthesis: an in vitro study, *Ann Plast Surg* 22:337, 1989.
6. Biggs TM, Yarish RS: Augmentation mammaplasty: retropectoral versus retromammary implantation, *Clin Plast Surg* 15:549, 1988.
7. Biggs TM, Yarish RS: Augmentation mammaplasty: a comparative analysis, *Plast Reconstr Surg* 85:368, 1990.

CHAPTER 13

Breast Augmentation: Transaxillary Retropectoral Approach

G. Patrick Maxwell
M. Dean Vistnes

The recent interest in surgical endoscopy within the field of plastic surgery has led to the development of a number of different procedures that may now be performed using this technology. These include endoscopic breast procedures of different types, facial rejuvenation procedures, harvesting a variety of autogenous graft materials, carpal tunnel release, and abdominoplasty. In the next several years, as with any new technology, some of these procedures will undoubtedly be abandoned for one reason or another in favor of preexisting or even newer techniques. Some of these endoscopic procedures, however, will find an established role in the field of plastic surgery, and perhaps even define a new standard. One procedure in particular that is likely to withstand the test of time is endoscopically assisted transaxillary retropectoral breast augmentation.

The traditional transaxillary approach to breast augmentation gained popularity among plastic surgeons and patients primarily because of the absence of scars on the breast. This blunt dissection technique, once learned, is considered by many to be quick, straightforward, and reproducible in terms of the surgical outcome. Other advantages of the transaxillary approach include minimizing loss of nipple sensation with a properly executed procedure and a theoretically decreased risk of periprosthetic infections by minimizing contact with the breast tissue.

The shortcomings of the traditional approach, however, are far from trivial. The anatomy of the axilla in the area of the initial dissection requires familiarity to consistently and easily develop the correct surgical plane without complications. Because the majority of the dissection is done blindly using blunt dissection, precise hemostasis and visualization of important anatomic structures can be difficult, if not impossible. Some people may criticize retropectoral implant placement because of the potential for muscular distortion of the prosthesis. But perhaps, most importantly, the blunt transaxillary approach considerably limits surgeons in their ability to precisely control the inframammary fold and lower pole of the breast. Consequently, patients with glandular ptosis or tight, constricted, inframammary folds are considered poor candidates for traditional transaxillary augmentation mammaplasty. Indeed, the inability to precisely manipulate and adjust the inframammary fold and adjacent tissues in these patients can result in irregularities, asymmetries, and suboptimal aesthetic results.

The usefulness of the blunt transaxillary approach in secondary breast augmentation or revisions is also limited. Again, the lack of direct exposure significantly limits surgeons in terms of their ability to alter the inframammary fold, surrounding fascia, glandular tissue, and prosthetic capsule, as is often required in this group of patients. In fact, patients undergoing traditional transaxillary breast augmentation were routinely counseled that revision surgery would almost certainly require an inframammary or periareolar incision for adequate access and exposure.

With *endoscopically assisted* transaxillary retropectoral breast augmentation, one is able to eliminate or significantly reduce many of the previously mentioned problems associated with the blunt technique. By incorporating surgical endoscopy into the procedure, bleeding vessels are easily seen and coagulated. Visualization of the entire pocket during the dissection allows significantly better control of the inframammary fold and lower pole breast tissue. The pectoralis major muscle can be divided either completely or partially under controlled visualization, which minimizes the risk of postoperative muscular distortion of the implant yet still allows muscle coverage of the implant. Similarly, the lower pole breast parenchyma and surrounding fascia can be surgically altered as required to obtain the desired result.

It is the ability to control the inframammary fold and the lower breast pole that is the primary benefit of using the endoscope during transaxillary retropectoral breast augmentation. This ability has elevated the transaxillary approach in primary breast augmentation to a significantly higher level of surgical sophistication. It has also improved the versatility and control of the operation and has made it possible to operate on selected patients with inframammary fold irregularities of pseudoptosis, as well as on patients undergoing secondary surgical procedures.

PATIENT EVALUATION

Augmentation mammaplasty should not be considered a trivial procedure where a generic surgical pocket is created into which an implant is then stuffed. This crude concept of breast augmentation should be replaced with one that blends artistic and aesthetic judgment with an objective analysis of the anatomic parameters that define breast shape and contour. This preoperative analysis should then be followed by an accurate, controllable, and reproducible surgical procedure to enhance the existing anatomy.

A complete and thorough discussion with the patient is prerequisite in determining the appropriate procedure and surgical approach for breast augmentation today. The decision on which approach to use (transaxillary, inframammary, or periareolar) in each patient should be based on a combination of physician judgment, patient desires, and anatomic considerations. A single technique or approach is neither appropriate nor ideal for all patients. Consequently, the surgeon should be comfortable with several techniques in order to offer the one that will give the best possible result and satisfy the patient at the same time.

A complete discussion of the risks and potential complications of any surgical procedure is mandatory. Any preexisting asymmetries of the inframammary fold, breast size, shape or position, and nipple–areola dimensions are documented and pointed out to the patient. Similarly, an analysis of the adjacent muscles, soft tissue, and skeletal structures is done in each patient. Limitations of the procedure must be discussed in detail with the patient, and she should have realistic expectations of what can be accomplished.

A three-dimensional analysis of the breasts, or dimensional analysis, is done on each patient preoperatively. This approach combines a subjective visual analysis with objective measurements. In particular, measurements are made of the specific parameters that define breast size and shape, and from these, preoperative markings are made to guide the surgeon during the operation. Every effort should be made to get away from thinking strictly in terms of volume, or "How many cc's should the implant be to get the result I want?" Instead, look at the various *aesthetic dimensions of the breast* and decide how these need to be changed to obtain the desired result. With this in mind, implants should be selected based on patient desires regarding changes in breast width, fullness, projection, and overall cup size, while taking into consideration the constraints imposed by the underlying anatomy.

Preoperative markings should be done with the patient awake, in a sitting or standing position. Start by marking the fixed anatomic landmarks: the sternal notch and the vertical midline. Measure the distance from the sternal notch or midclavicle to the nipple. This distance indicates the relationship of the nipples to each other, as well as the position of each breast mound on the chest wall. Measure the intermammary distance as the distance between the medial edges of the two breast mounds. Also note the distance from the vertical midline to the nipple on each side. The *base width* of each breast is measured from the medial- most aspect of the upslope of the breast mound to the lateral edge of the breast profile when viewed from the anterior. This is one of the most important dimensions to measure, since changing it can affect both the intermammary distance and the lateral projection or fullness of the breast. Question the patient regarding the amount of lateral and medial fullness (cleavage) she wants. Based on these desires and the overall change in size the patient wants, select an implant with the appropriate base dimension.

Choosing an implant with a wider base dimension than the existing breast width allows the surgeon to selectively and predictably increase medial and/or lateral fullness. Selecting such an implant will require pocket dissection beyond the borders that define the preoperative breast shape. When choosing to alter the medial or lateral fullness of the breast in this way, it is important to plan the proper pocket size and location, and to position the implant precisely within this pocket. Some patients, however, may not need or desire a change in the width in the breast, only a volume augmentation (such as a patient with postpartum involutional breasts). In these instances, select an implant corresponding to the existing base dimension, or even slightly smaller.

The location of the nipple–areola complex in relation to the inframammary fold is measured, as well as any differences in areola diameter. The level of the existing inframammary fold is marked, and any asymmetries in position are noted. The distance from the lower edge of the areola or nipple to the existing inframammary fold is measured on each side. The inframammary fold is then lowered as needed to maintain aesthetic balance with the other planned dimensional changes.

If the breast is to be enlarged by simply increasing the volume within the existing dimensions, lowering the inframammary fold may not be necessary. However, if the *base width* of the breast is to be significantly enlarged to accommodate a relatively large prosthesis, the inframammary fold must be lowered in proportion to the increase in medial and lateral dimensions. Failure to do so will result in an improperly positioned implant and unattractive upper pole fullness. As a general guideline, the new fold should be placed at a level such that the lower edge of the areola to inframammary fold distance is approximately 5.0 to 5.5 cm for B cup breasts, 5.5 to 6.5 cm for C cup breasts, and 6.5 to 7.5 cm for D cup breasts. These are approximate distances only and should be interpreted as such. What is important to realize is that as the breast volume and base width are increased, the distance from the nipple to the inframammary fold increases to maintain aesthetic proportions. In general, patients will rarely require lowering of the fold by more than 1.5 to 2.0 cm, unless they are requesting a very large change in breast dimensions or have a high, tight, inframammary fold as is found in the constricted breast deformity.

It is particularly important to pay attention to the inframammary fold area when a patient presents with a tight or high fold. Failure to address this specific anatomic variation during surgery can result in a "double-bubble" appearance postoperatively. In these instances, the fascia and/or breast parenchyma will usually need to be incised or scored to allow adequate release for expansion of the lower pole after placement of the implant. This task must be done under some type of visualization, either direct or with an endoscope.

Breast augmentation has evolved into a procedure that requires thoughtful preoperative planning followed by a surgical approach allowing versatility and control of the tissues that define breast shape. A combination of an objective dimensional analysis and a subjective evaluation based on aesthetic ideals is important, regardless of the surgical approach selected. Only by first understanding the individual components that determine aesthetic breast shape can breasts be surgically modified with any degree of consistency. Once these parameters have been analyzed and defined, a surgical plan and approach is selected that will allow predictable alteration of the breasts to achieve the desired shape and size. The use of the endoscope in transaxillary retropectoral augmentation gives the surgeon the ability to precisely control and alter those variables that will determine postoperative breast shape.

SURGICAL ANATOMY

To successfully perform the endoscopically assisted transaxillary retropectoral augmentation mammaplasty, the surgeon should be familiar with the anatomy in the area of the axillary incision, as well as the anatomy of the breast and adjacent tissues.

The pectoralis major muscle has broad origins from the clavicle, the sternum, and the first five to six ribs. In addition to the broad origins along the sternum and ribs, there are numerous small slips of muscle in these areas that also contribute to the origin of the pectoralis major muscle. Inferiorly, the pectoralis major muscle extends approximately 5 cm beyond the lower edge of the underlying pectoralis minor muscle. The lateral border of the pectoralis major muscle can be identified and marked by having the patient push her hands together on her hips.

The primary blood supply to the pectoralis major muscle is from the superiorly located thoracoacromial vessels, with the secondary supply coming medially from the deep perforator branches off the internal mammary artery. The motor innervation of the pectoralis major muscle is via the lateral pectoral nerve (innervating the upper, medial half of the muscle) and the medial pectoral nerve (innervating the lower, lateral half of the muscle).

Entering the correct surgical plane between the pectoralis major and pectoralis minor muscles is of key importance in the transaxillary augmentation procedure. The lateral border of the pectoralis minor muscle lies deep and just medial to the edge of the pectoralis major. As the pectoralis minor muscle courses cephalad toward its insertion on the coracoid process of the scapula, its investing fascia becomes more intimately associated with that of the overlying pectoralis major muscle. Identification of the fascia at the lateral edge of the pectoralis major allows one to enter the bloodless plane between the two muscles. This plane can be entered more easily through the caudal aspect of the axillary incision, rather than more cephalad where the fascia investing the two muscles becomes fused. Attempting to enter the retropectoral space higher up (cephalad) often results in entering the wrong plane under the pectoralis minor muscle. This becomes readily apparent by an excessively bloody dissection as one tries to develop the plane. Once in the correct plane between the pectoralis major and minor muscles, the dissection should proceed effortlessly and with little or no bleeding. *Careful control of hemostasis after making the incision and a bloodless operative field will simplify identification of the important anatomic landmarks.*

Care must be taken to avoid cephalad dissection in the axilla because numerous important anatomic structures can be injured in this area. The vector of dissection should proceed inferomedially from the axillary incision toward the lateral pectoral muscle border. Avoid dissection within the axillary fat pad to prevent injury to the intercostobrachial or medial brachial cutaneous nerves. These nerves, which supply sensation to the upper arm, course superficially within the subcutaneous tissues just posterior to the upper lateral border of the pectoralis major muscle. Dissecting higher within the axilla, or overaggressive cephalic retraction, can injure the brachial plexus and axillary vessels.

Once the correct surgical plane is identified and entered, care must be taken to avoid injuring the important neurovascular structures in this area. The medial pectoral nerve pierces the pectoralis minor muscle, then enters the pectoralis major muscle superiorly to innervate its lower portion. The thoracoacromial vessel with its pectoral branches along with the lateral pectoral nerve enter the pectoralis major muscle along its deep cephalic portion inferior to the clavicle. Although they are quite adherent to the deep surface of the muscle, they can be injured from overly aggressive dissection.

Blunt dissection of the inferolateral part of the pocket should be done gently with a medial-to-lateral motion to avoid avulsing or injuring the lateral intercostal nerves that are important in supplying nipple–areola sensation. This method of dissection stretches and pushes the nerves laterally without disrupting them. The medial parasternal internal mammary perforating blood vessels are also stretched, not disrupted, by sweeping medially and upward in this region.

As the dissection proceeds toward the inferior portion of the pocket, the lower border or costochondral origin of the pectoralis major muscle is encountered. Note that the inferior-most edge of the pectoralis major muscle is usually at or just above the inframammary fold. The fascia of the pectoralis major muscle continues inferiorly as the deep subcutaneous fascia of the anterior chest wall. Medially, this fascial layer is continuous with the anterior rectus sheath and fuses with it at the upper lateral border of the rectus abdominis muscle. Laterally, the prepectoral fascia continues inferiorly and is firmly adherent to the fascia of the serratus anterior muscle. This area of fascial continuity between the pectoralis major muscle, rectus sheath, serratus anterior muscle, and deep subcutaneous fascia extends along and below the inframammary fold medially to laterally.

Often existing as a dense, noncompliant layer, this fascia can create problems when the pocket dissection is extended deep into it in order to lower the inframammary fold. With blunt dissection techniques this fascial layer can often be disrupted enough to allow expansion of the lower pole of the breast, although this approach offers little in terms of precise surgical control. In many instances, this constricting sheet of fascia requires controlled release with direct scoring to allow the necessary expansion of the lower pole of the breast after a prosthesis is inserted.

INSTRUMENTATION AND EQUIPMENT

The following is a list of instruments and videoendoscopy equipment used in the endoscopically assisted transaxillary retropectoral breast augmentation procedure. This list is provided as a guide in instrument selection. Actual instrument selection may vary slightly according to the individual surgeon's preference (Figure 13-1).

- Small Maxwell flap retractor (Snowden-Pencer)
- 5-inch tenotomy scissors (Weck)
- Maxwell double-ended retractor (Snowden-Pencer)
- Maxwell small Deaver retractor (Snowden-Pencer)
- Right and left Agris-Dingman axillary dissectors (Padgett)
- Endoscopic breast retractor (Snowden-Pencer)
- Monopolar electrocautery cord (Wolf)
- Extended angled monopolar electrocautery (Snowden-Pencer)
- 10-mm, 30-degree angle, short-barrel endoscope (Snowden- Pencer)
- 3-chip endoscopic videocamera, Model 782 (Stryker)
- FRED (fog reduction and elimination device)
- Stryker 782 medical videocamera control unit
- Stryker quantum 4000 light source
- 20-inch color video monitor

Note the setup of the video tower with the color monitor positioned at the foot of the operating table (Figure 13-2).

A minimum of one assistant or scrub nurse should be standing either opposite or below the surgeon to assist in the endoscopic part of the pocket dissection. The initial sharp and blunt dissection of the pocket is done with the surgeon positioned *below* the patient's extended arm, directly across from the axillary incision. When the surgeon is ready to use the endoscope to continue the dissection, he or she should be positioned *above* the patient's arm, such that it is comfortable to direct the endoscope retractor inferiorly and view the monitor at the same time.

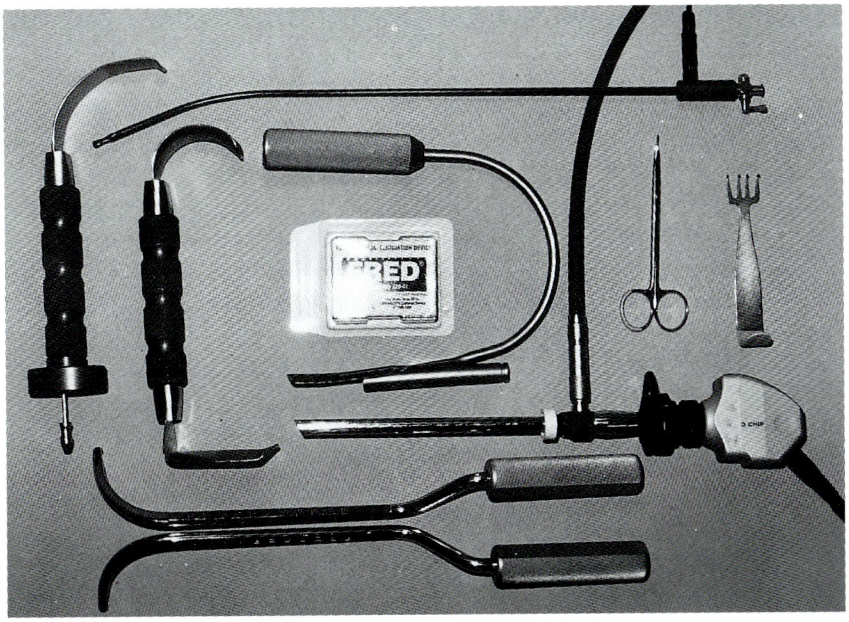

FIGURE 13-1
The essential surgical instruments for performing the endoscopically assisted transaxillary retropectoral breast augmentation procedure are shown. Note the extended angled electrocautery at the top, the endoscope and endoscope retractor in the middle, and the right and left Agris-Dingman axillary dissectors at the bottom.

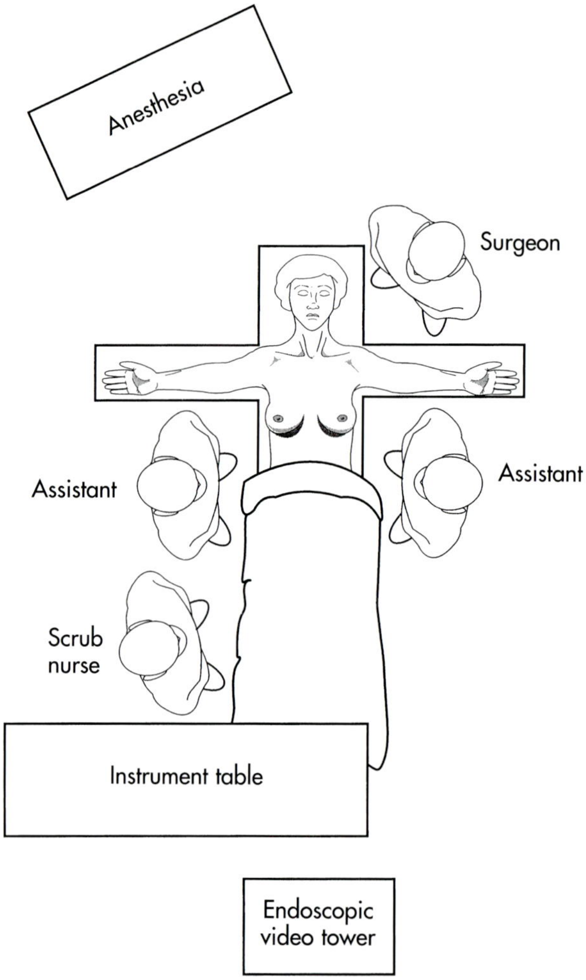

FIGURE 13-2
For the endoscopic part of the procedure, the surgeon should be positioned above the armboard, facing the video tower at the foot of the bed. This allows easy viewing of the monitor, while manipulating the endoscope and electrocautery.

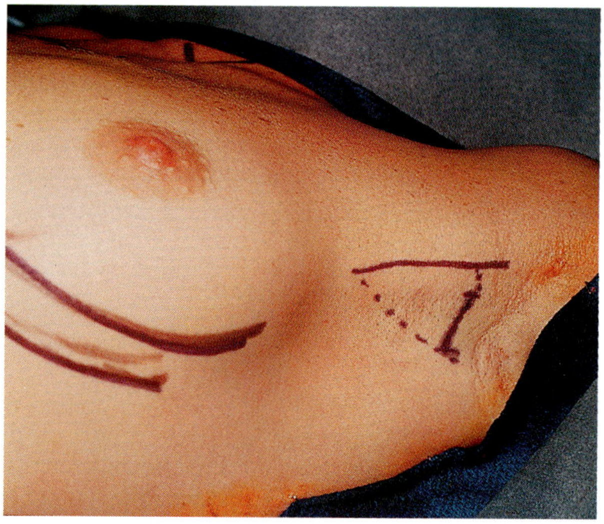

FIGURE 13-3
View of the left breast and axilla. The axillary incision and the lateral edge of the pectoralis major muscle have been marked. Dissection will proceed in an inferomedial direction in the area indicated by the dashed lines. The inframammary fold will be lowered as marked.

OPERATIVE PROCEDURE

PATIENT POSITIONING AND PREPARATION

Preoperative marking is done with the patient awake, in the upright sitting position. Care is taken to assure that the patient is sitting symmetrically, with the shoulders level and back straight. The vertical midline is marked, as are the existing inframammary folds. The new inframammary folds are marked if fold lowering is to be done, as are the medial and lateral limits of the proposed pocket dissection.

The lateral border of the pectoralis major muscle is identified by having the patient press her hands together on her hips, and a line is drawn along the anterior axillary fold corresponding to the lateral edge of the pectoralis major muscle. The axillary incision should begin 1.5 to 2.0 cm posterior to the lateral edge of the pectoralis major muscle, and extend approximately 3 cm in length toward the apex of the axilla. An effort is made to place the incision within a naturally occurring skin crease, if feasible (Figure 13-3). The incision should not be visible from either front or back with the arms fully adducted. Check all markings with a flexible tape measure to assure symmetry.

General anesthesia is typically used for this procedure due to surgeons' preference, although it may be done equally effectively using intravenous sedation with local or regional anesthesia.

The patient is positioned supine on the operating table with the arms abducted symmetrically to a 90-degree angle to allow easy access to the axilla. The arms are held securely and firmly to well-padded arm boards. This will prevent intraoperative neurapraxias and allow the patient to be elevated to a full sitting position on the operating table as necessary during the surgical procedure.

A fully electric operating table is used to allow rapid repositioning of the patient as needed during the procedure.

The patient is then prepared with a povidone-iodine preparation (Betadine), that is, scrubbed and painted. Draping is done in a manner that allows visualization of both shoulders, and the top of the drape is left unattached from anesthesia poles so the patient may be raised to the sitting position without tethering the drapes. After the patient is draped, the Betadine paint is wiped off with sterile saline, taking care to not wipe off the preoperative markings. These markings are then retraced as needed with a sterile surgical marking pen. An iced solution of 0.25% lidocaine (Xylocaine) with epinephrine (1:400,000) is infiltrated superficially in the area of the axillary incision and the subcutaneous tissues that will be dissected to reach the lateral edge of the pectoralis major muscle. The only other area of the breast that is injected is the region of the inframammary fold where the pectoralis major muscle will be divided and the fold lowered.

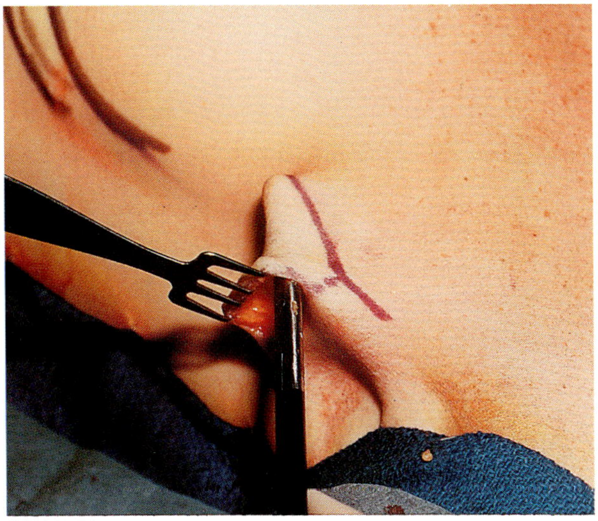

FIGURE 13-4
Subcutaneous scissors dissection has been performed to reach the posterolateral edge of the pectoralis major muscles. Note how the dissection is done in a superficial plane and in an inferomedial direction from the incision.

INITIAL SURGICAL DISSECTION

An axillary incision measuring approximately 2.5 to 3.0 cm in length is made with a No. 15 scalpel blade through the skin and just into the subcutaneous fat. Hemostasis is controlled with the cautery, then dissection proceeds with tenotomy scissors in the superficial subcutaneous plane. Avoid dissecting deeper within the axillary fat in this location, because the intercostal brachial and medial cutaneous nerves to the arm can be injured by doing so. A small Maxwell flap retractor is placed along the anterior skin edge to facilitate dissection toward the lateral edge of the pectoralis major muscle. Avoid using larger retractors or retracting toward the axillary contents because this can injure the brachial plexus and/or axillary vessels. Again, dissection should be just deep to the dermis and directed inferomedially toward the pectoralis major muscle (Figure 13-4). Meticulous hemostasis at this point is very important in order to easily identify the muscle edge. As the scissors dissection proceeds inferomedially, replace the small flap retractor with the small Deaver for better visualization.

Once the posterior lateral border of the pectoralis major muscle is identified, the subpectoral plane is entered using a spreading motion of the scissors tips. This plane is most easily entered lower along the edge of the pectoralis major muscle, rather than higher up in the axilla. Higher up, the fascia of the pectoralis major and minor muscles are more densely adherent to one another, and attempts to enter the desired plane here often result in dissecting under the pectoralis minor muscles. This, in turn, causes profuse bleeding, making it much more difficult to find the correct plane (Figure 13-5).

After the desired subpectoral plane has been identified, blunt finger dissection is used to partially dissect the pocket superiorly then inferiorly to just above the level of the nipple–areola complex (Figure 13-6). Care is taken to avoid injuring the thoracoacromial vessels and the pectoral nerves on the undersurface of the pectoralis major muscle superiorly. If pocket dissection at this point does not proceed effortlessly and with minimal bleeding, the thought must be entertained that the incorrect surgical plane has been entered. Avoid aggressive blunt dissection initially as this can cause bleeding within the pocket and make the endoscopic dissection much more difficult. Once this preliminary blunt finger dissection has been accomplished, it is time to proceed with the endoscopic part of the procedure.

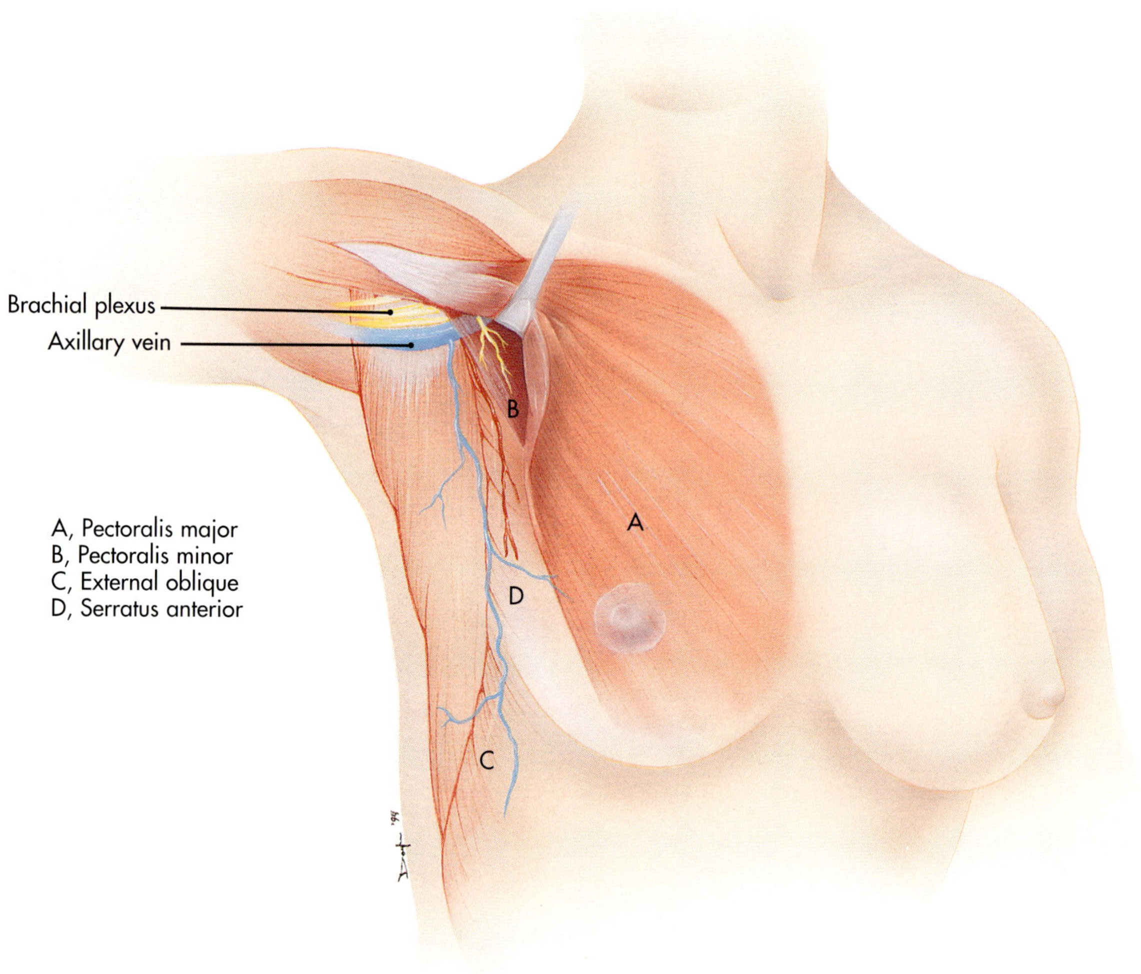

FIGURE 13-5
Enter the retropectoral plane by gently spreading the scissor tips along the fascia joining the pectoralis major and minor muscles. It is easier to enter the correct plane inferiorly, as indicated, than higher up in the axilla where the fascia between the muscles is more adherent.

FIGURE 13-6
Once the correct surgical plane has been developed between the pectoralis major and minor muscles, initiate gentle finger dissection of the upper portion of the pocket.

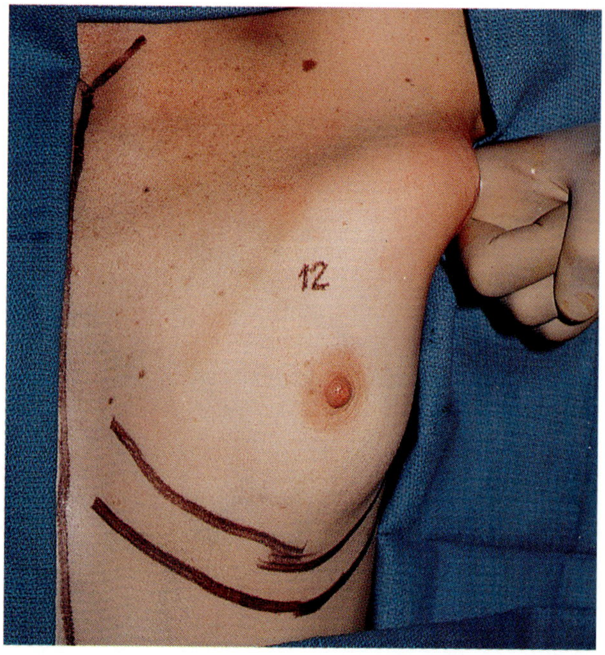

ENDOSCOPIC DISSECTION

At this point, the surgeon should move above the patient's abducted arm. This allows easy viewing of the monitor at the foot of the table, while manipulating the endoscope and electrocautery dissector. After coating the lens of the endoscope with a liberal amount of FRED, insert the endoscope and endoscope retractor through the incision and into the pocket. Position the scope within the retractor and the pocket so that a moderately wide angle, yet well lighted view, is obtained. Turn the overhead room lights down at this point to optimize the image on the monitor. The surgeon should hold the retractor-mounted endoscope with the nondominant hand, and the electrocautery dissector with the dominant hand.

If the correct plane has been entered, one should see the loose areolar tissue layer that joins the deep investing fascia of the pectoralis major muscle with the chest wall and pectoralis minor muscle. Under endoscopic guidance, use the extended electrocautery to divide this areolar tissue as the pocket dissection is carried medially and inferiorly. As the dissection reaches the inframammary fold, the origin of the pectoralis major muscle is encountered (Figures 13-7 and 13-8). Controlled release of the pectoralis major muscle is done at this point as follows.

An assistant gently places the fingertips on the patient's skin directly above the location of the cautery tip. The position of the cautery tip can be palpated through the subcutaneous tissue and muscle, and the endoscope light transilluminating from below can also be used as a guide to the cautery location. This is a very important step because as the muscle is divided, extreme care must be taken not to dissect too superficially and injure the overlying skin. The assistant moves the fingers along the skin, following the surgeon's dissection. If the surgeon releases the pectoralis major muscle right at the chest wall level, the risk of injuring the overlying skin is minimized (Figure 13-9).

Release the entire inferior edge of the pectoralis major muscle by dissecting through the muscle fibers until the subcutaneous fat is seen. This release will extend the pocket inferiorly toward the new inframammary fold marking. Stop the inferior cautery dissection approximately 1 to 2 cm *above* the level of the new inframammary fold, as the final dissection here will be done using the Agris-Dingman axillary dissectors. Continue to release the pectoralis muscle medially along the lower third of its medial sternal origin. At this point, division of the muscle may be done either totally or partially (Figure 13-10).

Full-thickness muscle division here will allow a maximum increase in the medial positioning of the implant to maximize cleavage and narrow the intermammary distance. The trade-offs and potential risks of full-thickness muscle division medially are a visible or palpable implant edge and synmastia, as the soft tissues in the presternal area tend to be very thin. Because of these potential problems, the medial pectoralis muscle is usually divided in a partial-thickness manner to allow modest expansion of the pocket medially, yet still provide adequate implant coverage. Some patients with a wide intermammary distance, however, may require full-thickness muscle division medially to create a pocket of the correct transverse dimension and attain the desired medial fullness. During the course of the endoscopic dissection, any bleeding vessels should be cauterized.

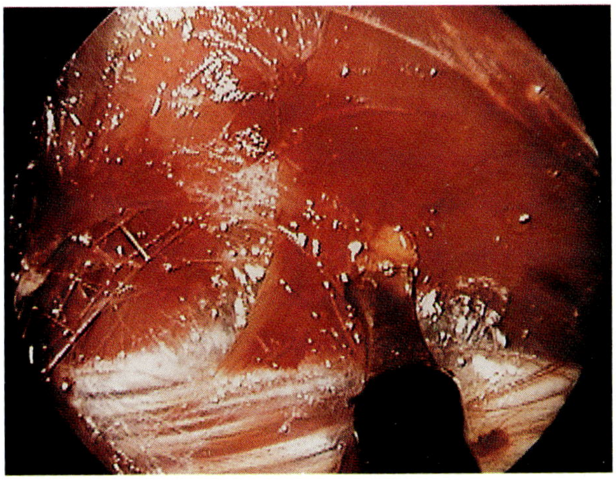

FIGURE 13-7
Endoscopic view showing the lower sternal origin of the pectoralis major muscle. Note one of the small individual slips of muscle to the left of the electrocautery tip.

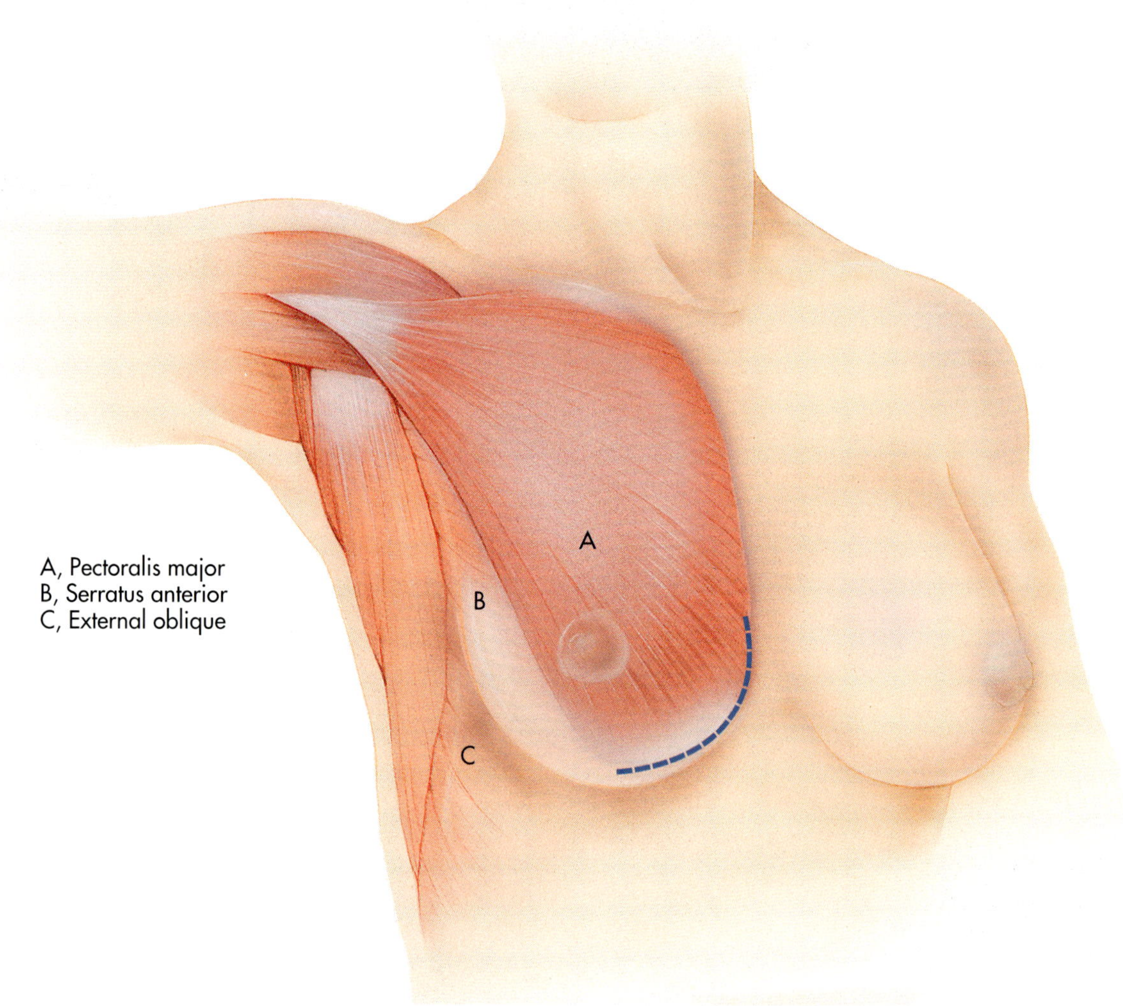

FIGURE 13-8
The sternocostal origin of the pectoralis major muscle is released with the electrocautery under endoscopic control, as indicated by the dashed lines. Inferiorly, full-thickness muscle division is done. Medially, partial-thickness muscle division is done, but under certain circumstances full-thickness division may be done.

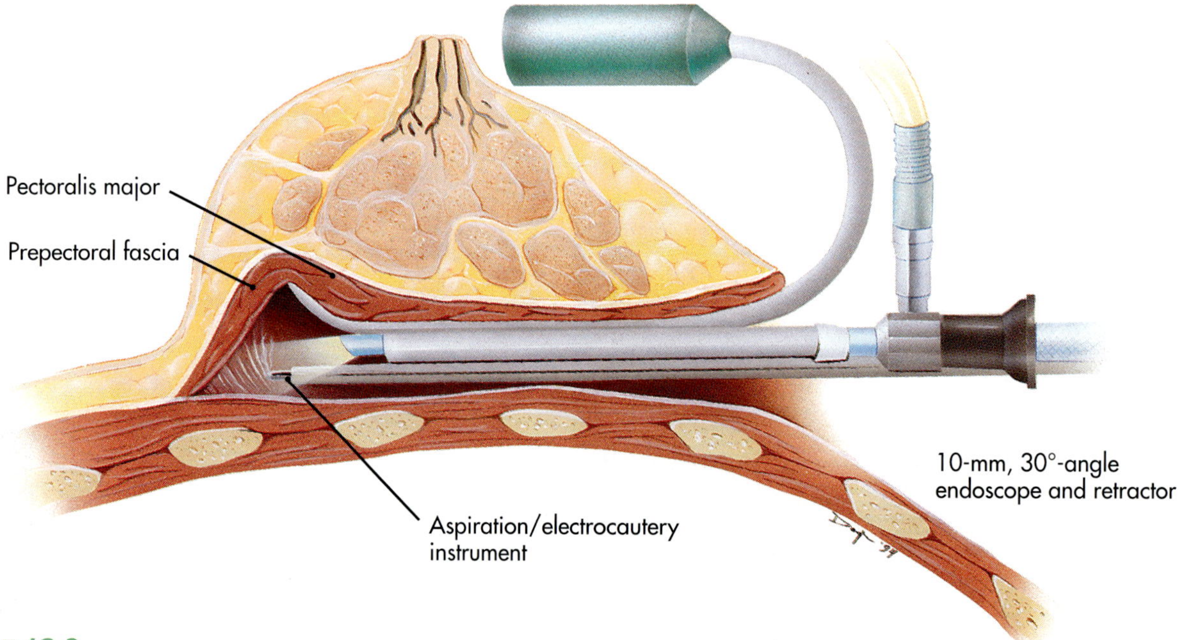

FIGURE 13-9
Diagrammatic representation showing endoscopic release of the pectoralis major muscle and the fascia just above the inframammary fold. Final dissection of the pocket to the new inframammary fold level will be done with the Agris-Dingman axillary dissectors. An assistant should palpate the progress of the dissection directly above the electrocautery.

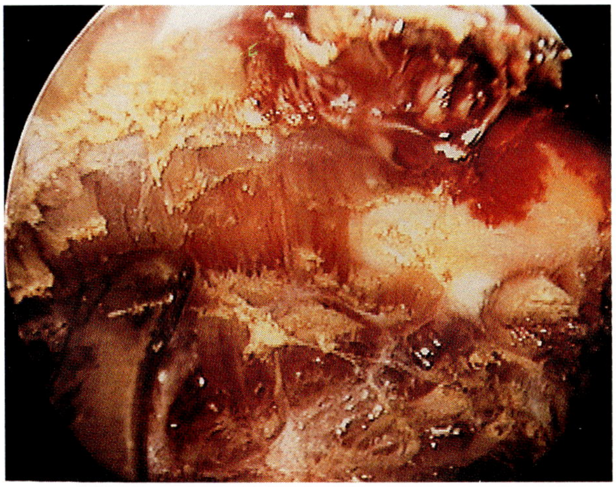

FIGURE 13-10
Endoscopic view showing electrocautery release of the origin of the pectoralis major muscle. *(Right)* Full-thickness release of the muscle is performed, and the subcutaneous fat is seen. *(Left)* Controlled partial-thickness release of the muscle is performed.

FINAL POCKET DISSECTION AND IMPLANT PLACEMENT

After the desired release of the pectoralis major muscle has been achieved and hemostasis has been controlled, final pocket dissection is done with the Agris-Dingman axillary dissectors. Insert the appropriate dissector into the pocket and sweep medially to laterally to dissect the lateral portion of the pocket. This is done with a gentle but firm motion, sweeping and stretching the neurovascular bundles laterally. The inferior and medial aspects of the pocket are also incrementally dissected to the preoperative markings. The motion here is down or medial, and outward toward the marked lines to stretch the released muscle and deep subcutaneous fascia. Be very careful not to extend the pocket beyond the preoperative markings, as it is infinitely more easy to gradually increase the pocket size than it is to correct an overdissected pocket (Figure 13-11).

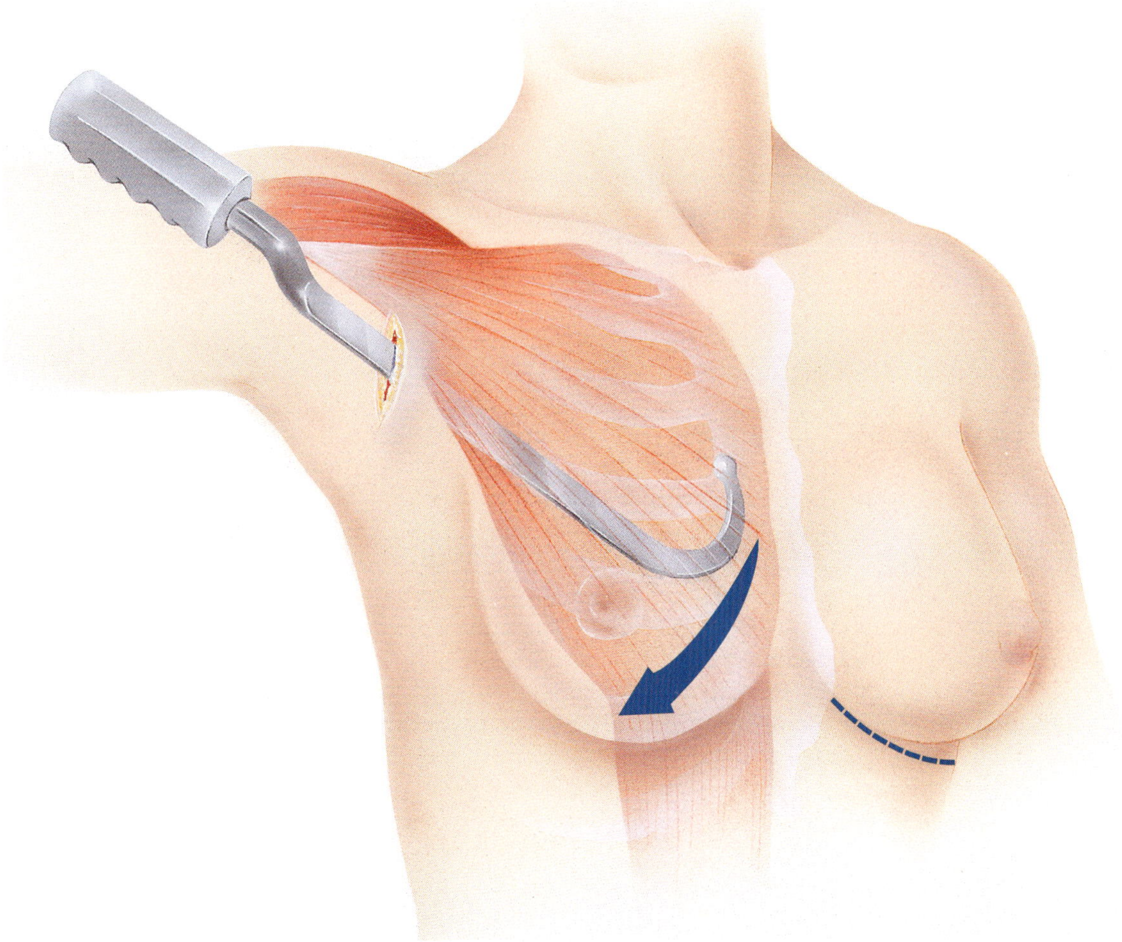

FIGURE 13-11
After releasing the origin of the pectoralis major muscle using the endoscope, the surgical pocket is extended incrementally to the preoperative markings with the Agris-Dingman axillary dissectors. The fascial, muscular, and parenchymal components of the pocket are gently stretched and made more compliant to accommodate the breast implant.

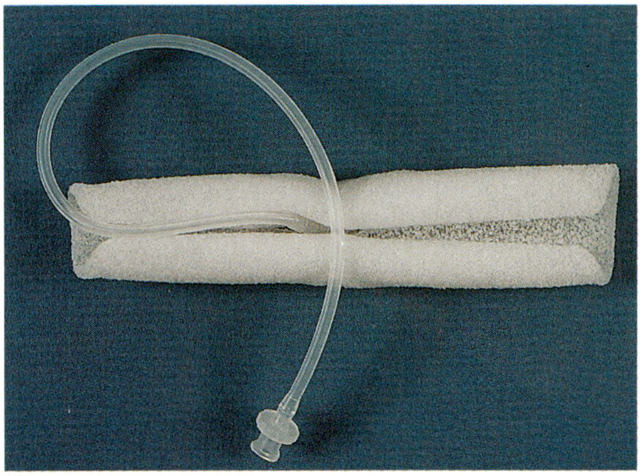

FIGURE 13-12
To insert the breast prosthesis, roll each edge toward the vertical axis of the device. Insert the device into the pocket with the vertical axis properly aligned, and the implant will unroll into its proper position.

At this point, irrigate the pocket with saline solution followed by antibiotic solution. We prefer a dilute solution of Betadine for final implant pocket irrigation. Prepare the selected implant according to the manufacturer's recommendations. If using an anatomically shaped augmentation implant, mark the vertical axis or an edge of the implant with a sterile marking pen for orientation purposes once the device is inserted. Evacuate all the air from the implant (assuming it is a saline-type device) and roll both edges of the implant toward the center to create a taco-shaped roll (Figure 13-12). When inserted in this fashion with the vertical axis in the center of the pocket, each edge will unroll toward its appropriate side. Position the implant at the lower edge of the pocket, and fill it to its recommended fill volume.

We do not find it necessary to use a sleeve or lubricant (such as a water-based jelly) for insertion of the emptied, rolled device, although both of these have been advocated in the literature. If the device is inserted with a significant amount of saline within, these measures may become necessary in order to get a textured-surface implant through a small incision. By rolling an empty implant as described, insertion is simple and quick, and the device can be positioned precisely within the pocket then filled via the fill tube. Presently, we use textured-surface devices (Biocell surface from McGhan or the Siltex surface from Mentor) for all breast augmentation procedures.

Saline implants are filled to the manufacturer's recommended fill volume or slightly overfilled if needed. *Avoid underfilling the device*, because this will predispose it to visible or palpable rippling and potential fold failure. Caution must be exercised when overfilling a device, because this will tend to make the implant more *spherical* in shape and firmer. Standard round implants can be overfilled by as much as 20% to 25% of the recommended fill volume. Exceeding this percentage can cause scalloping of the edges of the device. The new anatomically shaped implants tolerate less overfilling than standard round devices because of the distortion of the shape that can occur if significantly overfilled.

AESTHETIC EVALUATION AND WOUND CLOSURE

Sit the patient into the full upright position now and check for adequacy and symmetry of the pocket dissection. Press the implant inferiorly to evaluate the inferior pocket dissection. Similarly, press the implant medially and laterally to judge whether the pocket has been dissected evenly to the preoperative markings. Mark any areas on the skin that require further dissection or release. Note whether the pocket needs to be enlarged in certain areas, or if existing areas need to be released and made more compliant. Occasionally, the lower pole of the breast requires some fascial release to allow the implant to fill out this previously tight tissue. This can usually be accomplished by carefully reinserting the Agris-Dingman dissectors around the implant and bluntly stretching or dissecting the areas that require further release.

In patients with high, tight, inframammary folds or noncompliant lower pole soft tissues, scoring of the breast parenchyma or fascia should be done with the endoscopic cautery prior to insertion of the implant. If for any reason it becomes necessary to do further endoscopic work with the cautery, it is recommended that the implant be deflated and removed prior to doing so.

The same steps are then performed on the opposite breast. Before closure of the wounds, the patient should be sat upright again and viewed from the end of the table as well as from the sides. Check for symmetry of the folds and for symmetry of fullness and contour in each of the four breast quadrants. From a lateral view, check the symmetry and contour of the upper pole slope. Final adjustments are made as necessary to obtain symmetry and an appropriate aesthetic shape.

Wound closure is done by approximating the subcutaneous layers with a minimum number of

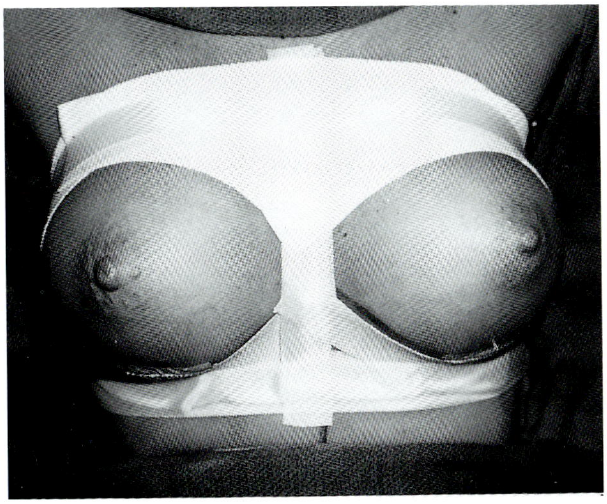

FIGURE 13-13
The inframammary folds are taped to help define their new position. Tape or an elastic bandage is placed superiorly to exert a gentle downward force on the implants.

absorbable polyglactin 910 (Vicryl) sutures, followed by a running intracuticular suture of Monocryl or polydioxanone sutures (PDS). No deep layers are closed, and *drains are rarely used.* Closure of the axillary incision is exact and precise to minimize any scarring in this potentially visible site. A longitudinally oriented Steri-Strip is placed over the incision. The inframammary folds are then taped with 1-inch Elastoplast tape to precisely define the new inframammary fold level. The implants are held down in the pocket by either taping the upper breast pole with 2-inch Elastoplast tape, or by using a circumferential 4- to 6-inch Ace bandage (Figure 13-13). This tape support is left in place for approximately 5 to 7 days. An Ace bandage is used as necessary for approximately 2 weeks postoperatively to exert and maintain a downward vectored force on the implants. Perioperative cephalosporin antibiotics are administered intravenously at the start of the surgery, and continued for 5 days postoperatively in an oral form.

POSTOPERATIVE CARE

Patients with primary breast augmentation generally require only minimal postoperative care, providing they do not experience any complications. Patients are discharged home on the day of surgery with oral narcotic-based analgesics as needed for pain control. An intramuscular injection of 60 mg of Toradol (a nonsteroidal antiinflammatory drug [NSAID]) is given to the patient after induction of anesthesia to help with immediate postoperative pain and to serve as a loading dose for subsequent oral Toradol dosing if desired. Because the pectoralis release and retromuscular dissection can sometimes be more painful than a retromammary dissection, patients will often be sent home on oral Toradol (10 mg orally four times a day with food) for 3 to 5 days to reduce their narcotic requirement and help with pain control. This combination of short-term oral Toradol with narcotic analgesics has yielded excellent control of postoperative pain in these patients.

Patients are seen in the office 5 to 7 days after surgery unless the need arises to see them earlier. At this time, the previously placed Elastoplast tape is removed. If the inframammary fold was lowered, as is usually the case, the patient is instructed to continue wearing an Ace bandage around the upper pole of the breasts for another week to keep a downward pressure on the implants. This prevents the implants from riding high in the pocket, which can produce both inframammary fold asymmetries and unattractive upper pole fullness. Thereafter, patients are seen weekly until the third week postoperatively, then monthly for 3 months, then on a regular basis every 6 months.

COMPLICATIONS

Endoscopically assisted transaxillary retropectoral breast augmentation is a straightforward surgical procedure that when performed correctly produces a minimal number of complications. Many of the complications common to the blunt transaxillary approach have been significantly reduced by incorporating the endoscope into the procedure. Other complications are common to both approaches as well as periareolar and inframammary approaches. These complications can be broken down into acute or early postoperative complications, and delayed complications.

ACUTE COMPLICATIONS

The acute or early postoperative complications include hematoma, seroma, infection, asymmetry, alterations in cutaneous sensation, pneumothorax, and injury to the overlying skin from the cautery dissection. Hematomas can occur unexpectedly in any patient even if hemostasis during the procedure was meticulous. The use of the endoscope reduces the risk of hematoma by allowing inspection of the entire pocket during and after the dissection to look for and control any bleeding vessels. Hematomas of any significant degree should be surgically drained, and the pocket should be irrigated of all clot with the implant removed. Drains may rarely be required after evacuation of a hematoma if the bleeding is diffuse and an isolated source cannot be detected.

Seromas are generally self-limiting in nature after a primary augmentation mammaplasty and require no surgical intervention. Reassuring the patient is the primary treatment in these instances. These seromas generally resolve with no untoward sequelae in 7 to 10 days. Taping the inframammary fold and applying tape or an Ace wrap to the upper pole helps reduce the potential dead space around the implant and may minimize the risk for seroma formation.

Infection can occur after transaxillary breast augmentation, as it can with any surgical procedure. These infections can be both superficial in the subcutaneous tissues or deeper at the periprosthetic space. The risk of a deep periprosthetic infection may be reduced in the transaxillary augmentation approach because contact with breast ducts and tissue is avoided. Fortunately, with correct surgical technique, perioperative and postoperative antibiotics, and pocket irrigation with antimicrobial solutions, infection following breast augmentation is rare. Nevertheless, patients should be instructed to be aware of any of the signs of an early infection and to call the office immediately if one is suspected. A superficial cellulitis, if caught early enough, should respond rapidly and completely with either short-term parenteral then oral antibiotics, or oral antibiotics alone. A true deep periprosthetic infection will likely require extended intravenous antibiotic therapy followed by oral antibiotics, and possibly implant removal. The axillary incision may also infrequently cause axillary folliculitis, a condition easily treated with a short course of oral antibiotics.

Implant asymmetry is far less common with the endoscopic transaxillary approach than when the same approach is taken without the endoscope. One must first be certain that the postoperative asymmetry is not something that existed preoperatively and has become more noticeable after surgery. If fluid accumulation is not the cause of the asymmetry, the most likely cause is either asymmetric pocket dissection, implant malposition, or implant volume discrepancy. The first two causes may be helped by a combination of selective inframammary fold taping, wearing an Ace wrap, and wearing a bra for a period of time to help the soft tissue envelope settle in the desired position relative to the implant. Breast asymmetry caused by improper selection of implant fill volume or base diameter will not resolve over time and will require a surgical solution if it is a major problem. These latter problems can be avoided by careful preoperative planning, which should lead to selection of the correct implant. Furthermore, care must be taken intraoperatively not to extend the dissection beyond the planned inframammary fold and medial and lateral borders. Dissection should be done incrementally in all directions, remembering that it is much easier to make the pocket larger than it is to make it smaller. Failure to remember this simple principle may result in the implant positioned in a location that fails to give the desired aesthetic shape.

Changes in cutaneous sensation following this procedure are a possibility in any patient, and the patient should be counseled about this before surgery. These changes can manifest as hypersensitivity, diminished sensation, or complete anesthesia. Most of these problems are transient in nature if care is taken during the procedure to remember the location of the important nerves both around the breast and within the axilla. Be particularly careful during the initial axillary dissection to avoid going deep into the axillary fat pad because injury of the cutaneous nerves to the upper arm can occur here. Keep in mind the location of the lateral intercostal nerves supplying the nipple–areola complex when using the axillary dissectors and the electrocautery in this area.

Pneumothorax is an extremely uncommon but possible complication of retropectoral augmentation mammaplasty. The most likely cause, aside from a needle injection for anesthetic placement, would be overaggressive use of the cautery to try to control a bleeder on the chest wall. Patients will typically present with dyspnea, tachypnea, and pleural pain in the recovery room or in the immediate postoperative period. An upright end-expiratory chest x-ray is diagnostic, with treatment (chest tube versus observation) depending on the volume of the pneumothorax.

The final acute complication that may occur as a result of endoscopically assisted transaxillary retropectoral breast augmentation is an electrocautery injury of the skin above the point of the pocket dissection. Because the surgeon holds the cautery in one hand, the endoscope in the other, and watches the dissection on the monitor, he or she is not able to feel the thickness of the soft tissue directly superficial to where the cautery dissection is being performed. This can lead to injury of the overlying skin in areas of thin subcutaneous tissue if care is not taken to avoid it. When the pectoralis major muscle is released medially and inferiorly, an assistant should place the fingertips directly on the skin above the cautery tip to constantly monitor the amount of intervening soft tissue. If the cautery tip becomes too superficial, it is easily palpated before any damage is done to the overlying skin.

Delayed Complications

Delayed complications can be broken down into problems associated with the implant itself and problems related to the soft tissues surrounding the implant. Soft tissue problems include axillary scar hypertrophy, capsular contracture, persistent implant contour irregularities, and muscular distortion of the implant. Although the axillary incision generally heals very well, a small percentage of patients may develop hypertrophic scar formation. Patients should be advised that the axillary scar may persist for the first several months, in a red, thickened state. This scar should mature over time such that by 6 to 12 months after surgery it is a fine linear scar (Figure 13-14). If scar hypertrophy persists or shows evidence of worsening, local steroid injections or scar revision may be required. Patients undergoing transaxillary breast augmentation should be counseled regarding a potentially visible axillary scar that may persist after surgery. This may be particularly important to women who wear sleeveless clothing or who are athletic.

Capsular contracture remains a problem with an elusive etiology. Speculation has abounded over the years as to the cause or causes of this problem, and the final answer will probably be multifactorial. The etiology and treatment of capsular contracture, in fact, is a topic unto itself. What is significant is that surgical treatment of capsular contracture by capsulotomy may now be done through the same axillary incision with an endoscope. Partial or total capsulectomy, however, should probably be done through an inframammary incision for optimal exposure and access.

Persistent contour irregularities may occur even if all possible attempts are made to correct them in the early postoperative period. The causes of these irregularities are essentially the same as for acute contour irregularities. These irregularities will require surgical correction if they are of significant concern to the patient. This can require fascial or parenchymal release of the lower pole of the breast to treat a "double-bubble" appearance, or further dissection of the implant pocket medially, laterally, or inferiorly. These adjustments can be done through the axillary incision under endoscopic visualization. If one or both inframammary folds have been lowered too far, the fold must be raised by using internal sutures to attach the capsule to itself at the correct level. While this is theoretically possible through the axillary incision using a long needle-holder and the endoscope, it would probably be faster, more precise, and easier through an inframammary incision.

Muscular distortion of the implant, caused by contracture of the overlying pectoralis major muscle, should rarely be a problem if the muscle is properly released with the cautery. Partial-thickness release of the muscle medially at the sternal origin will usually prevent this problem from occurring, while still offering the benefit of coverage of the

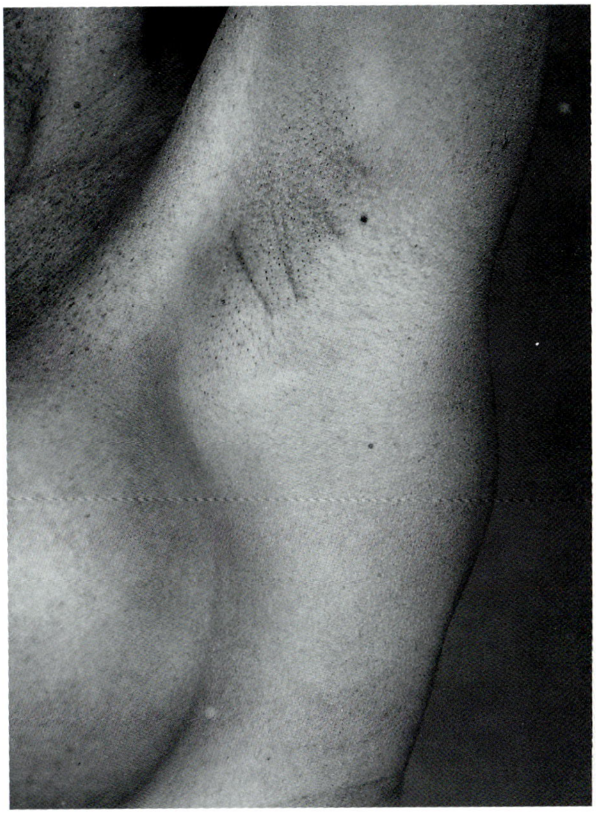

Figure 13-14
A typical well-healed, axillary incision 3 months postoperatively is shown.

medial edge of the implant. If this persists as a bothersome problem, the options include either further release of the implant pocket or replacing the implants in the retromammary position.

Delayed complications related to the implant itself include implant leakage or failure, palpable folds, and visible rippling. Most of these problems, if severe, require surgical treatment to obtain a satisfactory result. Leaking or deflated implants can be treated with the transaxillary endoscopic approach by removing the implant, doing capsule release as necessary, and replacing the defective implant with a new one. Palpable and visible folds are best *prevented* by avoiding underfilling saline implants and assuring adequate overlying soft tissue coverage. If these problems occur in patients who already have implants in the submuscular position, the options include accepting the deformity, adding volume to the existing implant, or in the case of saline-filled implants switching them to gel, if this is possible.

SUMMARY

A number of different surgical approaches are available to the plastic surgeon when considering a patient for breast augmentation. Each of these approaches differs from the others in terms of their specific advantages and disadvantages. Regardless of which approach is selected, it should be straightforward, reproducible, and predictable in terms of the surgical result. It should also allow versatility and surgical control of the parenchymal tissue, muscle, fascia, inframammary fold, and skin envelope if the approach is to be useful in a broad spectrum of patients with different breast types.

Until recently, the transaxillary retropectoral approach to augmentation has had limitations in several respects compared with the inframammary and periareolar approaches. Although predictable and relatively easy to perform in most patients, its main drawback was the inability to visualize and therefore directly control those soft tissue elements near the inframammary fold, which often required precise alteration. Consequently, suboptimal results were not uncommon, especially in patients with inframammary fold irregularities or pseudoptosis. Incorporating an endoscope into this approach has allowed a greater degree of surgical precision, versatility, and control of the variables that directly influence the final aesthetic result.

The advantages of the endoscopically assisted transaxillary retropectoral approach include (1) avoidance of a scar on the aesthetic breast unit, (2) preservation of sensation to the nipple–areola complex, (3) a theoretic decreased risk of periprosthetic infections, (4) direct control of hemostasis, (5) precise surgical control of the inframammary fold and lower breast pole glandular and fascial elements, and (6) controlled release of the pectoralis major muscle, which when properly done minimizes the likelihood of muscular distortion of the implant while still providing increased soft tissue coverage at the medial edge of the implant.

The important technical aspects of this procedure include (1) thorough and careful preoperative evaluation and marking, (2) selection of an implant based on a dimensional analysis of the patient, (3) proper placement of the axillary incision, (4) familiarity with the axillary anatomy to allow easy definition of the correct surgical plane, (5) dissecting the pocket with the endoscope *before* using the Agris-Dingman axillary dissectors, (6) releasing the pectoralis muscle and fascia with the endoscope, using an assistant to palpate the cautery tip through the overlying skin, (7) being careful not to extend the pocket dissection beyond the preoperative markings, (8) evaluating the augmented breast form and symmetry with the patient sitting fully upright on the operating table, (9) meticulous closure of the axillary incision, and (10) taping the inframammary folds if lowered and applying tape or an Ace wrap to the upper pole to prevent upward displacement of the implants.

The limitations of the endoscopically assisted transaxillary retropectoral augmentation approach are important to understand to avoid undesirable surgical results. Using the endoscope requires a certain degree of hand-eye coordination, but is a skill that is quickly and easily learned by most surgeons. That aside, this approach should be considered carefully before using it in patients who will require extensive soft tissue excision or scoring or in patients who would benefit from retromammary implant positioning. In particular, avoid using it in patients with severe tuberous breast deformities, where excision of the parenchyma under the nipple–areolar complex may be required. Similarly, secondary procedures requiring capsulectomy are best addressed by an inframammary approach. If patients with first-degree ptosis are to be treated by augmentation without mastopexy, retroglandular positioning of the implant may be most desirable to avoid the "double-bubble" appearance that can occur if the implant is placed retromuscularly.

In the appropriate surgical candidate then, with careful attention to preoperative planning and surgical detail, the endoscopically assisted transaxillary retropectoral augmentation procedure offers excellent results in a wide range of patients. The procedure is quick, easy to perform, reproducible, and allows considerable versatility and surgical control. When properly performed, it is very gratifying to both patient and surgeon (Figures 13-15 and 13-16).

A B

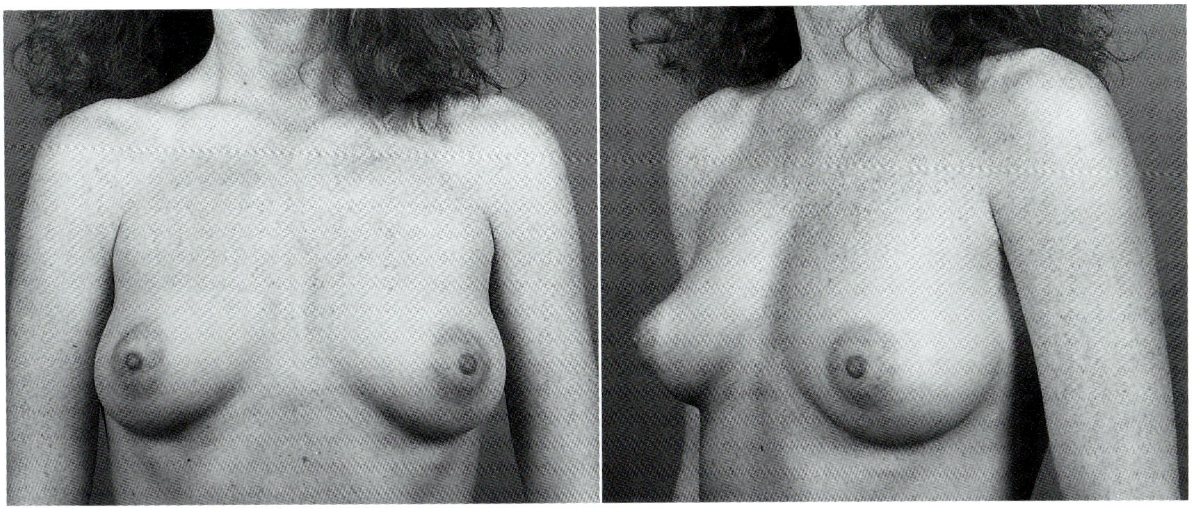

FIGURE 13-15
A and B, Preoperative views.

A B

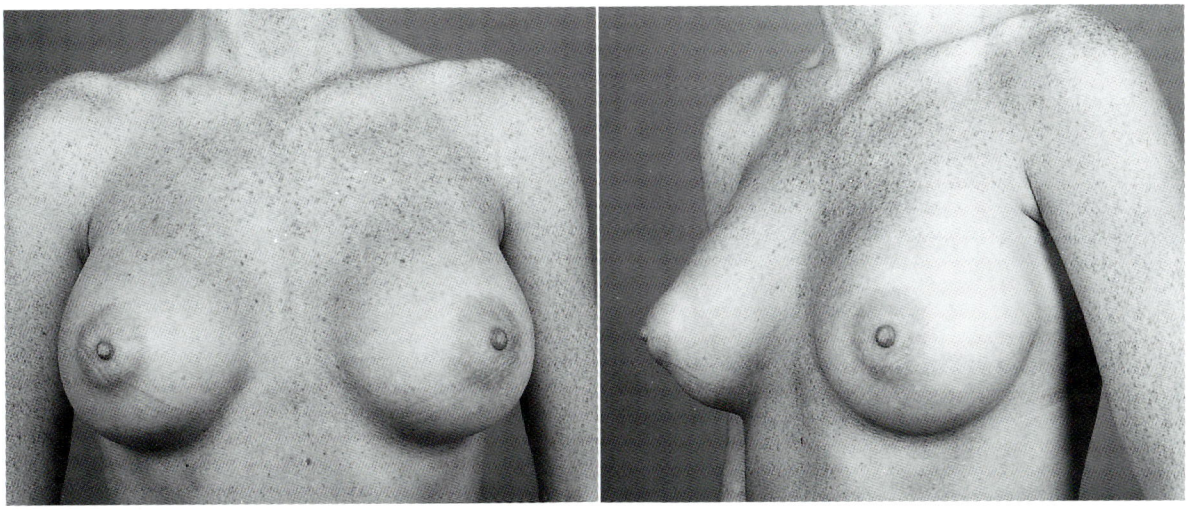

FIGURE 13-16
A and B, Postoperative views after endoscopically assisted transaxillary retropectoral augmentation mammaplasty.

Suggested Readings

Agris J, Dingman RO, Wilensky RJ: A dissector for transaxillary approach in augmentation mammaplasty, *Plast Reconstr Surg* 57:10, 1976.

Biggs TM, Yarish RS: Augmentation mammaplasty: retropectoral versus retromammary implantation, *Clin Plast Surg* 15:549, 1988.

Brody GS: Breast implant size selection and patient satisfaction, *Plast Reconstr Surg* 68:611, 1981.

Burkhardt BR, et al: Capsular contracture: a prospective study of the effect of local antibacterial agents, *Plast Reconstr Surg* 77:919, 1986.

Cole NM: Informed consent: considerations in aesthetic and reconstructive surgery of the breast, *Clin Plast Surg* 15:541, 1988.

Dowden RV, Anain S: Endoscopic implant evaluation and capsulotomy, *Plast Reconstr Surg* 91:283, 1993.

Eaves FE, Price CI, Bostwick J III, et al: Subcutaneous endoscopic plastic surgery using a retractor-mounted endoscopic system, *Perspect Plast Surg* 7(2):1, 1993.

Farina MA, Newby BG, Alani HM: Innervation of the nipple–areola complex, *Plast Reconstr Surg* 66:497, 1980.

Fisher J, Maxwell GP: *Selection of technique for augmentation mammaplasty.* In Noone RB, editor: *Plastic and reconstructive surgery of the breast,* Philadelphia, 1991, Mosby–Year Book.

Maxwell GP: *Basic principles in the management of complications following augmentation mammaplasty.* In Georgiade NG, Georgiade GS, Riefkohl R, Barwick WJ, editors: *Textbook of plastic maxillofacial and reconstructive surgery,* Vol 2, ed 2, Baltimore, 1992, Williams & Wilkins.

Maxwell GP: Discussion of Tebbetts, JB: Transaxillary subpectoral augmentation mammaplasty: long-term follow-up and refinements, *Plast Reconstr Surg* 47(5):648, 1984.

Maxwell GP: *Transaxillary subpectoral augmentation mammaplasty.* In Georgiade NG, Georgiade GS, Riefkohl R, editors: *Aesthetic surgery of the breast,* Philadelphia, 1990, WB Saunders.

Maxwell GP, Tornambe R: Management of mammary subpectoral implant distortion, *Clin Plast Surg* 15:601, 1988.

Papillon J: Pros and cons of subpectoral augmentation, *Clin Plast Surg* 3(2):321, 1976.

Pernkopf E: *Atlas of topographical and applied anatomy,* Vol II, ed 3, Baltimore, Munich, 1989, Urban and Schwarzenberg.

Peterson R: *Axillary approach.* In Regnault P, Danial RK, editors: *Aesthetic plastic surgery,* Boston, 1984, Little, Brown.

Puckett CL, Croll GH, Reichel C, et al: A critical look at capsule contracture in subglandular versus subpectoral mammary augmentation, *Aesth Plast Surg* 11:23, 1987.

Raynor A, Klein A, Habal M: Cosmetic advantages of augmentation of the hypoplastic breast via the transaxillary approach, *Aesth Plast Surg* 1:391, 1978.

Tebbetts JB: Transaxillary subpectoral augmentation mammaplasty: a 9-year experience, *Clin Plast Surg* 15(4):557, 1988.

Tebbetts JB: Transaxillary subpectoral augmentation mammaplasty: achieving facility, consistency, and reliability. Plastic surgery educational foundation instruction courses, vol 1, St Louis, 1988, Mosby–Year Book.

Tebbetts JB: Transaxillary subpectoral augmentation mammaplasty: long-term follow-up and refinements, *Plast Reconstr Surg* 47(5):636, 1984.

CHAPTER 14

Endoscopic Abdominoplasty

Gerald W. Johnson

In 1990 we began to consider ways to complete the xiphoid to pubis repair of the lax anterior abdominal wall, fascia, and muscle through a limited incision. This type of procedure is indicated in those patients who do not require excision of redundant skin but who need an effective repair of the muscle and fascia, occasionally combined with liposuction of the anterior abdominal wall.[1] We also set out a number of quality standards to serve as goals for the procedure as follows:

1. The acceptance of the procedure depends on the ease with which the technique can be learned and successfully performed by the surgeon who can do the standard "open" abdominoplasty.[2]
2. The quality of muscle and fascia repair must be at least equal to that obtained using the open technique. When no other scars are present on the abdomen, the endoscopic approach is ideal.[3]

From the inception of the concept of the no scar or limited incision abdominoplasty it was obvious that the use of the endoscope is required. Because we had no experience with the endoscope, we completed a course at the Houston Laser Institute in the fall of 1990. More thought was given to how we would be able to make a surgical approach through a 5-cm incision to allow dissection of the skin–subcutaneous pedicle cleanly away from the fascia. At the same time it would be necessary to be confident that hemostasis was secure as the dissection progressed.

Our initial concept was to use some type of fiberoptic laser that would give good dissection and hemostasis and that could also be used to coagulate the smaller caliber blood vessels. Since we had no experience in the use of the laser, we completed a laser gallbladder course at the Houston Laser Institute in December 1990. The course provided experience in the use of the fiberoptic laser and of the laser and the endoscope together.

In January 1991 a patient presented to our office requesting an abdominoplasty. She fit the requirements for the endoscopic abdominoplasty, and she also had a longer than normal suprapubic scar from a prior hysterectomy. The scar could be used to convert to an open technique and gain more exposure if we had technical difficulties with the endoscopic technique.[3]

In February 1991, using a 60-W yttrium-aluminum-garnet (YAG) laser and a 10-mm, 0-degree angle endoscope, with a 5-cm incision in the central portion of the existing suprapubic scar, our first attempted endoscopic abdominoplasty began. It quickly became obvious that dissection with the laser was no match for dissection with the electrosurgical unit on the large surface area of the abdominal fascia. We persisted with the laser, however, up to the level just below the umbilicus. At this point we extended the incision along the full length of the suprapubic scar and converted to an open approach, using the electrocautery. The electrocautery was about 5 times faster than using the YAG laser. Perhaps a more powerful laser would have made a better showing.

From this first attempt we also learned that there would be considerable technical difficulties in obtaining good exposure, hemostasis, smoke evacuation, fluid evacuation, keeping the tip of the scope clean to provide a continuous image, keeping the electrode tip or laser tip in position in view on the monitor to facilitate working with it, and doing all six of these things at the same time to enable functioning as a surgeon to perform the technical feat of an endoscopic abdominoplasty while watching television.

After this introduction to the endoscopic abdominoplasty we put on hold any second attempt until we had additional time for contemplation and to mentally work out a different technical approach.

We next decided to alter our approach and try to become proficient in each step or each part of the procedure by "practicing" each stage on our standard open abdominoplasties. The most difficult part of the endoscopic technique is the dissection. This requires the most hand-eye coordination. It also requires the maximal effort and attention of the surgeon, assistant, scrub nurse, and even a second assistant (if available).

When we had a patient for an open abdominoplasty we would first make our routine markings. Then we would make a 5-cm incision in the suprapubic area and begin the dissection using endoscopic techniques. As long as we were able to continue the dissection at about the same speed as with the open technique, we would continue with the endoscopic technique. Once we encountered technical problems of whatever nature so as to become 15 to 30 minutes behind, we would convert to the open technique so that the procedure would not run too long. This method of practice takes a little extra effort and adds a little more time to an open procedure; however, we feel that this is the most effective way for the surgeon and his team to become proficient in the endoscopic technique. By using this technique of 15 to 30 minutes of endoscopic practice on each open abdominoplasty, the surgeon and his team can soon accumulate several hours' experience.

The second most difficult part of the endoscopic abdominoplasty is the repair of the fascia. Initially we attempted placing sutures in the fascia through the 5-cm incision, and while technically this could be done it was very difficult to do and the time required was prohibitive. We then approached the Auto Suture Company about their fascial stapler. The company provided us with articles and references from the general surgery literature, which were very favorable and gave us the confidence to use the fascial staples on the abdominal fascia.

The staples come in a dispenser that is actually gun-shaped, with a 4-inch barrel. Each uncrimped staple is 1.4 cm wide. Each staple crimps down in the shape of a figure eight and is about 9 mm wide when closed down. Each gun has 20 staples, and on the average patient we use 2 guns, or 40 staples. We first used the staples on open abdominoplasties and very quickly learned that the best way to approximate the fascia and to allow the staples the best bite of fascia was to grip the fascia with a cervical tenaculum. Even though the fascial staples clinically gave a beautiful closure we initially did not feel secure enough using the staples alone; therefore, we reinforced the staple closure with a running suture of 1-0 Mersilene.

After using the staples on four open abdominoplasties as described above, on the next open procedure we completed all the dissection then temporarily closed the abdominal incision together with skin staples, leaving a 5-cm opening in the suprapubic area. We were now able to use this "incision" plus the circumumbilical incision as our endoscopic portals to practice the endoscopic repair of the abdominal fascia with the staples. After the repair was completed we could then remove the skin staples and have a perfect view of our endoscopic fascial repair with the staples. On the first four of these patients we also reinforced over the staples with 1-0 Mersilene. We no longer use reinforcement of the staple repair on any patient, and we now have sufficient clinical experience to convince us that the staple repair of the fascia is even stronger than any we obtained with sutures alone. We have continued to use the Auto Suture fascial staples on every abdominoplasty, both open and endoscopic. On the standard open abdominoplasty we have eliminated at least 15 to 20 minutes of surgical time from the procedure by using the fascial staples.

Days passed into weeks, weeks into months, and during this time we were also trying to work out a way to perform an augmentation mammoplasty from a remote location without leaving any scars on the breasts. This technique we knew would require the use of the endoscope. As an alternative to an endoscopic dissection under direct vision using the laser or electrocautery, we had been considering the possibility of using a tissue expander inserted through a small tunnel into a small pocket in the plane between the subcutaneous tissue and fascia, with intraoperative expansion, to accomplish the dissection. On October 3, 1991, we were performing an open abdominoplasty on a patient and also planned to do an augmentation mammoplasty through the open abdominoplasty approach.[4] We decided to make this our test case for the idea of creating the pocket by intraoperative tissue expansion. The technique worked beautifully and resulted in beautiful breast augmentation with good mobility.

Because of the outstanding ease and good results in creating the pockets in the endoscopic breast augmentations, the bright idea came to us of using the intraoperative tissue expansion technique to accomplish the dissection in the endoscopic abdominoplasty. We decided to use the "NBC peacock" technique. We specially ordered four sizes of tissue expanders shaped like hot dog buns, from the small size to the "foot-long" size, ordering two expanders of each of the four sizes. The two longest were placed on each side of the vertical, the two shortest on each side of the midline, and the other two sizes equally spaced in between to complete the arc to form a facsimile of the tail of the "NBC peacock."

We decided to practice this NBC technique on a patient scheduled for an open abdominoplasty in February 1992. In surgery we first made the 5-cm suprapubic incision and, using the endotube we designed for the endoscopic augmentation mammoplasty, we then made a tunnel on each side of the midline, one above the inguinal area on each side, and two on each side spaced evenly between the horizontal and the vertical. We then began inflation and found that because there is no rigid structure such as the rib cage behind the abdominal wall, we were unable to compress and manipulate the expander to help control development of the pocket, as we were able to do in the endoscopic augmentation mammoplasty. Therefore, we determined on the basis of this case that the expansion technique was not a satisfactory method to use in the endoscopic abdominoplasty.

Having tried different techniques and having developed a degree of skill in the endoscopic electrosurgical dissection and the endoscopic repair of the abdominal fascia with fascial staples, we elected to use this technique on our first "true" endoscopic abdominoplasty. We began to select from patients who came to the office requesting abdominal liposuction and/or abdominoplasty, those who would be candidates for the endoscopic abdominoplasty. We fully inform them about this new method or technique we will use to perform, with minimum scarring, a long-established procedure—the abdominoplasty. In our patient population probably no more than 5% to 10% of the patients are suitable for the endoscopic abdominoplasty. However, there is a very large population of women and men who are suitable for this procedure and it is likely that many more would be interested in having it done if they knew it could be done with only two essentially nonvisible incisions, one hidden in the umbilicus and one hidden in the pubic hair.

PREOPERATIVE EVALUATION

Our criteria for selecting patients for the endoscopic abdominoplasty are as follows:

1. Patient preference and motivation are the most important issues. If the patient simply will not accept the scar from an open abdominoplasty and your evaluation reveals the need for a muscle-fascia repair, then an endoscopic approach is the only choice.
2. The patient must not need a panniculectomy.
3. The patient must have enough diastasis recti abdominis and fascial laxity to benefit from the repair.
4. Should a patient have some loose skin, if in the surgeon's opinion the skin will shrink down with liposuction, the patient could be an endoscopic candidate.
5. Liposuction must be used as an adjunctive therapy in the majority of endoscopic abdominoplasties.
6. Just as a surgeon in any specialty who does endoscopic surgery will always inform the patient of the possible need to convert to an open technique if certain intraoperative complications arise, we as plastic surgeons must likewise inform our patients of the same possibility. We should also advise our patients that should postoperative complications arise, we may not be able to correct all complications via the endoscopic route. If the patient cannot accept this, then she or he is not a suitable candidate for this surgical approach.

7. Since endoscopic surgery is considered by the general public to be high-tech, the expectations of many patients may be unrealistic. Be certain to obtain an informed consent that is designed to engender *realistic expectations*.
8. Finally, we have always advised the patient of our level of expertise in any new procedure or technique that we have performed, until we have performed enough of a particular procedure that we possess reasonable skill and experience.

Once we have determined that a particular patient is a candidate for endoscopic abdominoplasty, we obtain preoperative photographs and videotape. The patient is allowed to have the surgery as an outpatient, unless multiple procedures are scheduled or other medical problems dictate that the patient needs to be an inpatient.[5] We obtain routine laboratory tests, electrocardiogram, and chest x-ray as indicated. We also have every patient tested for the human immunodeficiency virus.

INSTRUMENTATION

There are several good scopes and cameras on the market. The least expensive are the one-chip cameras, which cannot be sterilized and therefore are covered with a sterile sleeve. The three-chip cameras give the best images and can be soaked to sterilize them. They are also the most expensive ones. The three-chip cameras are studio quality, and on the high-quality monitors available in most operating rooms they give excellent images that greatly enhance hand-eye coordination. They also provide excellent videotapes. Any size scope can be used, but it needs to be approximately 30 cm long to allow good visualization up to the xiphoid process. A 10-mm scope is best because it allows more light to pass into the operative field and back through the camera and to the monitor, resulting in a better image.

In surgery we use the following:

SURGICAL SUPPLIES AND INSTRUMENTS

- Laparotomy pack
- Electrosurgical pencil
- Teflon Bovie blade
- Bovie blade extender
- Asepto syringe
- Suction tubing
- Lap sponges
- Antifog
- Raytecs
- No. 10 and No. 15 blades
- Marking pen
- 3M 1010 Steridrapes × 6
- Liposuction tubing and cannulas
- Suction drains × 2
- Methylene blue dye
- Plastic set
- Deaver retractor
- Harrington retractor
- Videocamera
- 10-mm scope
- Cervical tenaculum

SUTURES

- Fascial staples × 2
- Skin staples
- 3-0 Prolene PS-5 × 1
- 3-0 silk PS-2 × 1
- 2-0 polyglactin (Vicryl) FS-1 × 1

DRESSINGS

- Cottonball, benzoin, Steri-Strips
- Abdominal binder, 4 × 4 inch sponges
- ABDs × 4; Kerlix × 2

PATIENT PREPARATION

On the day of surgery the patient is seen preoperatively in the preanesthesia area. With the patient standing erect, the areas of the abdomen and flanks that need liposuction are marked.

The patient is taken to the operating room and placed under general endotracheal anesthesia. The hair over the abdomen and mons pubis is shaved. Antibiotics are administered intravenously. An indwelling Foley catheter is inserted. The abdomen is prepared and draped in the same manner as for the open abdominoplasty. Markings are then made from the suprapubic area out over the iliac crest, up the lateral flanks, across the lower costal margin and xiphoid process, and along the same areas on the opposite side (Figure 14-1).

A 5-cm-long mark is made for the suprapubic incision, and a 1-cm mark is made immediately to the left of the 5-cm mark for an incision to insert the endoscope (Figure 14-2). A second incision will be made in the umbilicus from the 12 o'clock

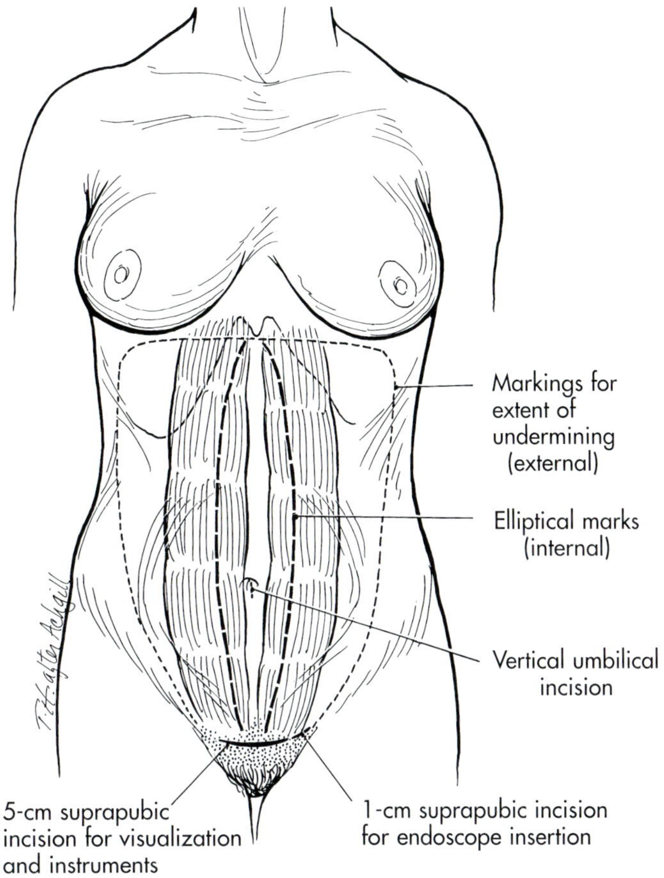

FIGURE 14-1
Markings for extent of undermining (external) are shown. Elliptical marks for extent of muscle plication (internal), vertical umbilical incision, suprapubic incision for insertion of endoscope, 1 cm, and suprapubic incision for visualization and instruments, 5 cm, are shown.

position to the 6 o'clock position. The incision may be extended along the umbilical rim from 12 to 9 o'clock and from 6 to 3 o'clock, if that is necessary to give more length to the incision (Figure 14-3). The umbilical incision must be able to stretch to at least 3 cm to allow the eventual insertion of the upper retractor and the electrosurgical pencil for dissection and the staple gun for closure of the fascia and muscle. The 1-cm suprapubic incision (Figure 14-2) is ideally located to place a 10-mm endoport or surgiport through which the 10-mm endoscope can be passed to keep it out of the way as one works with the retractor and electrosurgical pencil. The port is very useful to withdraw the endoscope into to prevent getting blood on its tip, blurring the image.

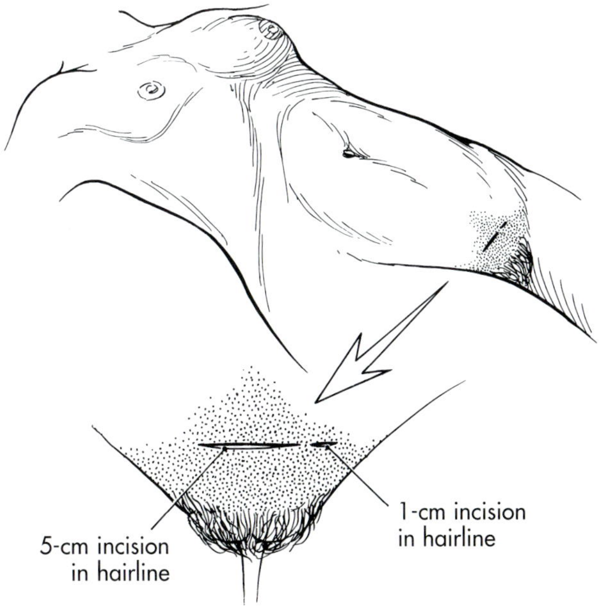

FIGURE 14-2
Incisions in hairline, 5 cm and 1 cm, are shown.

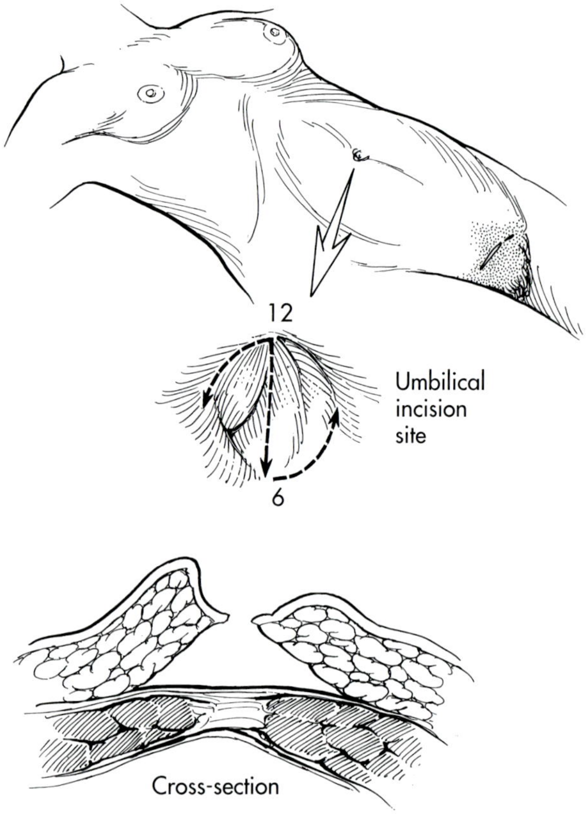

FIGURE 14-3
Dissection under umbilicus is shown *(top view and view from pubic area).*

OPERATIVE PROCEDURE

The surgery begins by making the 5-cm suprapubic incision inside the pubic hairline (Figure 14-2). The initial dissection can be done under direct vision using the electrocautery. Dissection is carried down to the rectus fascia, following the skin markings made on the abdominal skin (Figure 14-1) the pocket is developed as the skin and subcutaneous tissue are separated from the anterior abdominal fascia. It is very important to get a clean dissection of the fat and soft tissue off the fascia. If a clean dissection is not obtained, when the time comes for placement of the fascial staples the integrity of the muscle-fascial repair may be severely compromised.

Once we have opened the first few centimeters of the pocket, we then place the tip of the endoscope inside the pocket and continue the dissection using a combination of direct and endoscopic vision via the monitor. To carry out the dissection in the area below the umbilicus the surgeon needs two assistants. The right-handed surgeon standing on the patient's right side needs a scrub nurse or one assistant on the patient's left side, standing at or slightly below the level of the pubis. This assistant should be the one who holds and positions the scope and camera. As the dissection proceeds in a semicircle away from the incision and when the dissected pocket extends to 6 to 8 cm, we make the 1-cm incision approximately 1 cm to the left of the 5-cm suprapubic incision (Figure 14-2), insert the 10-mm port, and introduce the endoscope through the port. This allows the assistant to maintain satisfactory control of the scope and camera.

As long as the dissection remains below the umbilicus the surgeon can maintain most of the retraction with the left hand and can manipulate the electrosurgical pencil with the right hand. The second assistant is on the left side of the patient and assists the surgeon in holding the retractor. The two retractors we use (Harrington and Deaver) have both been modified with a metal suction tube that can be attached to wall suction and functions to keep the electrocautery smoke and vapors evacuated from the surgical area. Smoke evacuation is vital to maintain satisfactory visibility.

As our dissection approaches the umbilicus, we make the previously described vertical incision in the umbilicus. This divides the umbilicus into two halves, right and left. Each half is detached from the rectus fascia–umbilical stalk. This is done under direct vision. The dissection is continued underneath the divided and elevated umbilicus (Figure 14-3). Once we have completed the dissection to a level of 2 to 3 cm above the level of the umbilicus, we replace the Deaver retractor in the suprapubic incision with the Harrington retractor, we keep the endoscope passed through the port beside the suprapubic incision, and we relocate the Deaver retractor to the umbilical incision. The suction tubing can be attached to either retractor. We generally have it attached to the retractor closest to the area we are working on with the electrocautery.

At this point the surgeon must also have two assistants. One devotes his or her full attention to the placement and control of the endoscope. The other maintains retraction on the Harrington retractor in the suprapubic incision to keep the pocket open for visibility and to prevent contact of the flap and bloody tissue with the tip of the scope. It is possible for the surgeon using an extension tip for the electrocautery to continue to work on the dissection through the suprapubic incision. We find it, however, much easier and less stressful to dissect with the electrosurgical pencil passed through the umbilical incision. Changing from the suprapubic incision to the umbilical incision, while leaving the scope in the lower incision, causes the surgeon some minor adaptation of his hand-eye coordination, but the surgeon who has been able to accomplish the dissection from the pubis to the umbilicus will not have any great difficulty adapting.

We expose the fascia up to the xiphoid process, then laterally out over the rib cage far enough to be certain that the skin flap has room to spread out smoothly, rather than bunch up in the epigastric area when we begin the fascial plication. At this point we will have completed exposure of the fascia over the entire anterior wall in the area we planned and marked at the beginning of the operation. Once we have plicated the fascia we usually find that we need to do more dissection, especially in both lateral areas to allow for better redraping of the skin.[6]

If the fascia or the pocket is bloody we irrigate well and "dry" the surface of the fascia as much as possible with sponges. In an open abdominoplasty we are accustomed to seeing the exposed fascia dry if not kept moistened; however, with the endoscopic approach the fascia is not exposed and does not dry out during the procedure. We estimate how tightly we would be able to plicate the fascia if we were doing an open abdominoplasty, and using a Q-tip and methylene blue dye we mark an ellipse on the fascial surface that approximates the amount we think we should be able to plicate (Figure 14-1).

Fascial stapling begins in the epigastric area. Using the cervical tenaculum, the teeth on each side are imbedded into the fascia along the methylene blue-marked (internal) ellipse (Figures 14-4 and 14-5, *A*). The tenaculum is lifted as it is closed, thereby allowing the excessive fascia and muscle to imbricate (Figure 14-5, *B*). From the xiphoid to the pubis the first row of staples are placed approximately 6 cm apart (Figure 14-6, *A*). The second row of staples is used to produce some additional tightening of the fascia, where possible, as well as to fill in the spaces in the first row (Figure 14-6, *B*). When plicating the fascia with sutures the surgeon knows from experience and by the feel of the suture in his hands how much tension to apply. This feedback loop is absent when using staples, thus we use as the endpoint the amount of tension we can apply the point at which we begin to see the tenaculum's teeth tear through the fascia. Sometimes we can plicate the fascia 2 to 4 cm more than we estimated with our methylene blue markings, and other times we cannot quite approximate the blue marks together. In the third row of staples we may increase tension on the fascia a little more in some places, but basically the third row is used to fill in the gaps. Two guns, or 40 staples, are usually needed for each patient.

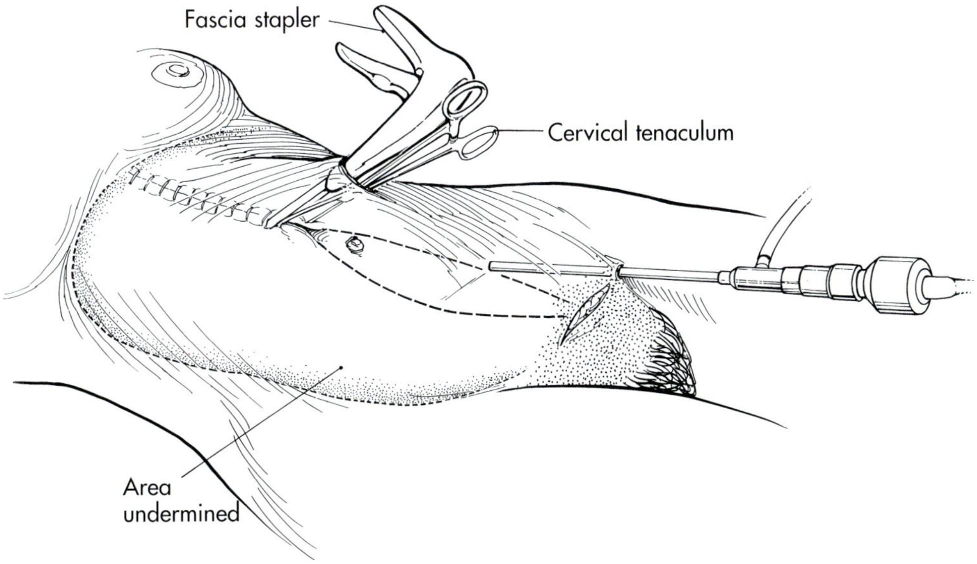

FIGURE 14-4
The use of cervical tenaculum, autosuture fascia stapler, and endoscope is shown.

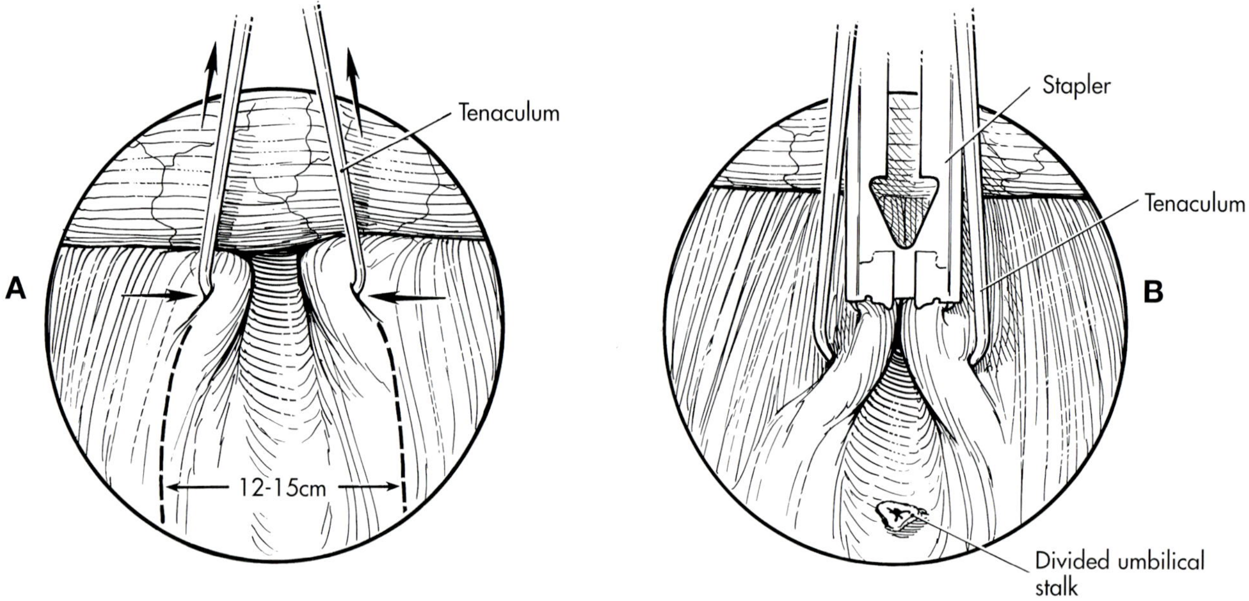

FIGURE 14-5
A, Elliptical (internal) markings 12 to 15 cm apart and cervical tenaculum are shown. **B,** Divided umbilical stalk and stapler adjacent to cervical tenaculum are shown.

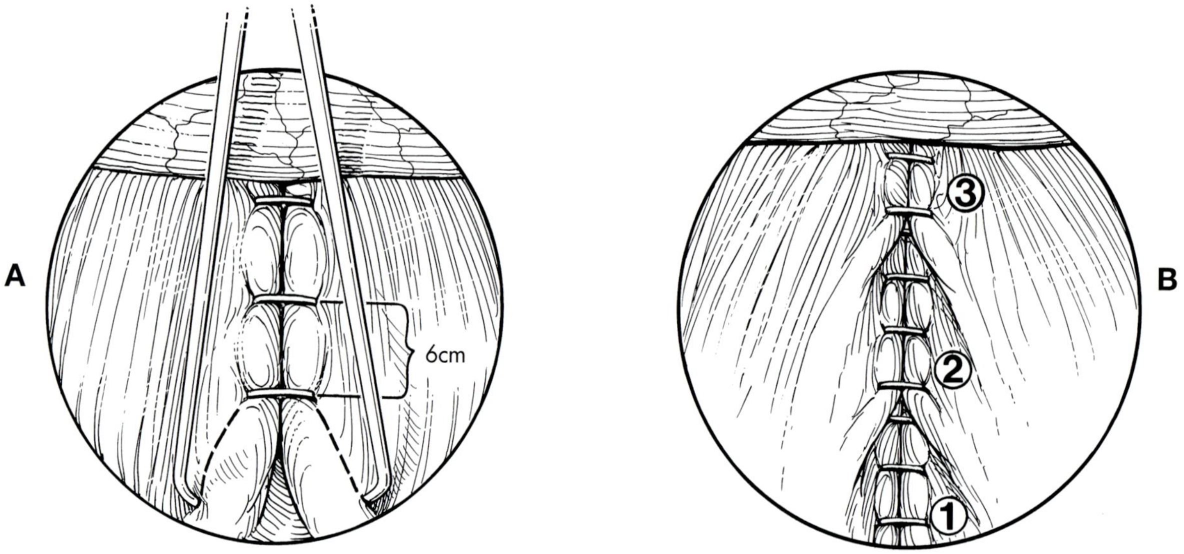

FIGURE 14-6
A, Placement of first row of staples is shown. **B,** A total of three stapled layers are shown. Forty staples are placed in an average patient.

Once the fascial imbrication has been completed, we usually find that we need to do some additional undermining, especially laterally, to allow for what we feel is sufficient release of the skin and subcutaneous tissue to effect skin redraping that will provide a satisfactory cosmetic result.

At this point we are ready to do whatever liposuction of the anterior abdominal wall and flanks that is necessary. The most important inferior epigastric blood supply to the lower anterior abdominal skin has not been interrupted by this endoscopic technique; therefore, we can effectively suction the entire abdomen and flanks if necessary without compromise of their vascular supply. We do not always infiltrate wetting solution with epinephrine before suctioning. After 1½ to 2 hours in

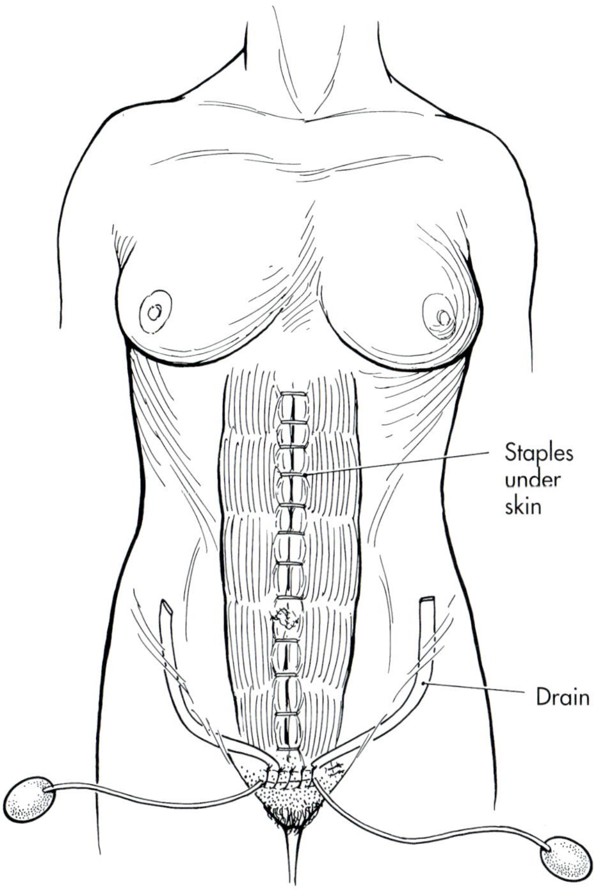

FIGURE 14-7
Placement of staples and drains under the skin is shown.

a cold operating room the abdominal flap is usually cool and vasoconstricted enough to perform liposuction without injection of epinephrine. We have found that doing liposuction at the beginning of the procedure causes serum, blood, and liquid fat to accumulate, which gets into the operative field and greatly compromises visibility. Therefore we do the liposuction after completing the endoscopic repair.

Closure of the umbilical incision is accomplished by suturing the right half of the umbilicus to the fascia with a suture of 2-0 Vicryl. The two halves of the umbilicus are then sutured together with a running suture of 3-0 Prolene. One 10-mm Jackson-Pratt drain is placed in each side and brought out through the suprapubic incision. This incision is closed with subcutaneous sutures of 2-0 Vicryl and skin staples. The drains are sutured in place with 3-0 silk. The 1-cm endoscopic incision is closed with one or two skin staples (Figure 14-7). Dressings of 4 × 4 inch gauze pads, Kerlix, and ABDs are applied and an abdominal binder is put in place.

POSTOPERATIVE CARE

The postoperative care is basically the same as with the standard open abdominoplasty. Patients feel very little need to bend forward postoperatively because there has been no skin excision resulting in a long, lower abdominal incision closed under tension. All our patients are given intraoperative antibiotics and are placed on oral antibiotics postoperatively. They are also given a strong oral analgesic for pain control; inpatients can receive intramuscular or intravenous medications. We leave the drains in place for 7 days, and the patients are instructed on how to empty the evacuation containers. It is extremely important that the patient is instructed how to loosen and reposition the binder no less than four times a day. A compressive bandage that folds, rolls, or makes ridges in a given place on the abdomen, if left in place too long, can produce permanent deformity just as garments or bandages applied after liposuction can.

COMPLICATIONS

It has been our experience over the past 20 years doing standard open abdominoplasties that we have an incidence of seroma formation that is at least equal to that reported in the literature. We have also found, as many plastic surgeons have reported, that the incidence of seroma formation in the limited incision or "mini" abdominoplasties, especially with associated liposuction of the abdominal pedicle, is frequently higher.[7] Therefore we were not surprised to learn from our early experience with the endoscopic abdominoplasty that we would have to be diligent to prevent or treat seroma formation. Even though we impress on the patient the need to reposition the binder frequently, we also emphasize our belief that the binder is necessary to help prevent swelling of the abdominal flap and hold it evenly in place so it can reattach to the fascia. We generally advise that the patient wear the binder for 3 weeks. We then recommend a good-fitting panty girdle for another 6 weeks, or until all swelling has subsided.

A

B

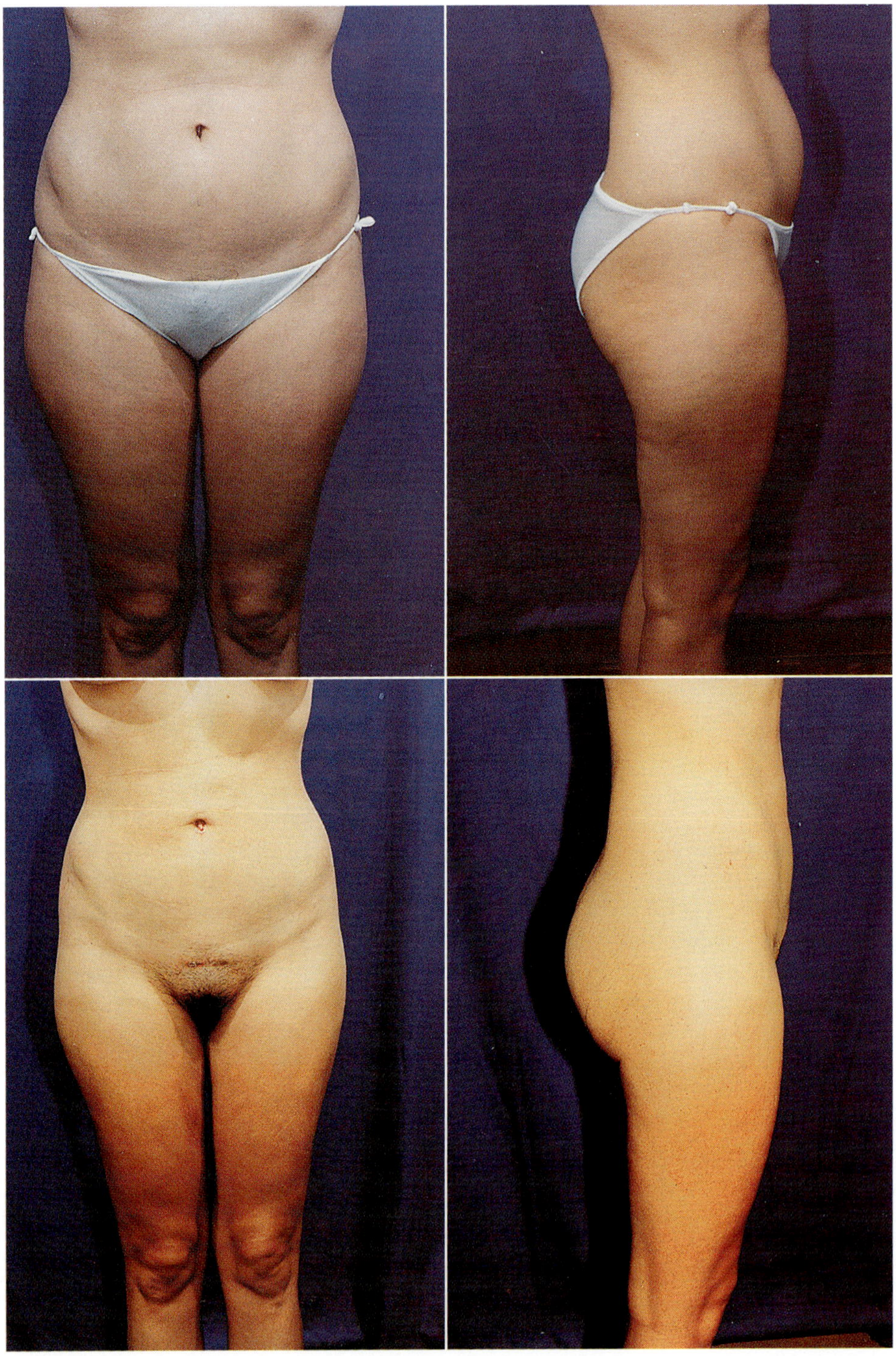

C

D

FIGURE 14-8
Case Study 1. **A and B,** A 30-year-old woman after two full-term pregnancies is shown preoperatively. **C and D,** One month postoperatively.

Continued.

E
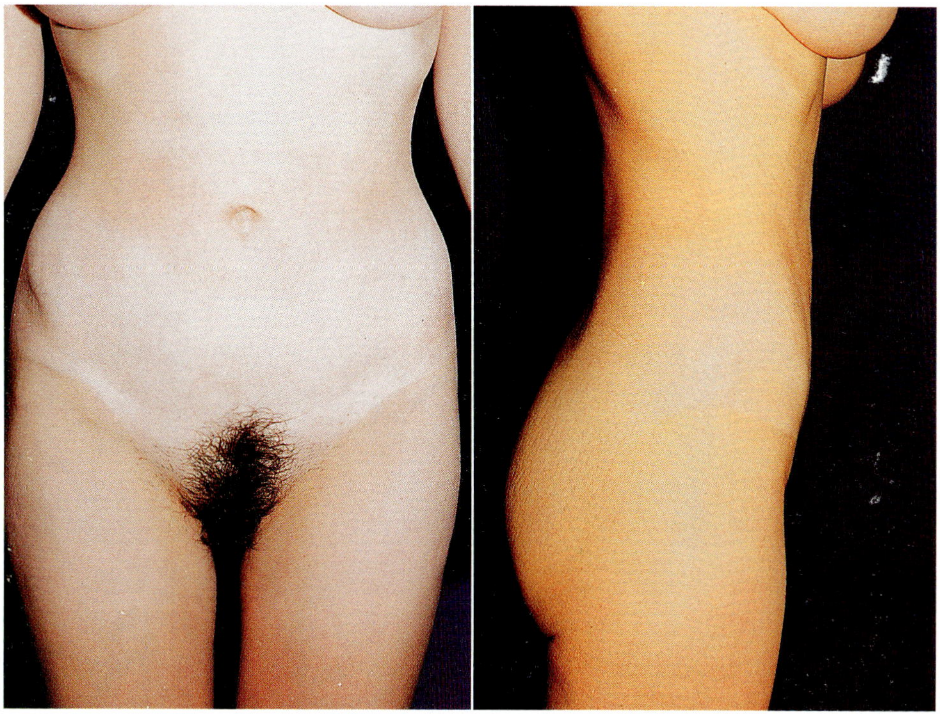
F

Figure 14-8, Cont'd.
E and F, Twenty months postoperatively.

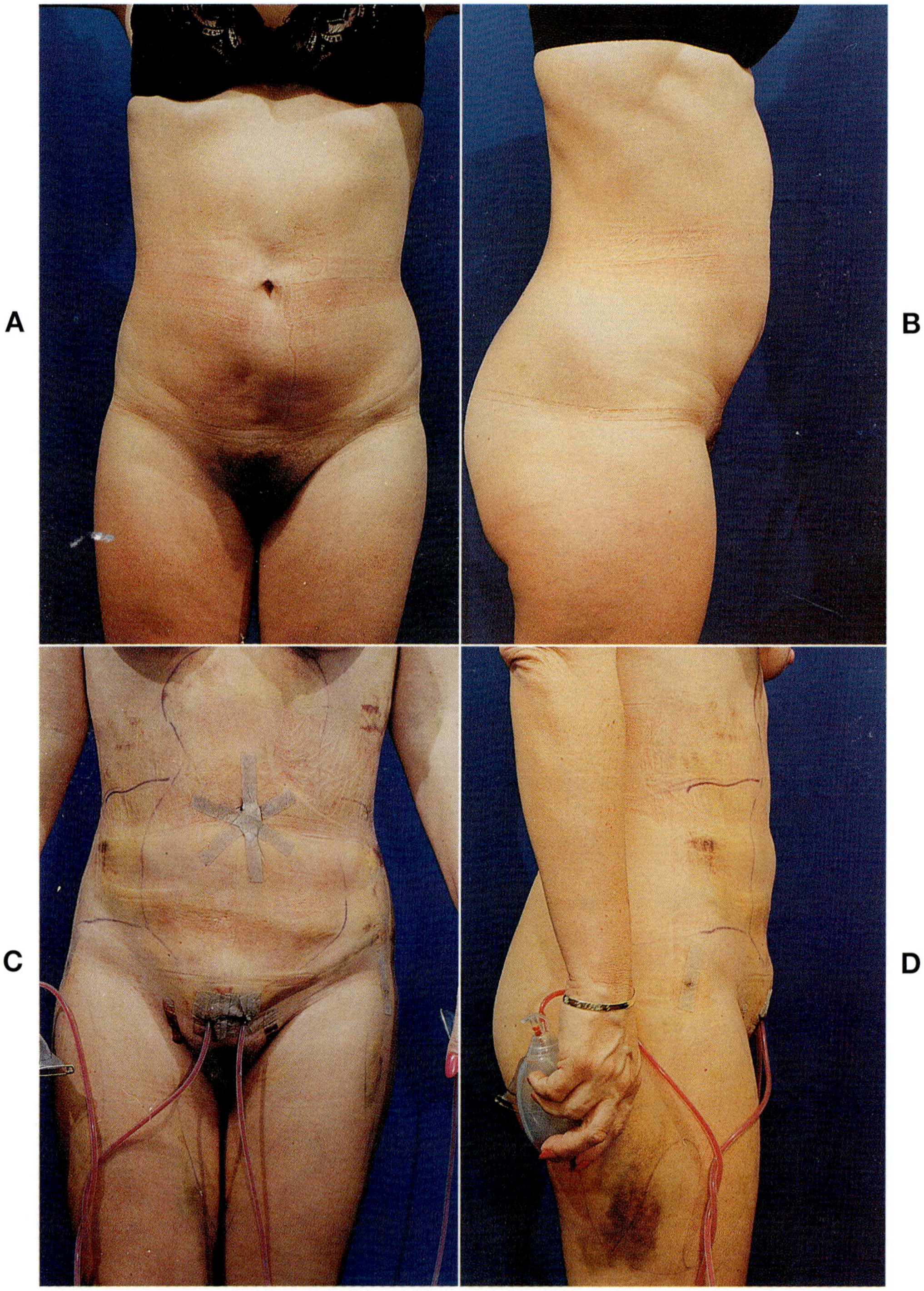

FIGURE 14-9
Case Study 2. **A and B,** A 38-year-old woman after two full-term pregnancies and a weight gain of 50 pounds with one of the pregnancies is shown preoperatively. **C and D,** One day postoperatively.

Continued.

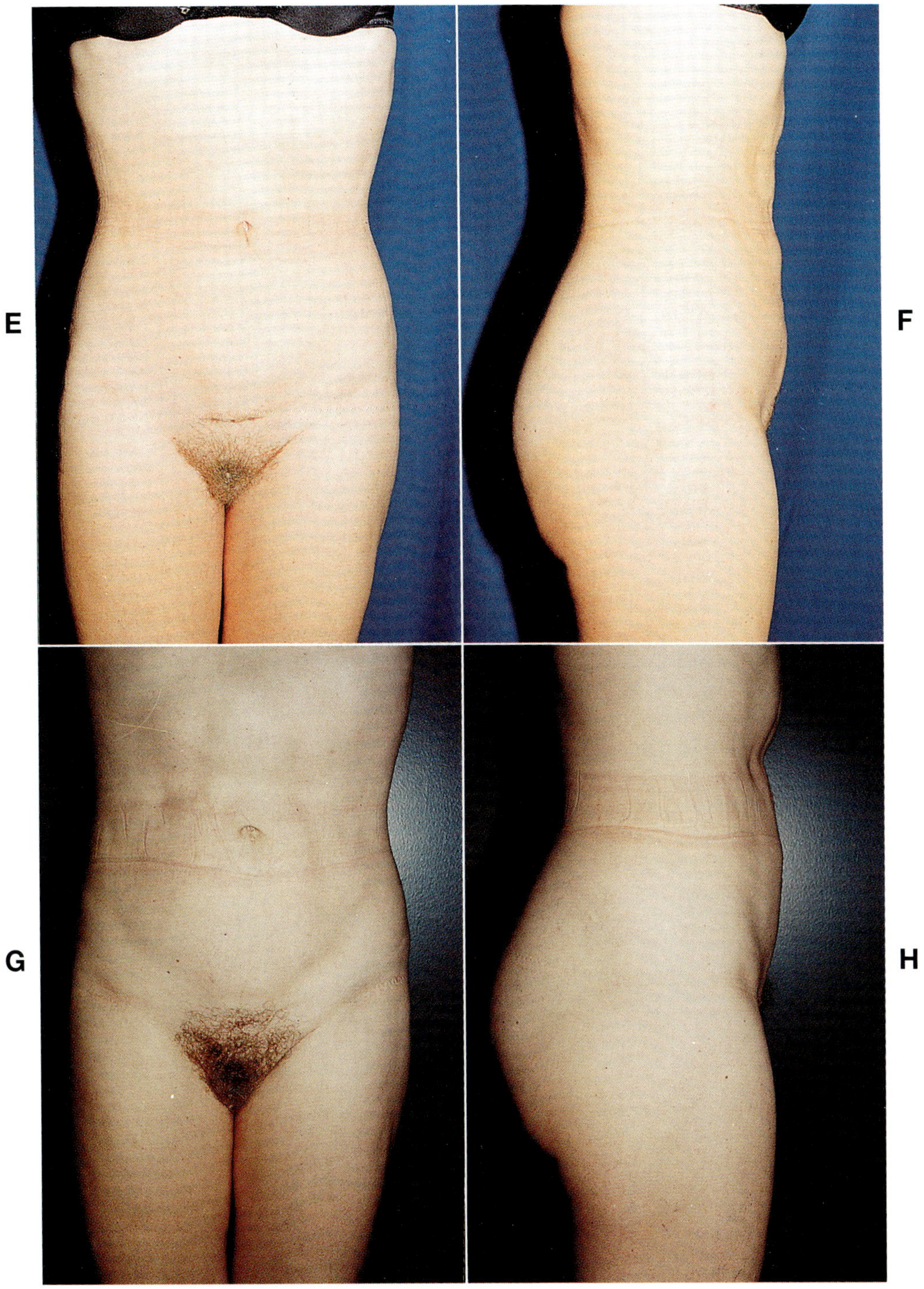

Figure 14-9, cont'd
E and F, Six weeks postoperatively. **G and H,** Twenty months postoperatively.

SUMMARY OF CLINICAL EXPERIENCE

To date we have a series of 20 patients who have undergone endoscopically assisted abdominoplasties. Of those 20, one was the first patient we attempted the endoscopic approach on using the YAG laser. Another patient was the one with whom we attempted to use the tissue expanders to undermine the abdominal flap. In both of these patients we had to convert to a "modified" open procedure to complete the surgery. Both patients had been informed preoperatively of the possible need to convert to an open approach. Both obtained a satisfactory result and did not complain about the need to change to a modified open approach to complete their surgery.

Six of the 20 patients were those on whom we practiced doing endoscopic dissection and fascial stapling and in whom a standard abdominoplasty incision was made to complete the surgery. These patients likewise had satisfactory results and no complications related to the endoscopic portion of their procedures.

Of the 12 patients who have to date undergone "pure" endoscopic abdominoplasties all have good results, with three relatively minor complications. One patient had minor surface irregularities caused by liposuction, which were treated by fat grafts. A second patient had more excess skin in the periumbilical area postoperatively than we expected, which was treated by periumbilical excision. This resulted in a hypertrophic scar which has again been revised. In another patient we inadvertently penetrated through the skin over the left iliac crest with the electrocautery; however, the wound healed well and she has an excellent result otherwise.

Certainly the endoscopic approach is technically difficult at first, as the neophyte is not used to the hand-eye coordination required with this approach. However, after acquiring endoscopic skills, perhaps through the learning steps described at the beginning of this chapter, results comparable to the ones shown could be obtained by any competent plastic surgeon.

REFERENCES

1. Wilkinson T, Swartz B: Individual modifications in body contour surgery: the "limited" abdominoplasty, *Plast Reconstr Surg* 77:779, 1986.
2. Converse J: *Reconstructive plastic surgery.* In Converse JM, McCarthy JG, editors: *Dermolipectomy of the abdominal wall, thighs, buttocks, and upper extremity,* ed 2, Philadelphia, 1977, WB Saunders.
3. Wilkinson T: Letter to the Editor, *Plast Reconstr Surg* 86:1039, 1990.
4. Barrett BM Jr: Combined abdominoplasty and augmentation mammaplasty through a transverse suprapubic incision, *Ann Plast Surg* 4:286, 1980.
5. Hester T Jr: Abdominoplasty combined with other major surgical procedures: safe or sorry? *Plast Reconstr Surg* 83:997, 1989.
6. Grazer F: Abdominoplasty, *Plast Reconstr Surg* 51:617, 1973.
7. Ersek R, Schade K: Subcutaneous pseudobursa secondary to suction and surgery, *Plast Reconstr Surg* 85:442, 1990.

INDEX

Note: "f" following page numbers indicates figures; "t" indicates tables.

N

O

P

R

S

T

U

V

Z

N-5-3 -4273.

BoxN-1

Box-15